AIDS and Obstetrics and Gynaecology

Edited by
C. N. Hudson and F. Sharp

With 26 Figures

Springer-Verlag
London Berlin Heidelberg New York
Paris Tokyo

Professor Frank Sharp, MD, FRCOG
Department of Obstetrics and Gynaecology, Northern General Hospital,
Herries Road, Sheffield S5 7AU

Christopher Neville Hudson, FRCS, FRCOG
Physician Accoucheur, Department of Obstetrics and Gynaecology,
St. Bartholomew's Hospital, West Smithfield, London EC1A 7BG.

ISBN 3-540-19540-8 Springer-Verlag Berlin Heidelberg New York
ISBN 0-387-19540-8 Springer-Verlag New York Berlin Heidelberg

British Library Cataloguing in Publication Data
Royal College of Obstetricians and Gynaecologists, *Study Group. (19th: 1988).*
AIDS in obstetrics and gynaecology: proceedings of the nineteenth study group of the Royal
College of Obstetricians and Gynaecologists, March 1988. 1. Gynaecology. Obstetrics.
Implications of AIDS. Man. AIDS. Implications for gynaecology & obstetrics.
I. Title II. Hudson, C.N. (Christopher N.) III. Sharp, F. (Frank), *1938–* . 618
ISBN 3-540-19540-8

Library of Congress Cataloging-in-Publication Data
Royal College of Obstetricians and Gynaecologists (Great Britain).
Study Group (19th: 1988)
AIDS and obstetrics and gynaecology: proceedings of the Nineteenth Study Group of the Royal
College of Obstetricians and Gynaecologists, March 1988/editors, C.N. Hudson, F. Sharp.
p. cm.
Bibliography: p.
Includes index.
ISBN 0-387-19540-8
1. AIDS (Disease) in pregnancy. 2. Gynecology—Practice—Safety measures. 3. AIDS
(Disease)—Prevention. I. Hudson, Christopher N. II. Sharp, F. (Frank) III. Title.
RG580.A44R68 1988 618.3—dc 19 88-39720

Typeset and Printed by the Peacock Press Ltd., Ashton-under-Lyne, Lancashire, England.

2128/3916-543210

Preface

Human immunodeficiency virus (HIV) is largely transmitted by sexual intercourse. Infection with this virus is particularly relevant to obstetric, gynaecological and perinatal practice. Although the true "heterosexual epidemic" of AIDS is mainly confined to intravenous drug abusers, the number of AIDS patients with heterosexual contact has been on the increase in recent years. If AIDS becomes prevalent throughout the general population, heterosexual spread is likely to increase further and the disease will no longer be restricted to specific so-called "high risk" groups.

For the obstetrician and gynaecologist, and perinatal specialist, a number of vital questions beg an answer. What is the effect of a pregnancy on HIV disease in a woman? What is the exact risk of HIV transmission from mother to child? What are the factors which influence the risk of perinatal transmission? Does the mode of delivery matter? What is the prevalence of HIV seropositive women attending antenatal clinics? What advice can be offered to the woman whose test is positive? What are the risks and consequences to herself and to her infant? How are they affected by breastfeeding? What are the special problems of HIV in the community in relation to gynaecological practice? What are the managerial implications of these matters, including the nature and cost of measures to minimise the risks to staff?

With these questions in mind, on 16th-18th March 1988 the Royal College of Obstetricians and Gynaecologists held its 19th Study Group, on AIDS and Obstetrics and Gynaecology, to discuss such problems. This volume represents the proceedings of that workshop, both the formal presentations which were made for consideration by the assembled clinicians and scientists and also an edited version of the discussion which took place. We also reproduce here the conclusions at which the group arrived, bearing in mind the rapidly changing state of our knowledge in this difficult area of medical practice and its social implications. This is borne out by the issue by the Department of Health and Social Security of the UK, within a month of the Study Group taking place, of important guidelines entitled "HIV Infection, Breast Milk and Human Milk Banking."[1]

Also, concerning the highly important area of the ethical considerations in relation to HIV and AIDS, on the 8th August 1988, all doctors in the UK were circulated with a statement on this matter by the President and the Chairman of the Standards Committee of the General Medical Council.[2] We strongly advise our readers to use these documents in conjunction with this volume.

Finally, we acknowledge the hard work and vigour of Diane Morgan, the RCOG Publications Officer, and Sally Barber, the Secretary of the Postgraduate Education Department of the RCOG, in helping to produce this record of the 19th Study Group within the year of its taking place.

RCOG, London   Mr C.N. Hudson
August 1988   Professor F. Sharp

REFERENCES
1. Anon. HIV infection, breastfeeding and human milk banking. PL/CMO(88)13 and PL/CNO(88)/7. London: DHSS, 1988.
2. Anon. HIV infection and AIDS: the ethical considerations. Statement from the General Medical Council. GMC, London, 8th August 1988.

Participants

DR R. ANCELLE-PARK
WHO Collaborating Centre on AIDS/IMET, Hôpital Claude Bernard, 10 Avenue de la Porte d'Aubervilliers, 75944 Paris Cedex 19, France.

MISS J. BRIERLEY
School of Midwifery, Mint Wing, St Mary's Hospital, London W2 1NY.

MISS E.M. CAMPBELL
Deputy Director of Nursing Services, Bangour General Hospital, Broxburn, West Lothian EH52 6LR.

DR J. CHIN
Chief of Surveillance, Forecasting and Impact Assessment Unit, Global Programme on AIDS, World Health Organisation, 1211 Geneva 27, Switzerland.

PROFESSOR A.A. GLYNN
Director, Public Health Laboratory Service, 61 Colindale Avenue, London NW9 5HT.

DR J. GREEN
District Psychologist, St Mary's Hospital, Praed Street, London W2 1NY.

MISS J. GREENWOOD
Nursing Officer (Midwifery), Room A620, DHSS, Alexander Fleming House, Elephant and Castle, London SE1 6BY.

MR M.J. HARE
Department of Obstetrics and Gynaecology, Hinchingbrooke Hospital, Hinchingbrooke Park, Huntingdon, Cambs.

DR D. HARVEY
Senior Lecturer in Paediatrics, Institute of Obstetrics and Gynaecology, Queen Charlotte's Maternity Hospital, Goldhawk Road, London W6 0XG.

DR B. HEDGE
Clinical Psychologist, Academic Department of Psychiatry, The Middlesex Hospital Medical School, James Pringle House, London W1N 8AA.

PROFESSOR P.W. HOWIE
Department of Obstetrics and Gynaecology, University of Dundee Medical School, Ninewells Hospital, Dundee DD1 9SY.

MR C.N. HUDSON
(RCOG Assistant-Convener of the Study Group), Department of Obstetrics and Gynaecology, St Bartholomew's Hospital, West Smithfield, London EC1A 7BE.

DR D.J. JEFFRIES
Division of Virology, Department of Medical Microbiology, Wright Fleming Institute, St Mary's Hospital Medical School, London W2 1PG.

MS E.A. JENNER
Senior Nurse, Infection Control/Research, St Mary's Hospital, Praed Street, London W2 1NY.

DR F.D. JOHNSTONE
Senior Lecturer, Department of Obstetrics and Gynaecology, Centre for Reproductive Biology, University of Edinburgh, 37 Chalmers Street, Edinburgh EH3 9EW.

DR H.J. LAMBERT
Department of Child Health, University of Newcastle upon Tyne, The Medical School, Framlington Place, Newcastle upon Tyne NE2 4HH.

DR A. LUCAS
MRC Dunn Nutrition Unit and University Department of Paediatrics, Downhams Lane, Milton Road, Cambridge CB4 1XJ.

MS M. McELWEE
Counsellor/Trainer AIDS, 93 Royal Crescent, South Ruislip, Middlesex HA4 0PL.

DR T.J. McMANUS
Consultant in Genito-Urinary Medicine, St Giles Hospital, St Giles Road, London SE5 7RN.

MISS S. McQUEEN
Senior Infection Control Sister, Hospital for Sick Children, Great Ormond Street, London WC1.

MR G.F. MEDLEY
Department of Pure and Applied Biology, Imperial College of Science and Technology, Prince Consort Road, London SW7 2BB.

DR A. MILLS
National Medical Officer, Family Planning Association, 27-35 Mortimer Street, London W1N 7RJ.

DR W.J. MODLE
DHSS, Room D1017, Alexander Fleming House, Elephant and Castle, London SE1 6BY.

DR J. MOK
Consultant Paediatrician, Community Health Services, 15-17 Carlton Terrace, Edinburgh EH7 5DG.

PROFESSOR N.F. MORRIS
16 Provost Road, London NW3 4ST.

PROFESSOR C.S. PECKHAM
Department of Paediatric Epidemiology, Institute of Child Health, 30 Guilford Street, London EC1N 1EH.

MR G.D. PINKER
President, Royal College of Obstetricians and Gynaecologists, 27 Sussex Place, Regent's Park, London NW1 4RG.

DR A. RAFFLES
Queen Elizabeth Hospital for Children, Hackney Road, London E2 8PS.

DR E.E. SCHOENBAUM
Assistant Professor, Department of Epidemiology and Social Medicine, Montefiore Medical Center, Albert Einstein College of Medicine, 111 East 210th Street, Bronx, NY 10467, U.S.A.

DR G.B. SCOTT
Division of Immunology and Infectious Diseases, Department of Pediatrics, University of Miami School of Medicine, Miami, FL 33136, U.S.A.

DR J.B. SCRIMGEOUR
Consultant, Department of Obstetrics and Gynaecology, Western General Hospital, Crewe Road, Edinburgh EH4 2XU.

PROFESSOR F. SHARP
(RCOG Convener of Study Groups), University of Sheffield Medical School, Department of Obstetrics and Gynaecology, Northern General Hospital, Herries Road, Sheffield S5 7AU.

MR A.J.W. SIM
Assistant Director, Academic Surgical Unit, Queen Elizabeth the Queen Mother Wing, St Mary's Hospital, London W2 1NY.

MR S.C. SIMMONS
57 Sheet Street, Windsor, Berks. SL4 1BY.

DR. J.W.G. SMITH
Director, Public Health Laboratory Service, 61 Colindale Avenue, London NW9 5DF.

MR W.P. SOUTTER
Reader in Gynaecological Oncology, Institute of Obstetrics and Gynaecology, Royal Postgraduate Medical School, Hammersmith Hospital, Ducane Road, London W12 0HS.

MRS A.M. SPIRO
Health Visitor, Harrow Health Authority, 66 Grange Gardens, Pinner, Middlesex HA5 5QF.

MR. S.J. STEELE
Director, Academic Department of Obstetrics and Gynaecology, The Middlesex Hospital, 4th Floor, Sir Jules Thorn Institute, Mortimer Street, London W1N 8AA.

PROFESSOR W. THOMPSON
Department of Midwifery and Gynaecology, The Queen's University of Belfast, Institute of Clinical Science, Grosvenor Road, Belfast BT12 6BJ.

DR J.P.P. TYLER
Integrated Fertility Services, 12 Caroline Street, Westmead, NSW 2145, Australia.

DR A. WHITELAW
Consultant Neonatologist, Hammersmith Hospital, Royal Postgraduate Medical School, Ducane Road, London W12 0NN.

PROFESSOR J.G. WHITWAM
Department of Anaesthetics, Hammersmith Hospital, Royal Postgraduate Medical School, Ducane Road, London W12 0NN.

MISS R.J. WILDAY
Director of Midwifery Services, Birmingham Maternity Hospital, Queen Elizabeth Medical Centre, Edgbaston, Birmingham B15 2TG.

PROFESSOR C.B.S. WOOD
Joint Academic Department of Child Health, Queen Elizabeth Hospital for Children, Hackney Road, London E2 8PS.

DR D.A. ZIDEMAN
Consultant and Honorary Senior Lecturer, Department of Anaesthetics, Hammersmith Hospital, Ducane Road, London W12 0NN.

Additional Contributors

DR A.E. ADES
Department of Paediatric Epidemiology, Institute of Child Health, 30 Guilford Street, London WC1N 1EH.

MR R.M. ANDERSON
Department of Pure and Applied Biology, Imperial College, London SW7 2BB.

DR V. CHOWDHURY
Department of Haematology, Royal Postgraduate Medical School, Hammersmith Hospital, Ducane Road, London W12 0NN.

DR J.A. CRITTENDEN
Department of Obstetrics and Gynaecology, Westmead Hospital, Westmead, NSW 2145, Australia.

MS K. DAVENNY
Department of Epidemiology and Social Medicine, Montefiore Medical Center, Albert Einstein College of Medicine, 111 East 210th Street, Bronx, NY 10467, U.S.A.

DR I. DE VINCENZI
WHO Collaborating Centre on AIDS/IMET, Hôpital Claude Bernard, 10 Avenue de la Porte d'Aubervilliers, 75944 Paris Cedex 19, France.

DR H. FRIESEN
Rubaga Hospital, Kampala, Uganda.

DR R.J.D. GEORGE
Senior Lecturer, Middlesex Hospital, London W1.

DR J.M. HOWS
Department of Haematology, Royal Postgraduate Medical School, Hammersmith Hospital, Ducane Road, London W12 0NN.

DR C. HUTTO
Division of Immunology and Infectious Diseases, Department of Pediatrics, University of Miami School of Medicine, Miami, FL 33136, U.S.A.

PROFESSOR W.P. PARKS
Professor of Pediatrics, Division of Immunology and Infectious Diseases, Department of Pediatrics, University of Miami School of Medicine, Miami, FL 33136, U.S.A.

MISS C. ROTH

School of Midwifery, Mint Wing, St Mary's Hospital, London W2 1NY.

DR P.A. SELWYN

Department of Epidemiology and Social Medicine, Montefiore Medical Center, Albert Einstein College of Medicine, 111 East 210th Street, Bronx, NY 10467, U.S.A.

DR Y.D. SENTURIA

Department of Paediatric Epidemiology, Institute of Child Health, 30 Guilford Street, London WC1N 1E4.

MR M.J. TURNER

National Maternity Hospital, Holles Street, Dublin, Republic of Ireland.

DR J.O. WHITE

Lecturer, Institute of Obstetrics and Gynaecology, Royal Postgraduate Medical School, Hammersmith Hospital, Ducane Road, London W12 0HS.

Contents

SECTION I

EPIDEMIOLOGY AND VIROLOGY

Virology

Dr D.J. Jeffries

INTRODUCTION

The acquired immune deficiency syndrome (AIDS) is caused by a human retrovirus, human immunodeficiency virus (HIV), which was discovered in 1983 by Barré-Sinoussi and her colleagues at the Institut Pasteur in Paris.[1] Confirmation was forthcoming the following year with the description of numerous isolations of the virus from patients with AIDS or AIDS-related complex (ARC) by Gallo and colleagues at the National Cancer Institute, Bethesda, USA.[2] In May 1986, an international expert committee, empowered by the International Committee on the Taxonomy of Viruses, introduced the term HIV to replace the previous terms (LAV, IDAV, HTLV-III and ARV) which had been used for the virus by different groups in France and the United States.[3] Discovery of a distinct, but related, human retrovirus in West Africa, which also causes AIDS and allied conditions[4] led to the introduction of the terms HIV-1 for the original AIDS virus and HIV-2 for the new virus. HIV-2 has now been reported as being present in several European countries and in one city in the United States, but this chapter is confined to HIV-1, the virus responsible for the global epidemic of AIDS, ARC, PGL (persistent generalised lymphadenopathy) and the related encephalopathy. This is appropriate as the genomic organisation, cellular tropism, transmission and clinical effects of HIV-1 and HIV-2 appear to be similar.

RETROVIRUSES

The retrovirus family (Retroviridae) are characterised by the production of a particle-associated enzyme RNA-directed DNA polymerase or reverse transcriptase.[5,6] This enzyme confers the unique property of reverse transcription in which the RNA of the viruses is converted to a complementary DNA copy which can then be inserted into the chromosomal DNA of an infected cell to create an integrated provirus.

There are three sub-families of retroviruses:

i) Oncoviruses

These include oncogenic viruses of animals and they are subdivided on morphological criteria into B-type (mammary tumour viruses), C-type (leukaemia viruses) and D type (Mason-Pfizer monkey virus).[7] Human T-cell leukaemia viruses (HTLV-II and III) are included with the C-type oncoviruses.

3

ii) Spumaviruses

The development of vacuolation in cell cultures derived from humans and other primates has occasionally been associated with the presence of retroviruses which have been termed spumaviruses. These agents have never been associated with disease formation in the original host.

iii) Lentiviruses

This term was introduced by Sigurdsson in 1954 following the discovery of visna/maedi virus which causes progressive degeneration of the nervous system or pneumonia in sheep.[8] Two other lentiviruses of ungulates have been identified: equine infectious anaemia virus (EIAV) and caprine arthritis encephalitis virus (CAEV).

HIV-1 and HIV-2 have been classified as lentiviruses on the basis of similarities in morphology, genetic structure and biological properties to visna virus.[9,10] Viruses isolated from different species of monkeys have been termed simian immunodeficiency viruses (SIV) and included in the Lentiviridae. Serological surveys have revealed that SIV infection is widespread in vervet monkeys in sub-Saharan Africa and this virus, which appears to be non-pathogenic in sooty mangabeys and vervets, has caused immunodeficiency (simian AIDS) in captive macaques.

STRUCTURE AND PROPERTIES OF HIV-1

The structure of the virion of HIV-1 is shown schematically in Figure I. The

Figure I

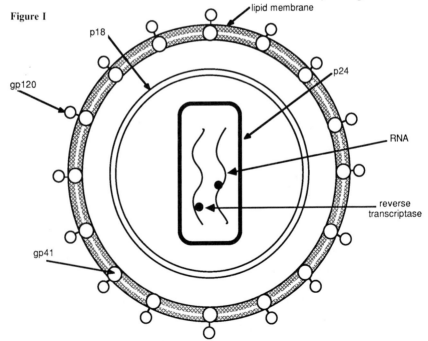

Schematic illustration of the structural organisation of HIV-1.

particle is roughly spherical with a diameter of approximately 100 nanometers. The viral core containing RNA and the associated reverse transcriptase is surrounded by an envelope which consists of a lipid bilayer membrane, derived from the plasma membrane of the host cell, into which viral-coded glycoproteins have been inserted. This basic structure is typical of all members of the Retroviridae, many of which have been studied since early in this century; this allowed confidence in predicting the physico-chemical properties of HIV-1. The glycoproteins of HIV-1 are in two components: gp41 spans the membrane and gp120 extends beyond it. The external glycoprotein contains the attachment site for the cell receptor for the virus, the CD4 antigen. Despite considerable variability in the genomes of different isolates indicating a high mutation rate, there appears to have been no change in affinity for the CD4 antigen indicating that the binding site is encoded from a conserved genetic sequence. This explains the consistent pattern of transmission and clinical effects of the virus since it was first recognised in 1981.

The physico-chemical nature of retroviruses was reviewed by Vogt in 1965.[11] Three groups reported that HIV-1, in high titre, was rapidly destroyed at 56°C.[12-14] However, Resnick and colleagues described a much slower rate of inactivation at this temperature with a reduction of only 3 log10 TCID 50 after one hour.[15] In this work, apparent total inactivation (loss of 7 log10 TCID 50) was only achieved after 5 hours, and they suggested that apparent differences in thermal inactivation characteristics between the studies may depend on variations in the testing systems and infectivity titrations being used. There is no doubt, however, that HIV-1 is much more thermolabile than many other viruses (e.g. Hepatitis B virus) and it is rapidly destroyed by boiling. HIV-1 is destroyed by exposure to high and low pH with inactivation occurring below pH2 and above pH13. Martin *et al.* demonstrated a reduction of infectivity of 3 log10 TCID 50 when virus was held for 10 minutes at pH6 compared to pH7.[13] The lipid-containing envelope confers properties on HIV-1 that are similar to those of other retroviruses. If the envelope is destroyed the virus is rendered non-infective. Thus HIV-1 is sensitive to the action of a wide range of chemical disinfectants and detergents including alcohols, acetone, hypochlorite, aldehydes, ethylene oxide, phenols, nonidet-P40 and hydrogen peroxide.[13,15] Relative resistance to ionising and ultraviolet radiation was reported by Spire *et al* with the retention of infectivity after exposure to less than 250 thousand rads of gamma rays and less than 5000 J/m^{2}UV.[12] This is, however, to be expected for a virus with the genomic size of the Retroviridae.

Knowledge of the nature of retroviruses and early studies of the inactivation characteristics of HIV-1 soon led to it being described widely as a fragile virus. This is largely true when HIV-1 is compared with viruses that lack the sensitive lipid-containing envelope. It is important to note, however, that the infectivity of the virus may persist at ambient temperatures for several days. It is likely that the lipid membrane surrounding the particle protects it against dessication. Resnick *et al*[15] demonstrated survival for up to 24 hours at room temperature after drying and infectivity was maintained for many days in aqueous preparations.

VIRUS-HOST RELATIONSHIPS

(i) Cellular tropism

The main target cell for HIV-1 is the helper/inducer subset of T lymphocyes which is characterised by expression on the cell membrane of the CD4 antigen. This antigen, which has been identified as the receptor for the virus, is also present in cells of monocyte/macrophage lineage in the blood, alveoli and brain, and infection is known to occur in these different cell types *in vivo*. Infection has been found in follicular dendritic cells in the lymph nodes of AIDS patients and HIV-1 has been shown to have the ability to infect neuroglial tissue and B lymphocytes transformed by Epstein-Barr virus. The cellular tropisms of HIV-1 have been reviewed by McClure and Weiss.[16] Studies on intestinal epithelium have indicated the possibility of direct involvement of the bowel in HIV-1 replication.[17] This pattern of distribution of infection at a cellular level is consistent with knowledge of the spectrum of diseases caused by HIV-1.

(ii) Replication

The replication cycle of HIV-1 is shown schematically in Figure II. Following attachment of the virus to the CD4 antigen, the particle is then internalised. The exact method of this process is unknown, but it is assumed to be achieved either by fusion of the viral envelope with the plasma membrane or by capture of the virus in an intracytoplasmic vesicle by endocytosis. Following uncoating of the virion, the naked, single stranded RNA is used as a template for reverse transcriptase to create a complementary DNA copy. The RNA is eliminated by RNase H activity thought to be encoded from the pol gene of the virus, and this then allows the formation of a second strand of DNA. The double strand of virally-derived DNA assumes a circular form and is integrated into the genome of the host cell by an endonuclease which is also encoded from the pol gene of the virus. The integrated DNA provirus may remain latent until the cell is activated. At this point the DNA is transcribed to mRNA and viral genomic RNA with the activity of host cell RNA polymerases. The mRNA is translated to form viral proteins by host cell ribosomes and the progeny viral RNA and proteins are assembled into new particles at the cell membrane. The virus is then released from the cell by budding. Unlike some human viruses (e.g. herpes simplex) which induce a rapid and permanent shut-down of cellular mechanisms, HIV-1 establishes a continuing relationship. This allows the cell to remain viable for a period of time which is likely to vary from one cell to another and to depend on the level of activity of the cell, whether it is in the immune system, and the state of activation of the virus. Several DNA viruses (herpes simplex virus type 1, polyoma viruses JC and BK and varicella zoster virus) have been shown to activate HIV-1 transcription *in vitro*.[18,19] Enhancement of virus production is thought to lead to destruction of the infected cell. Thus the original advice given to carriers of HIV-1, to lead a healthy lifestyle and avoid unnecessary contact with other infectious agents, would seem to have some substantiation from studies at a molecular and cellular level.

Figure II

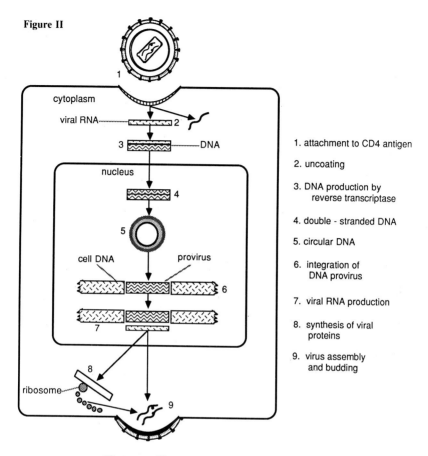

cytoplasm

viral RNA········· 2

3 ·········DNA

nucleus

4

5

cell DNA   provirus

6

7

ribosome······· 8

9

1. attachment to CD4 antigen

2. uncoating

3. DNA production by
   reverse transcriptase

4. double - stranded DNA

5. circular DNA

6. integration of
   DNA provirus

7. viral RNA production

8. synthesis of viral
   proteins

9. virus assembly
   and budding

Diagram to illustrate the replication cycle of HIV-1.

(iii) Pathogenesis

The pathogenesis of HIV-1 infection is not fully understood but the progressive destruction of the immune and/or central nervous systems is thought to be due to one or more of the following mechanisms.

a) cell fusion

The binding of the envelope glycoprotein (gp120) to the CD4 antigen on infected and uninfected cells causes the cells to aggregate. Fusion of plasma membranes then occurs by a process which requires the action of the transmembrane glycoprotein (gp41) and a multinucleated giant cell results. This process leads to the destruction of infected and uninfected cells and may partly explain the apparent discrepancy between the low numbers of infected cells and the marked depletion of CD4 cells *in vitro* and *in vivo*.

b) immunological mechanisms

The fact that peripheral blood lymphocytes can be killed by the virus *in vitro* in the absence of significant syncytium formation suggests other pathogenetic effects. The coating of CD4 lymphocytes (infected or uninfected) with gp120 may lead to their recognition as foreign and result in destruction and clearance by the immune system. In addition, HIV-1 infection may induce the formation of auto-antibodies directed against CD4 positive cells. Finally, changes in the HLA class II phenotype of HIV-1-infected cells may render them susceptible to immune clearance.

c) accumulation of virions or nucleic acid

There is evidence from studies of other lentiviruses that accumulation of unintegrated viral DNA is associated with cytopathic effects. In HIV-1 infection free DNA has been observed to persist in infected cells. The massive production of virions after activation of latently infected cells may also have cytocidal activity.

(iv) Viraemia

The sequence of events following post-natal infection with HIV-1 is described later. Once infection is established, however, the presence within circulating lymphocytes of the integrated proviral DNA of HIV-1 means that viraemia is persistent and anyone with a confirmed positive result on antibody testing must be assumed to be potentially infectious for the rest of their lives. In the period prior to seroconversion several workers have reported a period of marked plasma viraemia which subsides once the antibody responses have developed. The failure to demonstrate effective neutralising antibody in many patients suggests, however, that virus may continue to circulate in immune complexes comprised of non-neutralising antibody. There is now some epidemiological evidence to suggest that infectivity increases when the immune responses of an HIV-1 carrier start to fail and as AIDS or related conditions start to appear.

(v) Virus excretion

The routes of transmission of HIV-1 have been clearly defined by retrospective investigation of many thousands of AIDS cases and by carefully controlled studies of different types of contact situations. Blood has been shown to contain the highest titres of virus and transmission has been associated with transfusion of whole blood and plasma. Semen has also been shown to contain virus and transmission has occurred as a result of artificial insemination from an infected donor.[20] Virus has been grown from breast milk and the report of infection in a baby being breastfed from a mother who acquired HIV-1, post-natally from a blood transfusion, is evidence for transmission by this route.[21] Isolation of HIV-1 from female genital tract secretions[22] provides one possible explanation of female-to-male spread of infection but proof of transmission from this fluid is lacking.

Other body fluids known to contain virus on occasions are saliva, urine, tears, amniotic fluid, synovial fluid and cerebrospinal fluid. None of these has been shown to transmit infection to others. The possibility of transmission from saliva has caused considerable anxiety and, for this reason, studies have been conducted to assess the risks of kissing, biting and exposure to salivary contamination. Extensive follow-up of family contacts of AIDS patients and HIV-1 positive individuals in circumstances where intimate kissing, but not sexual contact, has been practised have failed to reveal evidence of transmission. Surveys of dental surgeons who are exposed to aerosols of saliva (and often blood) of HIV-1-infected patients have confirmed the lack of occupational transmission, and there has been no evidence of infection from bites received from HIV-1 carriers. In view of the fact that any body fluid may contain lymphocytes or frank blood it is normally recommended that infection control precautions should be designed to prevent contact with all body fluids.

Genomic structure of HIV-1

The genomic organisation of HIV-1 is shown in Figure III. As in other members of the Retroviridae, the three main genes of the virus, gag, pol and env, are flanked by long terminal repeat sequences (LTRs). The LTRs act as promoters of gene expression and contain specific enhancer elements on which viral proteins may act.

The gag gene encodes a precursor protein (55Kd) which is cleaved by a protease encoded from the pol gene to produce the three core proteins p15, p18 and p24. The pol gene encodes the reverse transcriptase, which is in 2 molecular sizes (51 and 66 Kd), and the endonuclease or integrase involved in integration of the provirus. The env gene products are the envelope glycoproteins (gp41 and gp120) which are derived from a precursor glycoprotein (160Kd). Towards the 3' end of

Figure III

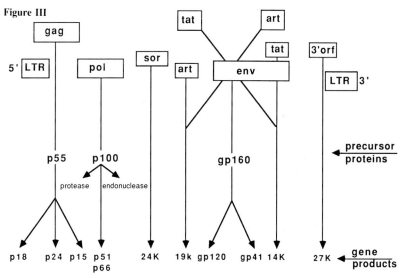

The genome of HIV-1. (See text for details.)

the genome there are a series of regulatory genes which are responsible for post-transcriptional regulation of HIV-1 replication. Deletion of the bipartite genes tat (transactivator of transcription) and art (anti-repression transactivator) results in a total inhibition of viral replication. Deletion of another small genetic sequence, the short open reading frame (sor) results in disablement of the virus with a severe reduction in virus production. In contrast the 3' open reading frame (3'orf) appears to have a suppressive effect on virus replication. The recognition of the importance of these regulatory genes in activating HIV-1 has led to cloning and expression of their products by recombinant DNA techniques and the possibility of developing antiviral therapy against these virus specific targets. The structure of the genome and the possible approaches to chemotherapeutic intervention have been reviewed elsewhere.[23] All of the gene products of HIV-1 have been characterised and have become available in pure preparations. This has allowed the development of sensitive and specific serological tests for the virus.

LABORATORY DIAGNOSIS AND PROGNOSTIC TESTS

HIV-1 can be cultured in the laboratory by separating out the mononuclear cells from heparinised blood and then cultivating them with permissive uninfected cells (peripheral blood mononuclear cells or lymphoblastoid cell lines). Following initial stimulation with phytohaemagglutinin, the growth of the cells is promoted with interleukin 2 and interferon responses are countered by adding antibodies to alpha interferon. The virus takes several days to grow and its presence is detected by the formation of syncytia, immunofluorescence or the presence of reverse transcriptase or p24 antigen in the supernatant medium. The technique of virus culture is laborious and costly and is not employed as a routine for the diagnosis of infection in adults. It is important for detecting virus in certain clinical situations, however, and it is the most reliable means of determining whether a neonate has become infected from an HIV-1-infected mother. Loss of antibody during the first year of life has been shown to be an unreliable index of freedom from congenital infection and virus has been isolated from babies who have become seronegative by all available tests.[24-25]

A variety of different antibody tests has been devised for routine screening for HIV-1 antibody[26] and these have been refined to yield high sensitivity and specificity. Purified antigens prepared by recombinant DNA technology have been incorporated into ELISA systems. Using these assays, sequential testing on HIV-1 infected adults has shown a pattern of antibody responses that correlates with prognosis. Although antibodies to the envelope glycoprotein (gp41) are maintained at high levels, loss of antibody to the core protein (gp24) correlates significantly with progression to disease.[27-28] The development of sensitive antigen assays for HIV-1 offers a method of detecting virus expression in serum and possibly other body fluids. Antigen can by detected in serum before the development of antibody[29] and the return of antigenaemia after the decline of core (p24) antibody provides another marker of impending disease.[30] The sequence of antigen and antibody responses following HIV-1 infection in an adult is shown schematically in Figure IV. If, as indicated earlier, infectivity of an individual increases with the decline of core antibody and the return of

Figure IV

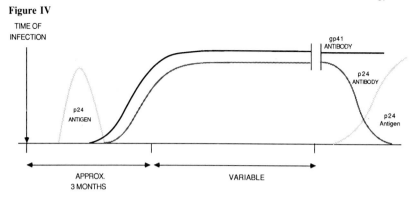

TIME OF INFECTION

gp41 ANTIBODY

p24 ANTIBODY

p24 ANTIGEN

p24 Antigen

APPROX. 3 MONTHS

VARIABLE

Antigen and antibody responses in blood following HIV-1 infection.

antigenaemia, application of these predictive tests to women in pregnancy may show a correlation between the stage of the infection and the risk of transmission to the fetus. Antigen detection has been used as a means of investigating the possibility of infection in the neonate. The sensitivity of the test in this age group requires further evaluation.

PREVENTION AND TREATMENT

Approaches to prevention in operation at present include attempts to educate the population towards lifestyle changes by reduction of contacts together with attempts to interrupt the transmission of the virus by safer sex counselling, condom usage and provision of clean syringes and needles to intravenous drug users. Donor screening has been introduced to prevent transmission of HIV-1 by blood transfusion and organ transplantation. Termination of pregnancy in those found to be HIV-1 carriers in the antenatal clinic will serve to reduce transmission to the next generation.

Vaccines are being developed in a number of centres and employing several different strategies. It remains to be seen whether these vaccines will confer protective immunity which will be efficient in stemming the spread of a virus which is showing a disturbing ability to mutate.

Antiviral drug development is offering some hope for AIDS patients and carriers of the virus. The reverse transcriptase inhibitor, zidovudine (azidothymidine, AZT) has been licensed for use on AIDS patients and has been shown to prolong their lives.[31] Zidovudine has marked toxicity on the bone marrow in these patients but pilot studies in asymptomatic carriers suggest that it may have less serious side effects in those who have minor symptoms or who are well. If drugs can be developed which are safe enough to use for suppression of virus replication in the large and increasing population of HIV-1 carriers, it may be possible to reduce or abolish their infectivity in addition to delaying or preventing disease onset.

CONCLUSIONS

The world has witnessed the appearance and spread of an epidemic with the human retrovirus HIV-1. No human members of this family have been recognised before the current decade and there is no record of a previous epidemic of this nature. It is fortunate that the appearance of HIV-1 has occurred at a time when recent developments in molecular biology and virology have allowed our understanding of the virus to progress at a remarkable rate. It is to be hoped that these advances will lead to the introduction of vaccines and antiviral drugs which will have impact on the escalation of the epidemic. In the meantime, there is a host of unsolved problems and many of these are related to our ignorance of human behaviour.

REFERENCES

 1. Barré-Sinoussi F, Chermann J-C, Rey F, Nugeyre MT, Chamaret S, Gruest J, Dauguet C, Axler-Blin C, Brun-Vézinet F, Rouzioux C, Rozenbaum W, Montagnier L. Isolation of a T-lymphotropic retrovirus from a patient at risk for acquired immune deficiency syndrome (AIDS). *Science* 1983; **220:** 868-871.
 2. Gallo RC, Salahuddin SZ, Popovic M, Shearer GM, Kaplan M, Haynes BF, Palker TJ, Redfield R, Oleske J, Safai B, White G, Foster P, Markham PD. Frequent detection and isolation of cytopathic retroviruses (HTLV-III) from patients with AIDS and at risk for AIDS. *Science* 1984; **224:** 500-503.
 3. Coffin J, Haase A, Levy JA, Montagnier L, Oroszlan S, Teich N, Temin H, Toyoshima K, Varmus H, Vogt P, Weiss RA. What to call the AIDS virus? (Letter) *Nature* 1986; **321:** 10.
 4. Clavel F, Guétard D, Brun-Vézinet F, Chamaret S, Rey M-A, Santos-Ferreira MO, Laurent AG, Dauguet C, Katlama C, Rouzioux C, Klatzmann D, Champalimaud JL, Montagnier L. Isolation of a new human retrovirus from West African patients with AIDS. *Science* 1986; **233:** 343-346.
 5. Baltimore D. Viral RNA-dependent DNA polymerase. *Nature* 1970; **226:** 1209-1211.
 6. Temin HM, Mizutani S. RNA-dependent DNA polymerase in virions of Rous sarcoma virus. *Nature* 1970; **226:** 1211-1213.
 7. Jeffries DJ. Virological aspects of AIDS. *Clinics in Immunology and Allergy.* 1986; **6:** 627-644.
 8. Sigurdsson B. Maedi a slow progressive pneumonia of sheep: an epizoological and pathological study. *Br Vet J* 1954; **110:** 255-270.
 9. Gonda MA, Wong-Staal F, Gallo, RC, Clements JE, Narayan O, Gilden RV. Sequence homology and morphologic similarity of HTLV-III and visna virus, a pathogenic lentivirus. *Science* 1985; **227:** 173-177.
10. Sonigo P, Alizon M, Staskus K, Klatzman D, Cole S, Danos O, Retzel E, Tiollais P, Haase A, Wain-Hobson S. Nucleotide sequence of the visna lentivirus: relationship to the AIDS virus. *Cell* 1985; **42:** 369-382.
11. Vogt PK. Avian tumour viruses. *Ad Virus Res* 1965; **11:** 293-385.
12. Spire B, Barré-Sinoussi F, Dormont D, Montagnier L, Chermann J-C. Inactivation of lymphadenopathy-associated virus by heat, gamma rays and ultraviolet light. *Lancet* 1985; **1:** 188-189.
13. Martin LS, McDougal JS, Loskowski SL. Disinfection and inactivation of the human T-lymphotropic virus type III lymphadenopathy-associated virus. *J Infect Dis* 1985; **152:** 400-403.
14. McDougal JS, Martin LS, Cort SP, Mozen M, Heldebrant CM, Evatt BL. Thermal inactivation of the acquired immunodeficiency syndrome virus human T-lymphotropic virus III/antihemophilic factor. *J Clin Invest* 1985; **76:** 875-877.

15. Resnick L, Veren K, Salahuddin SZ, Tondreau S, Markham PD. Stability and inactivation of HTLV-III/LAV under clinical and laboratory environments. *JAMA* 1986; **225:** 1887-1891.
16. McClure MO, Weiss RA. Human immunodeficiency virus and related viruses. In: *Current Topics in AIDS.* Eds. MS Gottlieb, DJ Jeffries, D Mildvan, AJ Pinching, TC Quinn, RA Weiss. Chichester: John Wiley, 1987; pp.95-117.
17. Nelson JA, Wiley A, Reynolds-Kohler C, Reese CE, Margarettan W, Levy JA. Human immunodeficiency virus detected in bowel epithelium from patients with gastrointestinal symptoms. *Lancet* 1988; **1:** 259-262.
18. Gendelman HE, Phelps W, Feigenbaum L, Ostrove JM, Adachi A, Howley PM, Khoury G, Ginsburg HS, Martin MA. Transactivation of the human immuno-deficiency virus long terminal repeat sequence by DNA viruses. *Proc Nat Acad Sci USA* 1986; **83:** 9759-9763.
19. Mosca JD, Bednarik DP, Raj NBK, Rosen CA, Sodroski JG, Haseltine WA, Pitha PM. Herpes simplex type-1 can reactivate transcription of latent human immuno-deficiency virus. *Nature* 1987; **325:** 67-70.
20. Stewart GJ, Tyler JPP, Cunningham AL, Barr JA, Driscoll GL, Gold J, Lamont BJ. Transmission of human T-cell lymphotropic virus type III (HTLV-III) by artificial insemination by donor. *Lancet* 1985; **2:** 581-584.
21. Ziegler JB, Cooper DA, Johnson RO. Postnatal transmission of AIDS-associated retrovirus from mother to infant. *Lancet* 1985; **1:** 896-898.
22. Wofsy CB, Cohen JB, Hauer LB, Padian NS, Michaelis BA, Evans LA, Levy JA. Isolation of AIDS-associated retrovirus from genital secretions of women with anti-bodies to the virus. *Lancet* 1986; **1:** 527-529.
23. Jeffries DJ. Human immunodeficiency viruses. In: *Recent Advances in Infection 3.* Eds. DS Reeves, AM Geddes. In press.
24. Mok JQ, Giaquinto C, De Rossi A, Grosch-Wörner I, Ades AE, Peckham CS. Infants born to mothers seropositive for human immunodeficiency virus. Preliminary findings from a multicentre European study. *Lancet* 1987; **1:** 1164-1168.
25. Borkowsky W, Kraskinski K, Paul D, Moore T, Bebenroth D, Chadwani S. Human-immunodeficiency-virus infections in infants negative for anti-HIV by enzyme-linked immunoassay. *Lancet* 1987; **1:** 1168-1170.
26. Mortimer PP, Clewley JP. Serological tests for human immunodeficiency virus. In: *Current Topics in AIDS.* Eds. MS Gottlieb, DJ Jeffries, D Mildvan, AJ Pinching, TC Quinn, RA Weiss. Chichester: John Wiley, 1987; pp.133-154.
27. Lange JM, Paul DA, Huisman HG, de Wolf F, van den Berg H, Coutinho RA, Danner SA, van der Noordaa J, Goudsmit J. Persistent HIV antigenaemia and decline of HIV core antibodies associated with transition to AIDS. *Br Med J* 1986; **293:** 1459-1462.
28. Weber JN, Clapham PR, Weiss RA, Parker D, Roberts C, Duncan J, Weller I, Carne C, Tedder RS, Pinching AJ, Cheingsong-Popov R. Human immunodeficiency virus infection in two cohorts of homosexual men: neutralising sera and association of anti-gag antibody with prognosis. *Lancet* 1987; **1:** 119-122.
29. Allain J-P, Laurian Y, Paul DA, Senn D. and members of the AIDS-Haemophilia French Study Group. Serological markers in early stages of human immunodeficiency virus infection in haemophiliacs. *Lancet* 1986; **2:** 1233-1236.
30. Forster SM, Osborne LM, Cheingsong-Popov R, Kenny C, Burnell R, Jeffries DJ, Pinching AJ, Harris JRW, Weber JN. Decline of anti-p24 antibody precedes antigenaemia as correlate of prognosis in HIV-1 infection. *AIDS* 1987; **1:** 235-240.
31. Fischl MA, Richman DD, Grieco MH, Gottlieb MS, Volberding PA, Laskin OL, Leedom JM, Groopman JE, Mildvan D, Schooley RT, Jackson GG, Durack DT, King D, and the AZT Collaborative Group. The efficacy of azidothymidine (AZT) in the treatment of patients with AIDS and AIDS-related complex. *N Engl J Med* 1987; **317:** 185-191.

The global patterns and prevalence of HIV infection in women

Dr J. Chin

INTRODUCTION

This paper provides some estimates of the current global dimensions of HIV infection among females. To place these estimates in proper perspective, it is first necessary briefly to describe the 3 global patterns of AIDS and HIV infections which currently exist.[1] The explanation for the existence of these patterns includes the likely date of HIV entry and/or period when HIV began to spread extensively in the population, the relative importance of the 3 modes of HIV transmission and details of sexual and other social risk behaviours in the population.

In areas with Pattern I, HIV probably began to spread extensively in the late 1970s. Most cases occurred among homosexual or bisexual males and urban intravenous (IV) drug users. Heterosexual transmission is responsible for only a small percentage of cases but is increasing. Transmission due to blood and blood products occurred between the late 1970s and 1985, but has now virtually been eliminated through the self-referral of persons with known risk factors/behaviour and by routine blood screening for HIV antibody. Unsterile needles, other than those used by IV drug users, do not constitute a large public health problem. The male to female sex ratio is generally about 10:1, and to date perinatal transmission is uncommon. Overall population seroprevalence is estimated to be much less than 1%, but has been measured at over 50% in some groups of persons practising high-risk behaviours such as men with multiple sex partners and IV drug users. This pattern is typical of industrialised countries with large numbers of reported AIDS cases, including North America, many Western European countries, Australia, New Zealand, and parts of Latin America.

In Pattern II areas, most cases occur among heterosexuals and it is likely that HIV began to spread extensively in the 1970s. The male to female ratio is approximately 1:1, and as a result perinatal transmission is common. IV drug use and homosexual transmission are either absent or occur at a very low level. In a number of countries, overall population seroprevalence is estimated at more than 1% and in some urban areas up to 20% of the sexually active age group is infected. Transmission through contaminated blood and blood products has been a significant problem and continues in those countries that have not yet

15

implemented donor screening. In addition, the use of unsterile needles and syringes for injection is considered an important public health problem. This pattern is observed in areas of central, eastern and southern Africa, and increasingly in some countries of Latin America, especially in the Caribbean.

In Pattern III areas, HIV was introduced in the early to mid-1980s and only small numbers of cases have been reported. Homosexual and heterosexual transmission have only recently been documented. Cases have generally occurred in persons who have travelled to Pattern I and II areas, or who have had sexual contact with individuals from such areas. Cases due to the use of imported blood products have been reported, and in a few Pattern III countries, these cases comprise the largest percentage of reported AIDS cases to date. This pattern is found in areas in Eastern Europe, the Middle East, Asia, and most of the Pacific (excluding Australia and New Zealand).

METHODS

Estimations of HIV-infected persons worldwide are currently made with very limited data. Such estimates are usually derived by extrapolating from serological data collected from a variety of selected population groups such as blood donors, pregnant women, sexually-transmitted disease clinic patients, female prostitutes, IV drug users, homosexual men, etc. The major problems with such extrapolations are that it is not known to what extent these surveys or studies (other than blood donors) are representative of the subpopulation group in question, and more importantly, what are the precise numbers in each of the subpopulations. Nevertheless, reasonable estimates can and must be made for planning or prediction purposes. Such estimates obviously will require revision as additional serosurvey data are collected.

This paper will review some of the published data on the prevalence of HIV infection in selected female populations. Estimates of total numbers of HIV-infected women globally, in the USA and in the UK, are derived from WHO estimates and from the known sex distribution of reported AIDS cases.

HIV INFECTION IN WOMEN WORLDWIDE

Global

Table 1 provides a very rough estimate of the number of HIV-infected women throughout the world. A reasonably conservative estimate of about 5,000,000 HIV-infected persons worldwide is used along with the observed male to female ratio of AIDS cases observed in each of the global pattern areas to arrive at a global estimate of about 1,500,000 HIV-infected females.

Table 1   **Estimation of the number of HIV-infected females, 1988**

Geographic Area	Estimated total HIV-infected persons	Observed M:F Ratio of AIDS	Estimated total HIV-infected females
Pattern I	2.5 million	9:1	250,000
Pattern II	2.5 million	1:1	1,250,000
Pattern III	10,000	1:1	5,000
TOTALS	> 5 million		1,505,000

Pattern III areas

In several of the Pattern III countries such as India, Thailand and the Philippines, where HIV serosurveys have been carried out, the findings show a large preponderance of infected females compared to males.[2] This seemingly surprising finding turns out to be not too surprising since the vast majority of HIV serosurveys carried out in these countries (aside from blood donor surveys) have been among registered female prostitute populations. Similarly, if HIV serosurveys are essentially restricted to homosexual/bisexual men, it would not be surprising to find a marked male preponderance. In general, the prevalence rate of HIV infection found among female prostitute populations in Pattern III areas is relatively low at the present time. They average approximately one in a thousand or less and their current rates are comparable to those of blood donor prevalence rates in some Pattern I areas.

Pattern II areas

In Pattern II areas, there have been numerous HIV serosurveys carried out over the past few years which indicate that the male to female ratio of both AIDS cases and of HIV infection is about one to one.[1] Relatively high prevalence of HIV infections is currently found among some female populations in some urban areas of central, eastern and southern Africa (P. Way, personal communication).

Table 2

HIV serosurveys of female prostitutes, Central Africa

City	Year	Number tested	Percent positive
A	1987	115	64.4
B	1985	376	27.0
C	1987	N/A	80.0

WHO 88375

Very high prevalence rates have to be expected among female prostitutes (Table 2), but the disturbing finding in these Pattern II area studies is the relatively high prevalence rate found among large numbers of populations of pregnant women (Table 3). However, these latter findings are consistent with blood donor studies in these same areas which indicate that up to 20% of sexually active adults in some urban areas are already HIV-infected. The only optimistic note is that preliminary survey results indicate that large portions of rural areas (where the majority of the population are) in Pattern II areas show a relatively low prevalence of HIV infection among the sexually active age group.[3]

Table 3

HIV serosurvey of pregnant women, Central Africa 1987

City	Number tested	Percent positive
A	2,910	2.7
B	6,000	5.7
C	170	24.0

WHO 88376

Pattern I areas

In Pattern I countries, the largest problem and the most documentation of HIV seroprevalence among selected female populations currently exists in the United States. The US Public Health Service, as part of what they have called "a family of serosurveys", has collected all of the available data on HIV serosurveys in the USA.[4]

Table 4

Summary of HIV-positive serosurveys of female prostitutes, USA 1985-1987

● These studies from 8 states involved incarcerated prostitutes, those in drug-treatment centres and community outreach programmes.

● The highest prevalence of 45.3% (82/181) was found in IV drug centres. The only survey which did not identify a seropositive was from a Southern State in 1985-1986 (0/76).

● Of the total of 3,474 prostitutes in these combined studies, 8.6% (299/3,474) were HIV seropositive.

WHO 88377

Female prostitute surveys in the USA, with the single exception of a survey among 76 prostitutes in the state of Tennessee during 1985-86, all revealed some HIV-infected prostitutes (Table 4). The major risk factor for these HIV positive women (in addition to their having multiple sexual partners) was that many, if not most of the seropositive prostitutes were also IV drug users or sexual consorts of male IV drug users. Overall, the percentage of HIV positive prostitutes among the circa 3,500 prostitutes tested in these surveys is 8.6%.

Table 5

HIV serosurveys of pregnant women or women in the childbearing age group, USA 1986-1987

	Number tested	Percent positive
Specified high-risk groups	625	15.2
Women from inner-city areas	3,220	2.6
General surveys	34,282	0.02*

*Virtually all the HIV seropositive women found were from large urban areas

WHO 88378

Of the more than 20 serosurvey studies of pregnant women or women of childbearing age from perinatal, prenatal or abortion clinics, these could be grouped into 3 categories as shown in Table 5. Where the population selected had some known HIV risk factor, such as IV drug use, the percentage found positive was relatively high at 15.2%. When pregnant women in hospitals or clinics in inner cities on the East Coast of the USA were sampled 2.6% were found to be HIV seropositive. At least 1 of these hospitals has a large number of women from Haiti. In the general surveys of women of childbearing age who were not in known risk groups or who were not in areas of high IV drug use, 0.02% were found HIV seropositive and virtually all the positive women were from large urban areas.

Estimating total numbers of HIV-infected pregnant women

One method for determining the number of HIV-infected pregnant women in a large area was recently published in the New England Journal of Medicine.[5] This method used the existing newborn screening system for PKU, which is required in many States, to survey the HIV seroprevalence in the general population of childbearing women. Detection of HIV antibody in blood collected from newborns can be used to monitor HIV infection rates in pregnant women. By unlinking personal identifying information, including the specific hospital of birth, the authors were able to guarantee complete anonymity. This method was never intended to be a case finding system, but was intended rapidly to identify those areas where HIV infections are detected in pregnant women, in order to direct specific programmes for individual HIV testing with informed consent and appropriate counselling to these areas.

Table 6

HIV seroprevalence rate in newborn blood samples according to hospital category
Massachusetts December 1986-June 1987

Hospital category	Number tested	Positive/ 100,000	Estimated annual number of sero-positive births
"Inner city"	3,741	800	43
Urban/suburban	16,870	250	84
Mixed	6,501	120	32
Rural	3,596	30	3
TOTALS	30,708	1,200	162

Table 6 summarises the findings from this study and is consistent with the known urban/rural distribution of HIV infections. Of particular value is the statistical estimation from their study that on an annual basis about 160 infants are born to HIV-infected women in the State of Massachusetts. Thus, in areas where there are no legal or ethical objections to such unlinked testing, such a system of statistically valid sampling can provide valuable information on the prevalence and trends of HIV infection in pregnant women.

Estimating the total number of HIV-infected women—USA

All the preceding studies of selected female populations in the USA do not provide for an estimation of the total number of infected women in the country. One indirect method which can be used is to distribute the estimated total number of HIV infections in the USA by age and sex according to the proportion of reported AIDS cases by age and sex. If an estimate of 1,250,000 HIV-infected persons in the USA as of early 1988 is accepted, and this total is distributed according to the age and sex distribution of reported AIDS cases, then an estimation of the number and age distribution of HIV-infected women can be derived. This number and distribution is shown in Table 7. About 100,000 HIV-infected women are estimated with the highest number in the 30-39 year age group.

If standard fertility rates are applied to the infected women of childbearing age, an estimate of close to 5,000 annual births to HIV-infected women, as of 1987-88, can be calculated. It needs to be emphasised that the distribution of HIV

Table 7

Estimated number and age distribution of HIV-infected females, USA

	Total	13-19 yrs	20-29 yrs	30-39 yrs	40-49 yrs	$\geqslant 50$ yrs
Population	99.88 million	12.91 million	21.36 million	18.43 million	12.90 million	34.28 million
Number infected	100,204	429	21,135	47,666	21,039	9,935
Number positive per 100,000	100	3	99	259	163	29
Estimated number of births to HIV-infected women	4,846	30	1,479	3,337	0	0

WHO 88380

infection in women in the USA varies tremendously by geographic area. New York, New Jersey and Florida have over 70% of all HIV-infected women in the USA and within these states virtually all the HIV-infected women are in the large urban areas.

Estimating the total number of HIV-infected women—UK

The number of HIV-infected women in the UK can also be estimated using this indirect method. At a recent WHO meeting on AIDS surveillance in Europe, estimates were made of the number of HIV infections in each European country.[6] The current estimate for the UK is 40,000. If this number of HIV-infected persons is used and distributed according to the distribution of reported AIDS cases, then the distribution of HIV infection in females in the UK can be estimated (Table 8). According to this extrapolation, there may be over 1,300

Table 8

Estimated number and age distribution of HIV-infected females, UK

	Total	0-14 yrs	15-24 yrs	25-44 yrs	45-64 yrs	$\geqslant 65$ yrs
Population	28.98 million	5.36 million	4.55 million	7.55 million	6.43 million	5.10 million
Number infected	1,366	308	340	580	104	34
Number positive per 100,000	4.7*	5.8	7.5	7.7	1.6	0.7

WHO 88381

*The estimated prevalence for the USA is 100/100,000

HIV-infected females in the UK with close on 1,000 of childbearing age. This estimated number could, on an annual basis result in about 50 to 100 infants born to HIV-infected mothers in the UK. Virtually all these infected women and births will be located in large urban areas. At the present time, the problem of HIV-infected females is about one-twentieth of the problem estimated in the USA, but the UK is probably several years behind the USA in the duration of the HIV epidemic. Thus, the UK has a great opportunity to react to this problem to minimise future increases in HIV infection.

CONCLUSION

A considerable amount of data and many estimates based on somewhat convoluted extrapolations have been presented. However, the conclusion which can be firmly drawn from these data and estimates is that whatever the actual numbers, the problem of HIV infection in women and thus of perinatal HIV infection leading to paediatric AIDS cases will be an increasing problem world-wide, especially in Patterns I and II countries.

REFERENCES

1. Piot P, Plummer FA, Mhalu FS, Lamboray J-L, Chin J, Mann JM. AIDS: An international perspective. *Science* 1988; **239:** 573-579.
2. *Virus information exchange newsletter—for South-East Asia and the Western Pacific.* Volume 4, No. 3. Nedlands: University of Western Australia, 1987.
3. World Health Organization. *Global Programme on AIDS*, unpublished data.
4. Human immunodeficiency virus infection in the United States: a review of current knowledge. In: Morbidity, Mortality Weekly Report (MMWR). Volume 36, No. 5-6, supplement; 1987.
5. Hoff R, Berardi VP, Weiblen BJ, Mahoney-Trout L, Mitchell ML, Grady GF. HIV seroprevalence in childbearing women: estimation by testing newborn blood samples collected on absorbent paper. *N Engl J Med* 1988; **318:** 525-530.
6. *Report of a Consultation on information support for the AIDS surveillance system, Tatry-Poprad:* 17-19 February 1988. World Health Organization, European Regional Office, Copenhagen.

Prediction of trends in AIDS incidence

Mr G.F. Medley and Mr R.M. Anderson

INTRODUCTION

This paper provides a brief review of the various approaches that can be adopted in the prediction of future trends in the incidence of HIV infection and cases of AIDS. In broad terms, past work in this area falls into two categories. The first is concerned with short-term prediction of the number of new cases that are likely to be reported over the coming few years. This approach is based on statistical extrapolation from past longitudinal trends in the incidence of infection or disease in defined or aggregated risk groups. The second approach is based on the development of simple or complex mathematical models of the epidemiological factors that determine the spread of infection and the biological processes that dictate the development of disease.

The former approach requires longitudinal data on infection or disease to make extrapolation possible. The latter requires a detailed understanding of the many factors that determine spread and influence disease progression in an individual patient. At present, our knowledge of detail in the case of HIV infection and progression to AIDS is somewhat limited. As such, mathematical models are of most use, firstly in highlighting areas in which our knowledge is inadequate for predictive studies, and secondly in investigating general concepts concerning the manner in which infection spreads at the population level.

The rate at which information accumulates on infection and disease is likely to be slow due to the long incubation period of AIDS, and the routes of transmission between people (i.e. sexual activity and needle-sharing). It is conceivable, for example, that the influence of infection on children born to HIV-infected mothers will not be fully understood until a cohort of such people have been studied for a period of the order of normal life expectancy (i.e. 72-75 years in the UK at present).

The construction of exploratory, simple, epidemiological models of the spread of HIV and the development of AIDS can help to pinpoint areas of ignorance. Probably the most important topics in this respect are:

i) the proportion of those infected with the virus that eventually contract the disease;[1]

ii) the length and distribution of the incubation period and the relative patterns and degrees of infectivity in both those who develop the disease and those who do not;[2-5]

23

iii) the detailed pattern of behaviour that permits transmission, for example: sexual and intravenous drug using habits;[6-7]
iv) the proportion of children infected perinatally and the pattern of childhood disease compared with that observed in adults.

Simple models can also help to clarify important general issues. For example, these models show that even if all transmission ceased today, the numbers of cases diagnosed would still continue to rise for some years due to the length and distribution of the incubation period.[2,8] It is also possible to obtain results that are insensitive to the actual values of the epidemiological parameters of a particular model. Thus, using simple demographic models, Anderson, May and McLean[9] have shown that it is possible for a disease with the epidemiological characteristics of AIDS to convert a positive population growth (such as found in many African countries) to a negative rate over a time span of a few decades. These models suggest that the ratio of children plus elderly people to economically productive adults (the dependency ratio) is fairly insensitive to change within wide limits of possible parameter values.

VARIABLE INFECTIVITY

There is evidence to suggest that people infected with HIV are not equally infectious to others throughout the long and variable incubation period. Part of this evidence comes from epidemiological studies of sexual partners of infected people. Such studies reveal great variability in the likelihood of transmission: some partners become infected after only a small number of contacts, while others remain uninfected after many sexual acts.[10-14] Taken in isolation such patterns could be evidence for variability between the infectivity of different people rather than variability within individuals over time. However, clinical and immunological studies indicate that antigenaemia varies throughout the incubation period in individual patients.[15-17] In particular, there appear to be 2 peaks in circulating antigen concentration: one immediately following infection and one preceding the development of ARC/AIDS. If one assumes that antigen concentration is positively correlated with infectivity then there appear to be 2 peaks of infectivity separated by a period of relatively low infectivity.

The epidemiological consequences of variable infectivity have recently been considered by Anderson[3] and Blythe and Anderson,[4] from which Figure I is taken. It shows the consequences of assuming different patterns of infectivity throughout the incubation period on the development of the epidemic in a given community. The different patterns are generated by varying the degree of infectivity in the 2 periods of infectivity, and by assuming an intervening period when an infected person is not infectious to his/her sexual partners. Generally, it is the degree of infectivity that follows shortly after infection that has the greatest influence on the form and magnitude of the epidemic curve.[3,4]

Studies of this nature emphasise the need for more and better data regarding the infectivity of infected patients throughout the incubation period. This requires more extensive clinical and immunological studies of the progression of disease in individuals following HIV infection. Although it seems likely that circulating antigen is correlated with infectivity for a virus with the

Figure I

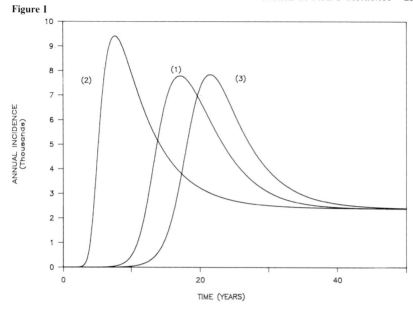

The effect of variable infectivity on the form of the epidemic as shown by the annual incidence rate.[4] The calculations assume an incubation period of 8 years, with (1) infectivity constant for the duration of the incubation period, (2) infectivity split equally between the beginning and end of the incubation period and (3) infectivity split unequally between the beginning and end of the incubation period, the later period having a higher infectivity than the early period. See Blyth and Anderson[4] for details.

transmission characteristics of HIV, it is known that these two phenomena do not necessarily coincide exactly in other viral infections.[18] Longitudinal sampling of semen and cervical secretions for virus would be a better indication of infectivity. It may be that the likelihood of vertical transmission from mother to child is related to the disease status of the mother, as in Hepatitis B.[19] This likelihood may be an indication of infectivity to sexual partners. The possible importance of the events immediately after infection would appear to indicate the need to obtain better data from "seroconverters"—people who are under observation through the early episodes of infection.

This particular example demonstrates the use of simple mathematical models of disease transmission to explore the manner in which a specific epidemiological process (variation in infectivity) influences the pattern of the epidemic. The results highlight the need for particular data to increase understanding.

INCUBATION PERIOD

Determining the incubation period distribution of AIDS is important if we are to interpret correctly the relationship between cases of AIDS and the number of people infected in the population. Clearly the manner in which the rise in infection precedes the rise in cases of AIDS is determined by the distribution of the incubation period. It also plays a crucial role in determining the general shape of the epidemic. It is necessary to talk about an incubation period distribution because the incubation period for AIDS is variable, some people developing the disease quickly, and others remaining seropositive for many years with no overt symptoms of disease. The causes underlying the observed variability are not fully understood at present.

The usual definition of the incubation period is the time between the point of infection and the point at which the diagnosis of the disease is made. However, there is a problem caused by imposing discrete points such as time of diagnosis on the continuous progression of the disease. It is conceivable, for example, that homosexual men in London tend to be diagnosed earlier in the natural history of AIDS than those in the remainder of the country because of referral of patients to hospitals with greater experience in the diagnosis and treatment of AIDS. This difference may well manifest itself as a regional difference during the incubation period, and perhaps also in the subsequent survival following diagnosis.

Data for the estimation of the incubation period distribution can come from 2 sources, namely: blood transfusion recipients and cohort studies. The blood tranfusion data have the advantage that the times of infection and diagnosis are known accurately, whereas cohort data consist of a period in which seroconversion has occurred and then either a date of diagnosis or a date at which the subject was last known not to have AIDS. The time between infection and seroconversion itself appears relatively long and variable and subject to measurement difficulties. This raises difficulties in the direct comparison of estimated period distributions from the 2 types of data.[20,21]

In both types of data it is not possible to link directly the risk of developing AIDS with the total numbers of cases diagnosed. In the case of blood transfusion data this arises because we do not know how many people will eventually be diagnosed. Figure II shows the US blood transfusion data set as of January 1987 with all diagnoses after June 1986 excluded. Although we can see that 4 people transfused with infected blood in 1979 were diagnosed in 1984, because the total number transfused in 1979 is unknown, we do not know what proportion the 4 people are out of the total. Therefore, we cannot directly estimate the associated risk. In the case of cohort data we face the same problem because we do not know the eventual proportion that will go on to develop AIDS. Thus Hessol *et al*[22] report that after 8 years of infection 40% of the total number of infected homosexual men in the San Francisco cohort have developed AIDS. However, because we do not know the eventual proportion of the total that will develop AIDS we cannot simply estimate the risk associated with carrying the virus for 8 years. On the other hand, cohort data provide the opportunity to estimate the proportion that will eventually develop AIDS.

A detailed analysis of blood transfusion data has attempted to overcome the problem of estimating the absolute risk by simultaneously estimating the incubation period distribution and the incidence of infective transfusions.[23-26] Figure III shows the incubation period distribution estimated from the data in Figure II, assuming that the incidence function is of exponential form, and that the incubation period has a Weibull distribution. The predictions depend strongly on the choice of function for the incubation period distribution. It should also be noted that the confidence limits for this curve are wide.[25]

Figure II

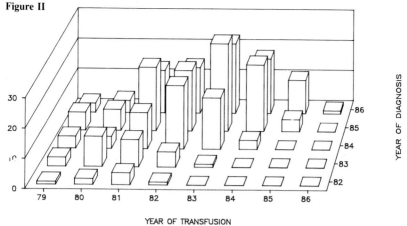

YEAR OF TRANSFUSION

The US blood transfusion data as kindly supplied by T.A. Peterman, CDC, Atlanta, Georgia, USA. The data consist of cases diagnosed prior to July 1986 and reported to CDC prior to January 1987 (297 cases). The data were divided on the basis of month for analysis.[23,24]

Figure III

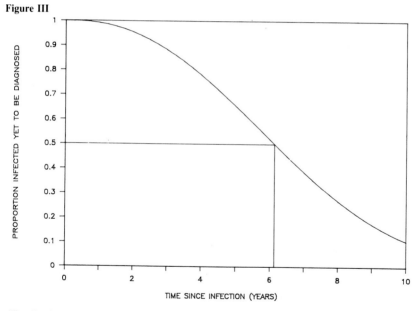

TIME SINCE INFECTION (YEARS)

The distribution of the incubation period of AIDS as estimated from the data in Figure II. The method of estimation is outlined in the text and Medley *et al*,[23,24] and assumed an exponential growth in infective transfusions and a Weibull incubation period. The graph shows the expected proportion of an infected cohort still to be diagnosed as a function of time since infection. The median of the distribution (marked) is the expected time taken for half the infected people to develop AIDS and is estimated to be 6.14 years (the mean is 6.33 years).

For these reasons, many authors have used non-parametric methods which do not require the choice of a function to estimate the changing risk of developing AIDS as time since infection passes. However, as pointed out above, these estimated risks are only relative, not absolute. Furthermore, it is fairly obvious from Figure II that most of the infective transfusions occurred toward the later end of 1979-1986. Tranfusion recipients therefore have been at risk for only a relatively short period. The observations at present are concentrated around the left-hand end of the distribution in Figure III. In order to estimate statistics such as median time of the incubation period it is necessary to extrapolate beyond the observation time of the majority of the data. This problem will remain until more of the incubation period has been observed in the coming years.

The analyses would be greatly improved if some independent estimate of the distribution could be used to "tie down" the incubation period to a particular value at a particular time. It has been suggested that data from cohort studies be used for this purpose. However, we are wary of using any method that mixes the data from the blood transfusion recipients with those from groups infected by other routes of transmission. There is no reason to believe that the incubation periods in different risk groups are similar. Analyses could be strengthened if

Figure IV

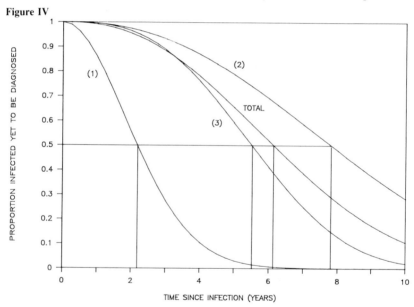

The difference in the estimated incubation period distribution for different age groups (the curve from Figure III is included for comparison marked "total"). The age groupings are (1) less than 5 years old at infection, (2) older than 4 years but younger than 60 years and (3) 60 years and older. The median times between infection and the diagnosis of AIDS for the three groups are 2.18 years, 7.80 years and 5.51 years respectively. The influence of age group is statistically significant, but the difference between the older age groups (2 and 3) is less well established than the fact that the youngest age group convert from infection to AIDS faster than in the older age groups.

independent estimates of the number of (infective) transfusions given (stratified by time of transfusion, age and sex of recipient) were available.

Figure IV displays the results of considering different incubation period distributions for different age groups. The shorter average incubation period in children compared to adults is statistically significant. The difference between the adult and elderly age groups is less significant. It should be borne in mind when designing data collection protocols and interpreting data that explanatory variables such as route of transmission and age may influence the incubation period.

SHORT-TERM PREDICTION

Accurate predictions of numbers of AIDS patients that can be expected to be diagnosed in the future are of obvious value to ensure that adequate resources will be available for patient care. In planning terms, an excess of resources is almost as bad as a dearth. In practice, this can only be achieved over the short-term, say, up to 5 years ahead. In order to make such predictions it is necessary to estimate some incidence function which describes the numbers of diagnoses made over time. However, this function is not observed directly, but only after a reporting lag.

The Communicable Disease Surveillance Centre (CDSC), part of the Public Health Laboratory Service (PHLS), at Colindale requests clinicians to report the diagnosis of an AIDS case. The resulting data, together with results of blood tests from PHLS laboratories, can be used to chart the progress of the epidemic in the UK. Tillett *et al*[27] describe the available data, their completeness and the problems associated with their interpretation. An inevitable consequence of the reporting procedure is the delay between the diagnosis being made, and the report eventually reaching CDSC—the reporting lag. This lag makes estimation of the actual incidence of diagnoses (rather than notifications) difficult. The problem has been discussed with particular reference to the UK by Healy and Tillett.[28]

Unpublished studies by Cox and Medley attempt to estimate the reporting lag distribution and the incidence function of diagnoses simultaneously from the notifications collected by CDSC. It should be noted that the reporting lag as it is observed directly is biased against the longer lags, as the length of the lag is not observed until the notification is received. This is particularly important as most of the diagnoses have been made recently due to the exponential growth of the epidemic. Therefore, the majority of diagnoses have had only a limited period in which to be reported. Interestingly, this problem is statistically equivalent to the estimation of the incubation period distribution. The reporting lag distribution corresponds to the incubation period distribution as some lag between the incidence function (either diagnoses or infective transfusions) and observation of the incidence (either notifications or diagnoses).

The method is capable of describing the available incidence data (Figure V) and of predicting the total number of cases reported to a reasonable degree of accuracy (see Table 1). However, it is the total number diagnosed, and not only those notified, that is required, together with some form of confidence limits for

Table 1.   **Projections of cumulative notifications and diagnoses**

End of quarter	Observed	Reported	Diagnosed
Dec 87	1227	1227	1611
Mar 88	1429	1437	1859
Jun 88		1665	2122
Sept 88		1909	2398
Dec 88		2168	2686
Dec 89		3314	3913
Dec 90		4567	5205
Dec 91		5868	6521

N.B. An increasing number of cases will be diagnosed but unreported in the future.

The predicted total cumulative number of notifications compared with the actual numbers received by CDSC, and the predicted numbers diagnosed, but not yet reported.

Figure V

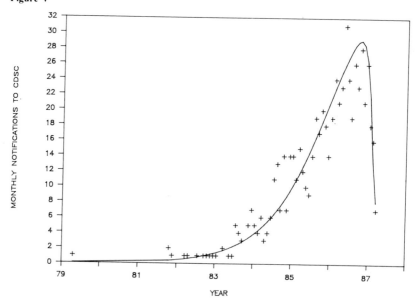

The points are the monthly reports of AIDS cases (monthly incidence) received by CDSC up to April 1987. The down-turn at the end of the observation period is due entirely to the effect of the reporting lag. The line is that expected when an incidence function of logistic form and a reporting lag of mixed gamma form are fitted to the data. Although this method gives a good description of the observed data, it does not guarantee a high degree of accuracy in predictions. Table 1 compares prediction with observation.

the prediction. In order to be of use to health care planners, it will be necessary to extend this work to stratify the predicted cases by a number of explanatory variables. In particular, the region of residence of the patient and perhaps the risk group or the major clinical features of the disease at diagnosis should be considered. Furthermore, the number of patients alive at any point could be estimated using a combination of the incidence of diagnoses and results of survival analysis. Such survival analysis attempts to estimate the distribution of deaths following diagnosis for different explanatory variables.[29-31] Ideally, some data for the health care costs of different patient groups could also be used to predict explicitly the resources that will be needed.

A further application of this work is the prediction of the changes to the notifications that can be expected as a result of, for example, altering the reporting lag or changing the case definition.

Given the problem of estimating the incidence function, the major source of error regarding predictions comes from the choice of the functional form for the changes in incidence through time (i.e. the growth of the epidemic). Generally, forms that are derived from epidemiological theory such as the logistic equation, should be preferred to completely empirical forms, such as exponential or polynomial functions.

CONCLUSIONS

Well defined mathematical models can go some way towards increasing our understanding of the processes that govern the spread of HIV and the development of the AIDS epidemic. However, it is the collection and analysis of good quality data that will make prediction feasible. Increased epidemiological understanding can then be used to plan effectively, and to provide clinicians and counsellors with detailed, accurate information on the basis of sound predictions. Appropriate resources need to be allocated to epidemiological study and data collection to facilitate the planning process.

We can identify 3 areas of data collection that require urgent attention. Firstly, the degree of spread of HIV within defined populations, and its continued monitoring must be determined. This can be achieved only by periodically screening sections of the population such as those attending STD clinics and antenatal clinics. Secondly, sociological aspects relating to behaviours which influence transmission of HIV, especially intravenous drug use and sexual activities need to be assessed. Thirdly, the natural history of the disease (including infectiousness), and the manner in which it varies with age, sex, route of transmission, etc. requires further study. The collection of these data requires long-term, large-scale cohort studies on groups such as haemophiliacs. The European Perinatal Study[32] and the European Heterosexual Study[33] are examples of the type of investigation required. To our knowledge there is no equivalent study of the thousand or so known seropositive haemophiliacs in the UK. Because of the time scale of data acquisition, it requires investment of resources now if we are to experience the benefit of such strides in future health care planning and the design of central policies.

ACKNOWLEDGEMENTS

We wish to thank CDSC and T.A. Peterman for access to data. We acknowledge financial support from the MRC. Much help and advice on statistical matters has been generously provided by David Cox of the Department of Mathematics at Imperial College. We also thank Drs S.P. Blythe, A.R. McLean and S. Blower of the Department of Biology at Imperial College for advice and criticism.

REFERENCES

1. Anderson RM, Medley GF, May RM, Johnson AM. A preliminary study of the transmission dynamics of the human immunodeficiency virus (HIV), the causative agent of AIDS. *IMA J Math App Med Biol* 1986; **3**: 229-263.

2. Anderson RM, Medley GF, Blythe SP, Johnson AM. Is it possible to predict the minimum size of the acquired immunodeficiency syndrome (AIDS) epidemic in the United Kingdom? *Lancet* 1987; **1**: 1073-1075.

3. Anderson RM. The epidemiology of HIV infection: variable incubation plus infectious periods and heterogeneity in sexual activity. *J Roy Stat Soc* 1988; **151**: 66-97.

4. Blythe SP, Anderson RM. Variable infectiousness in HIV transmission models. *IMA J Math App Med Biol* 1988; **5**. In press.

5. Blythe SP, Anderson RM. Distributed incubation and infectious periods in models of the transmission dynamics of the human immunodeficiency virus (HIV). *IMA J Math App Med Biol* 1988; **5**: 1-19.

6. Anderson RM, Johnson AM. *Rates of sexual partner change in homosexual and heterosexual populations in the United Kingdom*. 1988. Report to Kinsey Institute AIDS Meeting, Bloomington; December, 1987.

7. Johnson AM. Social and behavioural aspects of the HIV epidemic—a review. *J Roy Stat Soc* 1988; **151**: 99-126.

8. Brookmeyer R, Gail MH. Minimum size of the Acquired Immunodeficiency Syndrome (AIDS) epidemic in the United States. *Lancet* 1987; **2**: 1320-1322.

9. Anderson RM, May RM, McLean AR. Possible demographic consequences of AIDS in developing countries. *Nature* 1988; **332**: 228-234.

10. Burger H, Weiser B, Robinson WS, Lifson J, Engleman E, Rouzioux C, Brun-Vézinet F, Barré-Sinoussi F, Montagnier L, Chermann J-C. Transmission of lymphadenopathy-associated virus/human T-lymphotrophic virus type III in sexual partners. Seropositivity does not predict infectivity in all cases. *Am J Med* 1986; **81**: 5-10.

11. Darrow WW, Echenberg DF, Jagge HW, O'Malley PM, Byers RH, Getchell JP, Curran JW. Risk factors for human immunodeficiency virus (HIV) in homosexual men. *Am J Pub Health* 1987; **77**: 479-483.

12. Padian N, Marquis L, Francis DP, Anderson RE, Rutherford GW, O'Malley PM, Winkelstein W. Male to female transmission of human immunodeficiency virus. *JAMA* 1987; **258**: 788-790.

13. Winkelstein W, Lyman DM, Padian N, Grant R, Samuel M, Wiley JA, Anderson RE, Lang W, Riggs J, Levy JA. Sexual practices and risk of infection by the human immunodeficiency virus: the San Francisco men's health study. *JAMA* 1987; **257**: 321-325.

14. Winkelstein W, Samuel M, Padian N, Wiley JA, Lang W, Anderson RE, Levy JA. The San Francisco men's health study: III. Reduction of human immunodeficiency virus transmission among homosexual/bisexual men, 1982-1986. *Am J Pub Heal* 1987; **76**: 685-689.

15. Pedersen C, Neilsen CM, Vestergaard BF, Gersfoft J, Krogsgaard K, Neilsen JE. Temporal relation of antigenaemia and loss of antibodies to core antigens to development of clinical disease in HIV infection. *Br Med J* 1987; **295**: 567-572.

16. Zolla-Pazner S, Des Jarlais DC, Friedman SR, *et al.* Non-random development of immunological abnormalities after infection with HIV: implications for immunologic classification of the disease. *Proc Nat Acad Sci* 1987; **84:** 5404-5408.

17. Jeffries DJ. Virology. In: *AIDS and obstetrics and gynaecology.* Eds. C Hudson, F Sharp. London: Royal College of Obstetricians and Gynaecologists/Springer-Verlag, 1988; pp.3-13.

18. Carter MJ, ter Meulen V. Measles. In: *Principles and Practise of Clinical Virology.* Eds. AJ Zuckerman, JE Banatvala, JR Pattison. Chichester: John Wiley, 1987. pp.291-314.

19. Zuckerman AJ. Viral hepatitis. In: *Principles and Practise of Clinical Virology.* Eds. AJ Zuckerman, JE Banatvala, JR Pattison. Chichester: John Wiley & Sons, 1987. pp.135-158.

20. Ranki A, Valle S-L, Krohn M, Antonen J, Allain J-P, Leuther M, Franchini G, Krohn K. Long latency precedes overt seroconversion in sexually transmitted human immunodeficiency virus infection. *Lancet* 1987; **2:** 589-593.

21. Saah AJ. Latency preceding seroconversion in sexually transmitted HIV infection. *Lancet* 1987; **2:** 1402.

22. Hessol NA, Rutherford GW, O'Malley PM, Doll LS, Darrow WW, Jaffe HW. The natural history of HIV infection in a cohort of homosexual and bisexual men: a 7yr prospective study. *III International Conference on AIDS, Washington* 1987, Abstract M.3.1.

23. Medley GF, Anderson RM, Cox DR, Billard L. Incubation period of AIDS in patients infected via blood transfusion. *Nature* 1987; **328:** 719-721.

24. Medley GF, Billard L, Cox DR, Anderson RM. The distribution of the incubation period for the acquired immunodeficiency syndrome (AIDS). *Proc Royal Soc Lond, Ser B.* 1988; **233:** 367-377.

25. Kalbfleisch JD, Lawless JF. Estimating the incubation period for AIDS patients. *Nature* 1988; **333:** 504-505.

26. Medley GF, Anderson RM, Cox DR, Billard B. Reply to Kalbfleisch and Lawless. *Nature* 1988; **333:** 505.

27. Tillett HE, Galbraith NS, Overton SE, Porter K. Routine Surveillance on AIDS and HIV infections in the UK: a description of the data available and their use for short-term planning. *Epidemiol Infect* 1988; **100:** 157-169.

28. Healy MJR, Tillett HE. Short-term extrapolation of the AIDS epidemic. *J Roy Stat Soc* 1988; **151:** 50-65.

29. Marasca P, McEvoy M. Length of survival of patients with acquired immunodeficiency syndrome in the UK. *Br Med J* 1986; **292:** 1727-1729.

30. Rothenberg R, Woelfel M, Stoneburger R, Milberg J, Parker R, Truman B. Survival with the acquired immunodeficiency syndrome. *Engl J Med* 1987; **317:** 1297-1302.

31. Reeves G, Overton SE. Preliminary survival analysis of UK AIDS data. *Lancet* 1988; **1:** 880.

32. Peckham CS, Senturia VD, Ades AE. Infants born to mothers seropositive for HIV: results from the ongoing European Collaborative Study. In: *AIDS and obstetrics and gynaecology.* Eds. C Hudson, F Sharp. London: Royal College of Obstetricians and Gynaecologists/Springer-Verlag, 1988; pp.77-82.

33. Ancelle-Park R, De Vincenzi I. Heterosexual transmission of HIV. In: *AIDS and obstetrics and gynaecology.* Eds. C Hudson, F Sharp. London: Royal College of Obstetricians and Gynaecologists/Springer-Verlag, 1988; pp.39-47.

Discussion

Chairman: Professor C.S. Peckham

SOUTTER: I would like to direct a question to Dr Chin. He said that the evidence is that HIV spreads in a manner similar to that of Hepatitis B. Does he derive any reassurance from that knowledge, keeping in mind that Hepatitis B is extremely common in the homosexual community, but extremely uncommon in the heterosexual community in the developed countries?

CHIN: Yes, I do take some consolation in that finding. In general, HIV is much less infectious in terms of unit of exposure than Hepatitis B, but the types of exposure are almost identical.

GLYNN: You may have seen the letter in the *Lancet* a couple of weeks ago[1] which stated that the incidence of Hepatitis B continues to fall in recent years in this country even among sub groups. One possible reason is the incubation period for Hepatitis B which is very much shorter. So perhaps it will take a period of years to see the effect of HIV.

CHIN: The cohort studies show a certain incidence of uterine infections, especially in San Francisco where the greatest incidence in the cultural and bi-ethnic group has declined and the incidence of new infections has just plummeted.

MILLS: We need more detailed knowledge about the way the virus is absorbed when it is transmitted by sexual intercourse. Do we have any general evidence that the virus can attach itself to the vaginal mucosa or sperm?

JEFFRIES: We know from studying very common viruses in the past how difficult it is to know exactly how a virus affects one individual or another. In San Francisco where certainly they demonstrated that virus was present in the colonic epithelium there is also some evidence that the virus will infect the trans-formed colonic carcinoma cells *in vitro*, but I think it is pure speculation that the virus will establish a primary infection on the colonic mucosa. There is no evidence that the cells of the female genital tract are infected. What I didn't go into was the known infectious body fluids such as seminal fluid, with a large question mark on breast milk, but we can also assume that female genital tract secretions are infectious. The sort of evidence that we would like in terms of which parts of the genital tract are vulnerable to infection just isn't forthcoming.

GREEN: I would just like to ask Dr Chin about this issue of cohort studies in general. There seem to be two problems. Firstly, that being involved in a cohort study *per se* may cause people to change their behaviour. Secondly, the individuals who enrol in these cohorts are probably completely atypical of the population from which they are drawn since they are usually volunteers attending STD clinics and other unusual subcohorts.

CHIN: There are problems with any kind of epidemiological study, whether we are talking about AIDS control studies, cross-sectional studies or cohort studies. Regardless, I think that the data that you obtain from cohort studies probably are as good as any.

JOHNSTONE: Could I ask Dr Jeffries a question? I think we would all agree that it seems very reasonable that when individuals have antigenaemia they become more infectious both to their sexual partners and to their babies. But apart from the data on haemophiliac men, very small numbers in the States, and perhaps the European collaborative study on babies, what actual data are there to support this?

JEFFRIES: What I said is that I thought that there may be a difference, not that there was a crucial difference in terms of the transmission of AIDS at any given time. It becomes remarkably easier to isolate the virus in those later stages than in the middle asymptomatic phase. The data that I was thinking of are based on a compilation of the haemophiliac data and on the evidence from your own part of the world of the apparent lack of sexual transmission between intravenous drug users and their partners once they get into the asymptomatic phase.

CHIN: There are some data coming out of Africa on pregnant women. There is good correlation there between a depressed T cell ratio and transmission to their infants.

ANCELLE: We have a multi-centre heterosexual study going on in the EEC community, and the data coming out of this study show that there is a statistical link between the clinical phases. The later the phase and the more advanced the disease is in the clinical stage, the higher the rate of transmission.

PECKHAM: We talked a lot about the incubation period, and how important this is for your model. You mentioned that in children the incubation period was much shorter. Is that based on children who have received transfusions, or is it based on children who have acquired the infection from their mothers?

MEDLEY: In children under 5 who have received a single transfusion of blood, and subsequently have been exposed to no other risk, so that specifically excludes having an HIV positive mother.

PECKHAM: The transmission rates in those groups are very high indeed, aren't they, in terms of the number infected per exposure?

MILLS: Do we have any information on the incubation periods in the adult groups? Do they vary very much?

MEDLEY: As far as I know, I do not think that anyone has seriously tried to extrapolate the data, and to estimate what the incubation period is.

MOK: I would like to ask Dr Jeffries to comment on the neonate who might have been infected early and who was unable to respond to HIV in terms of enteral reduction or tolerance.

JEFFRIES: I would use the word "tolerance" because there are precedents in terms of animal intrauterine virus infections with viruses, which in animals can live within the immune system, in which there is clearly a state of partial tolerance. In particular the animal model in this would be choriomeningitis. In that situation it is rather difficult in that the newborn animal is tolerant from the point of view of cell-mediated immune responses, although they do produce circulating antibody. We do not know the immunological responses in the neonatal form of HIV infection; we do know that some of them in Berlin which have yielded virus have been totally seronegative. Bearing in mind that at the present time, the number of babies that we have seen in the European study who have become ill in the first year appear to be a lot less than we would expect from listening to people who have just been looking at ill babies in other parts of the world; the question arises if infection occurs early *in utero* can the baby accept foreign antigens in a tolerable state?

CHIN: Some of those early studies were based on looking at reverse transcriptase, and when the studies were subjected to further review it turned out not to be virus positive.

PECKHAM: Has this phenomenon been reported in others who are known to have seroconverted? Have they lost antibody despite the fact that they are all immunologically involved?

JEFFRIES: Certainly if one reads some of the earlier literature, it did appear. Now we have better serological tests I cannot think of any cases of AIDS in which the patient has died as a result.

SCRIMGEOUR: Dr Chin; you made the comment that the prevalence of HIV positive women in the UK is one-twentieth of that in the United States. I just wondered how you had come to that particular figure. If we are not sure of the prevalence of the disease in the UK, how does Dr Medley suggest that we go about finding it?

CHIN: I did adjust those absolute numbers, basically cutting out the total number of HIV infected women in the United States. My calculations and extrapolations yielded roughly overall 1 per 1,000 for the US. Again by a route of convoluted extrapolation I came up with about 1 per 20,000 for the UK. So it is one-twentieth.

PECKHAM: How did you obtain your numbers for the HIV infected women in this country? Was that from laboratory reports?

CHIN: Again, the method is relatively straightforward. You first take an estimate of the total number of HIV affected persons there are in your area—in the United States, 1,500,000. In the UK the estimate is 40,000. Once you have that number you then take the numbers of reported distribution of AIDS cases by age and sex, and then apply that distribution to this 1,000,000–1,500,000 estimated HIV infections in the United States. That is at least one method of distributing the infections. You can have problems with that in developing other alternative distributions, but I think that that would give a conservative estimate.

MEDLEY: The only way in which you could estimate the prevalence rate in the entire population is to take a random sample of reasonable size from the general population being tested.

HOWIE: I would like to ask Dr Chin to what extent the problem of false positive results might confound the prevalence data as quoted for pregnant women if they were using anonymous testing.

CHIN: False positives are going to have to be considered as very important when dealing with individual testing. When doing surveys, I think that the error of false positives is relatively small compared to all the other errors found in the survey.

REFERENCE
1.   Polakoff S. Decrease in acute Hepatitis B incidence continued in 1987. (Letter) *Lancet* 1988; **1:** 540.

Heterosexual transmission of HIV

Dr R. Ancelle-Park and Dr I. De Vincenzi

Since 1983 countries in the WHO European Region have taken part in the surveillance of AIDS in Europe by reporting their data to the WHO Collaborating Centre on AIDS. The cases of AIDS recorded fulfil the CDC case definition published in the Morbidity and Mortality Weekly Report in September 1982[1] and revised in June 1985.[2] One source per country, recognised by their respective national health authorities, provides the information. The national data are noted on standard tables, and each source is responsible for the quality of the data provided.

EUROPEAN AIDS SURVEILLANCE DATA

By 31st December 1987, a total of 10,181 cases of AIDS had been reported to the WHO Collaborating Centre on AIDS by 28 countries (Table 1), an increase of 124% (5,632 new cases) since December 1986.

Between September and December 1987, the greatest increases in the number of reported cases were noted in France (550, or 42-43 per week); Italy (307, or 23-24 per week); Germany, F.R. (269, or 20-21 per week); Spain (165, or 12-13 per week); United Kingdom (160, or 12-13 per week); Switzerland (56, or 4-5 per week); and Netherlands (50, or 3-4 per week). AIDS cases per million population have been calculated for each country from 1987 population estimates (INED, Paris) (Table 1). The highest cumulative incidence rates per million population were noted in France (55.3), Switzerland (53.8) and Denmark (44.7). By way of comparison, the rate in the USA was 216 per million population.[3]

Among the 9930 adult AIDS cases in the WHO European Region, 5865 (59%) were homosexuals or bisexuals, 1944 (20%) were intravenous (IV) drug users, and 609 (6%) were presumed to be infected by heterosexual contact (Table 2). The male: female sex ratio was 8.9:1. The sex ratio was nearer unity in the following transmission groups: IV drug users (2.8:1), heterosexual contact (1.8:1), transfusion recipients (1.4:1); 51.5% of the female cases have been reported among IV drug users and 50% in the 20 to 29 year age group.

Although cases reported in Table 2 are those diagnosed in the European region their distribution by transmission groups is the reflection of an epidemiological pattern. In Europe all groups are represented, with a majority of cases reported among homosexuals. In Africa and the Caribbean Islands, few cases are reported in the major European groups and the majority of patients are found in the "heterosexual contact" group showing a typical African pattern.

Table 1

Cumulative AIDS cases reported by 28 European countries and estimated cumulative incidence rates per million population
31st December 1987

COUNTRY	Dec. 86	Mar. 87	June 87	Sept. 87	Dec. 87	Rate per million[*]
Austria	54	72	93	120	139	18.3
Belgium	207	230	255	277	277	28.0
Bulgaria	—	—	1	1	1	0.1
Czechoslovakia	6	7	7	7	8	0.5
Denmark	131	150	176	202	228	44.7
Finland	14	19	19	22	24	4.9
France	1221	1632	1980	2523	3073	55.3
German Dem. Rep.	1	3	4	4	6	0.4
German Fed. Rep.	826	999	1133	1400	1669	27.4
Greece	35	41	49	78	88	8.8
Hungary	1	3	5	6	8	0.8
Iceland	4	4	4	4	4	20.0
Ireland	14	19	19	25	33	9.4
Israel	34	38	39	43	47	10.7
Italy	523	664	870	1104	1411	24.6
Luxemburg	6	7	7	8	9	22.5
Malta	5	5	6	7	7	17.5
Netherlands	218	260	308	370	420	28.8
Norway	35	45	49	64	70	16.7
Poland	1	2	2	3	3	0.1
Portugal	46	54	67	81	90	8.7
Romania	2	2	2	2	3	0.1
Spain	264	357	508	624	789	20.2
Sweden	90	105	129	143	163	19.4
Switzerland	192	227	266	299	355	53.8
United Kingdom	610	729	870	1067	1227	21.6
USSR	1	3	3	3	3	0.0
Yugoslavia	8	10	11	21	26	1.1
TOTAL	4549	5687	6882	8508	10181	

Source: WHO Collaborating Centre on AIDS.

The percentage representation of heterosexual intravenous drug abusers (IVDA) among European AIDS cases has increased sharply from 1% in December 1984, to 7% in December 1985, 14% in December 1986 and 20% in December 1987. These cases are concentrated particularly in southern Europe, 87% of them having been reported collectively by Italy, Spain or France. Heterosexual IVDA accounts for 59% and 52% of AIDS cases in Italy and Spain, respectively. The seriousness of this situation has been frequently stressed: heterosexual IVDA is a key link for the spread of HIV in the heterosexual population, and to children through mother-to-child transmission. As observed in Table 3, children of IVDA mothers are more frequently reported in countries where AIDS cases among IVDAs prevail.

The specific contribution of HIV-infected heterosexual IVDAs to the challenge of AIDS should be emphasised.[4] A number of characteristics stand out when separate analysis of AIDS surveillance data related to heterosexual IVDA is undertaken. Although the AIDS epidemic began in Europe in 1981, cases among

Figure I
AIDS cases reported in Europe among IVDA and other transmission categories by half-year of diagnosis—31st March 1987.

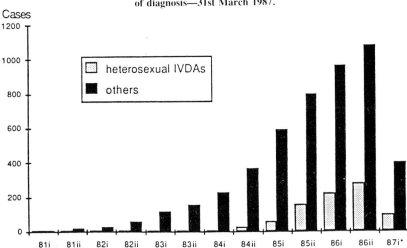

heterosexual IVDAs began to appear only during the second part of 1984. The continuous increase in the relative percentage of these cases indicates rapid spread of the disease in this group (Figure I). Heterosexual IVDAs with AIDS are reported significantly more often in the clinical group with opportunistic infections (759/826 or 91%) than in other AIDS patients (3235/4861 or 67%). This difference, as observed in the USA, is related to the high frequency of Kaposi's sarcoma in HIV-infected homosexual males. The distribution of cases according to age differs remarkably between heterosexual IVDAs and the others. 76% of heterosexual IVDA patients with AIDS are under 30 years of age, whereas 78% of the other AIDS cases are aged 30 or over. Heterosexual IVDAs account for 42% of cases in the 20 to 29 year age group. Moreover, even though sexual transmission remains the main route of spread of HIV infection throughout the world, the young age of most heterosexual IVDAs with AIDS means that AIDS information campaigns directed at adolescents in Europe should pay particular attention to education on drug abuse.

PREVALENCE OF HIV INFECTION IN HETEROSEXUAL POPULATIONS
The prevalence of HIV infection in the general population in the Northern hemisphere remains very low, as suggested by 1986 HIV seroprevalence rates of 17 per 100,000 blood donors collected at the Paris centre. In contrast to numerous surveys of homosexual men, fewer studies have been reported on HIV seropositivity rates in heterosexual populations at risk for sexually-transmitted diseases. The seroprevalence rates in Europe and North America are fairly near to zero, whereas among African men with sexually-transmitted diseases up to 29% had HIV antibodies.[5-6]

Table 2

Cumulative AIDS cases in adults by transmission group and geographic origin for 28 European countries*
31st December 1987

Transmission Group	Geographic Origin				Total	
	Europe	Africa	Caribbean	Other/Unknown	No.	%
Homo-/bisexual	5585	31	9	240	5865	59
IV drug user	1918	19	2	5	1944	20
Homosexual IV drug user	247	3	1	8	259	3
Haemoph/coag. disorder	348	0	0	1	349	4
Transfusion	331	21	4	3	359	4
Heterosexual	364	209	32	4	609	6
Other/unknown	371	99	61	14	545	5
TOTAL	9164 (92%)	382 (4%)	109 (1%)	275 (3%)	9930	100

*Austria, Belgium, Bulgaria, Czechoslovakia, Denmark, Finland, France, German D.R., German F.R., Greece, Hungary, Iceland, Ireland, Israel, Italy, Luxemburg, Malta, Netherlands, Norway, Poland, Portugal, Romania, Spain, Sweden, Switzerland, United Kingdom, USSR, Yugoslavia.
Source: WHO Collaborating Centre on AIDS.

Table 3

Cumulative paediatric AIDS cases* by transmission group and country of diagnosis—18 European
countries
31st December 1987

Country of Diagnosis	Mother with AIDS or at risk for AIDS:				Haemo- philiac	Trans- fusion	Other/ Unknown	Total
	IV	Trs	Het	Oth/Unk				
Austria	1	0	0	1	1	1	0	4
Belgium	0	0	0	8	0	0	3	11
Denmark	1	0	1	0	1	0	0	3
France	19	3	18	19	4	15	2	80
Germany, F.R.	10	1	2	1	6	5	0	25
Greece	0	1	0	1	0	0	0	2
Ireland	2	0	0	0	1	0	0	3
Israel	0	0	0	0	1	0	0	1
Italy	39	0	4	1	4	5	0	53
Luxemburg	0	0	0	0	1	0	0	1
Malta	0	0	0	0	1	0	0	1
Netherlands	1	0	1	0	0	6	0	8
Portugal	0	0	0	0	2	0	0	2
Spain	14	0	0	0	12	2	0	28
Sweden	0	0	1	0	1	0	0	2
Switzerland	3	0	1	3	0	0	0	7
United Kingdom	0	5	6	2	2	4	0	19
Yugoslavia	0	0	0	0	1	0	0	1
TOTAL	90	10	34	36	38	38	5	251

*Children under 15 years
IV: Intravenous drug user; Trs: Transfusion recipient;
Het: Heterosexual contact; Oth: Other; Unk: Unknown.
Source: WHO Collaborating Centre on AIDS.

Data on female prostitutes, another high risk group for sexually-transmitted diseases, are given in Table 4, with only non-intravenous-drug-abusing prostitutes being considered.[7] In Europe HIV infection in this population still seems to be very uncommon. Variable HIV seroprevalence rates have been found in North America, with none of 535 Nevada prostitutes having antibodies, but up to 30% of 27 non-intravenous-drug-abusing prostitutes in south Florida being infected. Among African prostitutes, HIV seropositivity rates of up to 88% have been reported. However, substantial geographical variations also exist in infection rates in female prostitutes in Africa. This may reflect differences in intensity of exposure or a more recent introduction of HIV in a given area.

The fulminant rise in HIV seroprevalence among a particular group of Nairobi prostitutes between 1981 and 1985[8] demonstrates the rapid dissemination of HIV infection in a population of very promiscuous heterosexuals, similar to that observed among promiscuous homosexual men in the United States.

Table 4

Prevalence of HIV antibodies in non IVDU female prostitutes

Continent	City/Area	Year	Number studied	% postive
Europe	Amsterdam	1986	84	0
	Antwerp	1987	60	1.7
	Athens	1986	270	0.7
	London	1986	50	0
	Paris	1986	50	0
America	Nevada	1986	535	0
	Seattle	1986	92	5
	South Florida	1986	27	30
	Santo Domingo, Dominican Rep.	1985	68	10
Africa	Meiganga, Cameroon	1985	221	8
	Abidjan, Ivory Coast	1986	101	20
	Nairobi, Kenya	1985	286	61
	Blantyre, Malawi	1986	265	56
	Butare, Rwanda	1984	33	88
	Arusha, Tanzania	1986	42	0
	Dar es Salaam, Tanzania	1986	225	29
	Kinshasa, Zaire	1985	377	27
	Equateur, Zaire	1986	283	11
Asia	Madras, India	1986	102	6

Source: Piot P. Heterosexual transmission of HIV. *AIDS* 1987; **4**: xxx.

RISK FACTORS FOR HETEROSEXUAL TRANSMISSION

HIV has been isolated from semen of seropositive men and cervical and vaginal secretions of seropositive women, and it has been demonstrated that bidirectional heterosexual transmission occurs. However, the mechanics of heterosexual transmission have not yet been elucidated.[9-12]

The risk of male-to-female and female-to-male heterosexual transmission has been estimated from studies of stable heterosexual couples in the United States and Europe (Table 5). The prevalence of HIV antibodies in the wives of seropositive haemophiliacs has ranged from 7 to 17%. In cases of blood transfusion-associated HIV infection, the risk of husband-to-wife heterosexual

Table 5

HIV heterosexual transmission rates

Author (Country, Date)		Index case Population	Male-to-female No.	%	Female-to-male No.	%
Allain	(France 86)	Haemophiliac	148	6.8		
Bardin	(France 86)	"	17	11.7		
Jason	(USA 86)	"	33	6.0		
Goedert	(USA 87)	"	24	17.0		
Miller	(UK 87)	"	30	3.3		
Smyley	(USA 87)	"	32	15.6		
France	(UK 88)	IVDU	34	15.0	7	14.0
Steighigel	(USA 87)	ARC/AIDS patients	88	47.0	12	58.0
Fischl	(USA 87)	AIDS patients	28	50.0	17	71.0
Johnson	(Haiti 87)	"	279	53.0	53	55.0
Katzenstein	(Africa 87)	Sero(+) subjects	75	60.0		
Taelman	(Africa 87)	"	38	81.0	10	60.0
Luzi	(Italy 85)	"	22	59.0	6	33.3
Padian	(USA 87)	"	97	23.0		
Weber	(USA 87)	"	60	36.6	11	27.2
Peterman	(USA 88)	Transfusion	55	18.0	25	8.0

transmission was 18% and of wife-to-husband transmission 8%. In a study in San Francisco, 14% of female partners of seropositive bisexual men were seropositive.[13] In heterosexual partners of AIDS patients and partners with AIDS-related complex in the USA, the prevalence of HIV antibodies was 47-50% in women and 58-71% in men. In a prospective study of spouses of AIDS patients, seroconversion occurred in 42% of husbands and 38% of wives during a 1-3 year period, suggesting that the efficacy of heterosexual transmission may be similar in both directions.[11]

Several important co-factors for HIV transmission have been identified. There is accumulating evidence that sexually-transmitted diseases (STD), which result in genital tract ulceration with resultant disruption of the integrity of the mucosal epithelium, may potentiate sexual transmission of HIV. In surveys of HIV prevalence in high-risk heterosexual populations in Africa, seropositivity has been associated with a history of genital ulcers and a positive serological test for syphilis.[14-15] Although sexually-transmitted diseases such as herpes or syphilis may simply be markers for sexual promiscuity, the associations between HIV antibody and genital ulcer in these studies persisted after controlling for confounding factors such as the number of sexual partners, suggesting that certain sexually-transmitted diseases are independent risk factors for HIV acquisition.

A second co-factor for sexual transmission of HIV may be the degree of virus expression and/or immunosuppression in the seropositive "donor". In a recent study of 24 wives of seropositive haemophiliacs,[16] 4 women developed HIV antibodies. The husbands of the women who became infected tended to have a lower absolute T4 count than the husbands of the women who remained uninfected, suggesting that a seropositive individual's infectivity increases with severity of disease.

It was demonstrated by a study of recipients of infected semen during artificial insemination that exposure to the female cervical and vaginal epithelium to HIV is sufficient for transmission to occur but specific sexual practices like receptive anal intercourse (the major risk factor for HIV infection in male homosexuals) also appears to be a risk factor for heterosexual transmission.[14,17-19]

A prospective multicentre European study on the risk of heterosexual transmission, co-ordinated by the WHO Collaborating Centre in Paris, was set up in 1987.[20] The aims of the study are to determine rates of infection from male to female (M-F) and female to male (F-M), and to investigate risk factors. Nine centres from 6 countries are currently participating. Preliminary results do not allow comparison of rates of transmission between M-F (42/147 or 29%) and F-M (6/42 or 14%) couples because of differences in recruitment. Various risk factors for transmission were evidenced from the analysis of M-F couples. Multivariate analysis of M-F couples showed that transmission was linked to the clinical state of the infected partner, a history of STD in the receptive partner and the practice of anal sex. No association was found with length of relationship or frequency of sexual contacts. Different classes of risk were established from these results (Table 6), showing that only 7% of the couples were infected when none of the factors were present and 67% when 2 or more were present.

Table 6

Male to female transmission
HIV prevalence in partners for different classes of risk

	HIV+ partners (N)	HIV− partners (N)	HIV+ (%)
History of STD (for female partner)	6	20	23%
Index case: AIDS	3	4	43%
Anal sex	13	16	45%
2 or 3 of the above risks	12	6	67%
None of the above risks	4	56	7%

(Clinical status unknown for 7 index cases)
Source: WHO Collaborating Centre on AIDS.

The association between oral contraception pill use and HIV, was observed in a prospective study of Nairobi prostitutes[21] and other risk factors yet unknown could be linked to genetic, or biological characteristics. To date it is clear that the probability of sexual transmission of the HIV is not constant but dependent on characteristics of patients and their sexual practices.

CONCLUSION

Sexual transmission of HIV represents the major mode of dissemination of this virus throughout the world. In Europe the increase in the number of infected IVDAs represents a threat to the heterosexual population. Although it is now clear that the probability of heterosexual transmission is not constant but depends on characteristics of the infected patient and partner, further studies are needed to define rates of transmission from male to female and from female to male.

ACKNOWLEDGEMENTS

AUSTRIA—Federal Ministry of Health and Environmental Protection, Vienna; BELGIUM—Conseil Supérieur de l'Hygiène Publique, Ministère de la Santé, Brussels; BULGARIA—Institute of General and Comparative Pathology, Sofia; CZECHOSLOVAKIA—Czech S.R.: Institute of Hygiene and Epidemiology, Prague; Slovak S.R.: Ministry of Health, Bratislava; DENMARK—Statens Serum Institute, Copenhagen; FINLAND—National Board of Health, Helsinki; FRANCE—Direction Générale de la Santé, Paris; GERMAN, D.R.—Ministerium für Gesundheitswesen, Berlin; GERMANY, F.R.—Robert Koch Institute, West Berlin; GREECE—Ministry of Health, Athens; HUNGARY—National Institute of Hygiene, Budapest; ICELAND—General Direction of Public Health, Reykjavik; IRELAND—Department of Health, Dublin; ISRAEL—Ministry of Health, Jerusalem; ITALY—Ministry of Health, Rome; LUXEMBOURG—Ministère de la Santé, Luxembourg; MALTA—Department of Health, Valletta; NETHERLANDS—Staatstoezicht op de Volksgezondheid, Rijswijk; NORWAY—National Institute of Public Health, Oslo; POLAND—National Institute of Hygiene, Warsaw; PORTUGAL—Instituto Nacional de Saude, Lisbon; ROMANIA—Ministère de la Santé, Bucharest; SPAIN—Ministerio de Sanidad y Consumo, Madrid; SWEDEN—National Bacteriological Laboratory, Stockholm; SWITZERLAND—Office Fédéral de la Santé Publique, Berne; UNITED KINGDOM—Communicable Disease Surveillance Centre, London; USSR—Ministry of Health of the USSR, Moscow; YUGOSLAVIA—Federal Institute of Public Health, Belgrade.

REFERENCES

1. Centre for Disease Control. *Morbidity and Mortality Weekly Report*. 1982; **31:** 507-514.
2. Centre for Disease Control. *Morbidity and Mortality Weekly Report*. 1985; **34:** 373-375.
3. Centre for Disease Control. *AIDS activity*. 28th December 1987.
4. Ancelle-Park R, Brunet JB, Downs AM. AIDS and drug addicts in Europe. *Lancet* 1987; **2:** 626-627.
5. Piot P, Caraël M. Epidemiological and sociological aspects of HIV-infection in developing countries. *Br Med Bull* 1988; **44:** 68-88.
6. Wallace JI, Christonikos N, Mann J. HIV exposure in New York City streetwalkers (prostitutes). Abstract THP.55, *Third International Conference on AIDS*, Washington DC, June 1-5, 1987.
7. Piot P, Kreiss JK, Ndinya-Achola JO, Ngugi EN, Simonsen JN, Cameron DW, Taelman H, Plummer FA. Heterosexual transmission of HIV. *AIDS* 1987; **4:** 199-206.
8. Piot P, Plummer FA, Rey MA, Ngugi EN, Rouzioux C, Ndinya-Achola JO, Vercauteren G, D'Costa LJ, Laga M, Nsanze H, Fransen L, Haase D, Van der Groen G, Ronal AR, Brun-Vézinet F. Retrospective seroepidemiology of AIDS virus infection in Nairobi populations. *J Infect Dis* 1987; **155:** 1108-1112.
9. Piot P, Quinn TC, Taelman H, Feinsod FM, Minlangu KB, Wobin O, Mbendi N, Mazebo P, Ndangi K, Stevens W, Kayembe K, Mitchell S, Bridts C, McCormick JB. Acquired immunodeficiency syndrome in a heterosexual population in Zaire. *Lancet* 1984; **2:** 65-69.
10. Peterman TA, Stoneburner RL, Allen JR. Risk of HTLVIII/LAV transmission to household contacts of persons with transfusion-associated HTLVIII/LAV infection. Abstract S22b, *Second International Conference on AIDS*, Paris 23-25 June 1986.

11. Fischl MA, Dickinson GM, Scott GB, Klimas N, Fletcher MA, Parks W. Evaluation of heterosexual partners, children, and household contacts of adults with AIDS. *JAMA* 1987; **257:** 640-644.
12. Piot P, Mann J. Bidirectional heterosexual transmission of human immunodeficiency virus. *Ann Inst Past Virol* 1987; **138:** 125-132.
13. Padian NS, Winkelstein W, Rutherford GW, O'Malley PM, Marquis L, Echenberg DF. The heterosexual spread of AIDS virus in San Francisco: female partners of bisexual men. Poster 212, *Second International Conference on AIDS*, Paris, 23-25 June 1986.
14. Kreiss JK, Koech D, Plummer FA, Holmes KK, Lightfoote M, Piot P, Ronald AR, Ndinya-Achola JO, D'Costa LJ, Roberts P, Ngugi EN, Quinn TC. AIDS virus infection in Nairobi prostitutes: spread of the epidemic to East Africa. *N Engl J Med* 1986; **314:** 414-418.
15. Cameron DW, Plummer FA, Simonsen JN, Ndinya-Achola JO, D'Costa LJ, Piot P *et al.* Female to male heterosexual transmission of HIV infection in Nairobi. Abstract MP 91, *Third International Conference on AIDS*, Washington DC, June 1-5 1987.
16. Goedert JJ, Eyster ME, Biggar RJ. Heterosexual transmission of human immunodeficiency virus (HIV): association with severe T4-cell depletion in male hemophiliacs. Abstract W.2.6., *Third International Conference on AIDS*, Washington DC, June 1-5, 1987.
17. Bonneux L, Taelman H, Cornet J, Van Der Groen G, Piot P. Case control study HIV-seropositive versus HIV-seronegative European expatriates in Africa. Abstract W.2.4., *Third International Conference on AIDS*, Washington DC, June 1-5, 1987.
18. Denis F, Barin F, Gershy-Damet G, Rey J-L, Lhuillier M, Mounier M, Leonard G, Sangare A, Goudeau A., M'Boup S, Essex M, Kanki P. Prevalence of human T-lymphotropic retroviruses type III (HIV) and type IV in Ivory Coast. *Lancet* 1987; **1:** 408-411.
19. Steigbigel NH, Maude DW, Feiner CJ, Harris CA, Saltzman BR, Klein RS *et al.* Heterosexual transmission of infection and disease by the human immunodeficiency virus (HIV). Abstract W.2.5., *Third International Conference on AIDS*, Washington DC, June 1-5, 1987.
20. De Vincenzi I, Ancelle-Park R, and the European multicentre study group. Heterosexual transmission of HIV: a European Community multicentre study. Poster 4024. *IVth International Conference on AIDS*, Stockholm, June 1988.
21. Plummer FA, Simonsen JN, Ngugi EN, Cameron DW, Piot P, Ndinya-Achola JO. Incidence of human immunodeficiency virus (HIV) infection and related disease in a cohort of Nairobi prostitutes. Abstract M.8.4, *Third International Conference on AIDS*, Washington DC, June 1-5, 1987.

Effects of human seminal plasma on the lymphocyte response to viral infection

Mr W.P. Soutter, Mr M.J. Turner and Dr J.O. White

INTRODUCTION

Immunosuppression by human seminal plasma

Human seminal plasma suppresses various components of the immune system *in vitro* and *in vivo*. The proliferative response of both T and B lymphocytes to mitogen or antigen;[1,2] recognition of target antigens by macrophages and polymorphonuclear leucocytes;[3] recognition and destruction of tumour or viral infected cells by natural killer cells (NK) and cytotoxic T cells;[2,4] and phagocytosis by macrophages[5] can all be inhibited by seminal plasma *in vitro*. Mouse prostatic fluid inhibits complement-mediated haemolysis.[6] Most of these effects can be achieved with very low concentrations of seminal plasma (0.05-0.1% by volume) and can be demonstrated with seminal plasma from several mammalian species.[6]

Although there are fewer data from experiments *in vivo*, pooled extracts of mouse epididymis, prostate and seminal vesicles inhibit both the primary and the secondary antibody response to subcutaneous injections of bovine serum albumin or epididymal sperm.[5] The instillation of rabbit seminal plasma into the rectum of male rabbits impaired the response of circulating T lymphocytes.[7] The growth of transplanted, methyl cholanthrene-induced tumours in syngeneic mice may be enhanced by seminal plasma.[8]

Identity of immunosuppressive factors in human seminal plasma

Human seminal plasma contains a variety of immunosuppressant factors. The true identity of these agents has not yet been elucidated. This may be because small molecules bind reversibly to higher molecular weight components, or because of aggregation of smaller molecules. The proposed candidates include zinc, prostaglandins, polyamines, transglutaminase and several unidentified proteins ranging up to 720KD in size.[9] The many different effects of seminal plasma on the immune system are unlikely to be due to a single factor and may come from the prostate, seminal vesicles and the epididymis.[5]

Rationale for current study

The study on which this paper is based was originally stimulated by the knowledge that cervical cancer is associated with sexual activity, immunosuppression and viral infection.[8] However, it is readily apparent that AIDS is associated with sexual activity, that immunosuppression is a prominent feature of the disease and that viral infection is the primary cause. It therefore seemed possible that the immunosuppressive effects of seminal plasma might play some part in the pathogenesis of these diseases. However, in spite of its many different immunosuppressive effects, it was not known at that time if seminal plasma would affect the lymphocyte response to viral infection. This study set out to examine the effect of dialysed seminal plasma on the lymphocyte response to infection with Epstein-Barr virus (EBV).[9]

METHODS

Seminal plasma was obtained from healthy men attending the hospital's infertility clinic. Repeated seminal analysis had been normal, the men were disease-free and there was a known female factor responsible for the infertility. The seminal plasma was dialysed twice against 1 litre of phosphate buffered saline to remove small molecules such as prostaglandins and spermine but retain small proteins of higher molecular weight. The dialysed seminal plasma (DSP) was stored at $-70°C$ until further use.

An established lymphocyte regression assay[10] was used to test the effect of DSP on the lymphocyte response to infection with EBV. In the assay, DSP was used at a final concentration of 0.5mg per ml. The same concentration of bovine serum albumin (BSA) was used as a control in parallel cultures. Cyclosporine (Sandoz Products Ltd), which inhibits T lymphocyte function, was used at a concentration of 1 µg/ml as a positive control. Venous blood was collected in preservative-free heparin from healthy EBV-seropositive donors. Mononuclear cells prepared by centrifugation through Ficol-Hypaque were incubated at 37°C for one hour with EBV from the B95-8 cell line.[10] The medium used throughout was RPMI 1640 supplemented with glutamine, 2% fetal calf serum and a 1% penicillin-streptomycin mixture (supplemented RPMI) as similar incorporation of ^3H thymidine was observed using 2% and 10% fetal calf serum. The infected lymphocytes were placed in 5 replicate microtest wells at two concentrations (1 and 2×10^6 per ml).

The lymphocytes were cultured in supplemented RPMI alone or in the presence of DSP or BSA or cyclosporine. DSP from 6 subjects was used. The cultures were incubated at 37°C in 5% CO_2 in air and fed with fresh supplemented RPMI alone every 5 days for 4 weeks. Every well was observed regularly for enlarging foci of proliferating lymphocytes and for the subsequent regression of the foci (Figure I). In those conditions which allowed proliferation to continue for 4 weeks, some of the foci of proliferating cells were removed from the microwells and subcultured in fresh supplemented RPMI where they could be maintained in culture indefinitely.

Normally, EBV-infected lymphocytes from EBV-seropositive donors will proliferate for 10-14 days before the foci regress due to the cytotoxic action of memory T lymphocytes. Once regression has begun, these foci cannot be subcultured.[11] In contrast, lymphocytes from seronegative donors or those whose

Figure I(a)

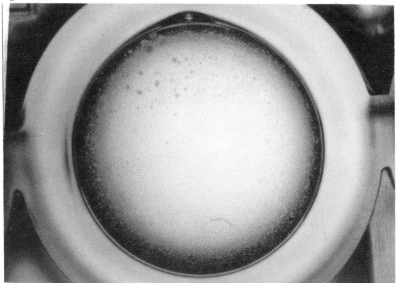

A control well showing regression of the proliferating foci after 4 weeks in culture.

cytotoxic T cell function has been inhibited do not undergo regression and the foci can be subcultured. The establishment of permanent lymphoblastoid cell lines infected with EBV forms the basis for confirming transformation of the infected cells.[12]

Lymphocytes successfully subcultured were assayed for Epstein-Barr Nuclear Antigen (EBNA) using a 3-layer anticomplement immunofluorescence assay.[13] Using the peroxidase-antiperoxidase method,[14] the lymphocytes were also examined with pan-B and pan-T monoclonal antibodies and polyclonal antibodies to kappa and lambda light chains (Dakopatts).

In a separate series of experiments, lymphocytes were grown in supplemented RPMI to which DSP was added at several different concentrations. On day 21, ^{3}H methyl-thymidine (1μCi per well) was added. After 4 hours, the DNA was precipitated with trichloroacetic acid and collected on Whatman GFC filters. Free thymidine was removed by repeated washing and the incorporated label on the filter was measured by liquid scintillation counting.

RESULTS

The results of the lymphocyte cultures are summarised in Table 1. The number of wells are shown in which no regression of proliferating foci occurred (i.e. lymphocyte response inhibited). The results obtained from 5 replicate wells in 5 separate experiments with seminal plasma from 6 subjects are combined. The results shown were obtained at a lymphocyte concentration of 1×10^6/ml. Similar results were seen at a lymphocyte concentration of 2×10^6/ml. In supplemented RPMI

Table 1

Results of lymphocyte cultures

	Number of wells	
	No regression observed	Total
RPMI alone	1	25
BSA	0	20
Cyclosporine	20	20
Seminal plasma subject 1	15	15
Seminal plasma subject 2	13	15
Seminal plasma subject 3	10	10
Seminal plasma subject 4	5	5
Seminal plasma subject 5	4	5
Seminal plasma subject 6	5	5

alone and in supplemented RPMI plus BSA the foci regressed as expected (Figure Ia) and could not be subcultured. In the cyclosporine cultures the foci persisted as expected and could be subcultured. In all 5 experiments and with seminal plasma from every one of the 6 donors the lymphocytes in the wells containing DSP continued to proliferate (Figure Ib and Table 1). These were readily and repeatedly subcultured, thus confirming the inhibition by DSP of the normal regression of proliferating foci.

Figure I(b)

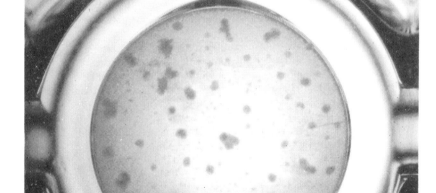

Lymphocytes grown in the presence of seminal plasma continue to proliferate after 4 weeks in culture. Culture wells with foci of EBV-infected proliferating lymphocytes (14 times magnification).

In cultures of lymphocytes that were not infected with EBV, DSP did not induce proliferation nor did it reduce cell viability as measured by the trypan blue exclusion test.

Immunohistochemical staining confirmed that the cells in the foci were B lymphocytes. These cells stained with both the lambda and kappa light-chain antibodies, confirming their polyclonal nature. EBNA was identified in the subcultured cells thus identifying them as being infected with EBV.

The thymidine incorporation experiments confirmed the increased DNA synthesis in the wells containing proliferating foci. The dose-response curve demonstrated a half-maximal effect at a DSP protein concentration of 12.5μg/ml (Figure II).

Figure II

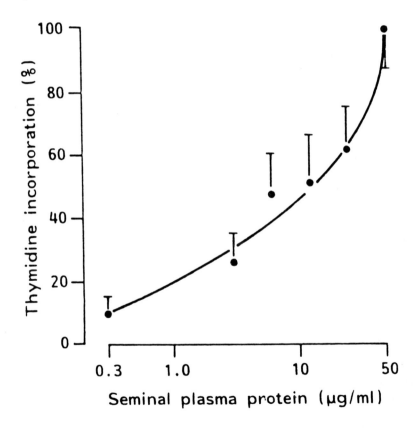

Thymidine incorporation into the DNA of proliferating lymphocytes on Day 21 of culture in the presence of different protein concentrations of DSP is shown. Maximal incorporation of thymidine was observed in cultures with the highest concentrations of DSP (50-500μg protein/ ml).

DISCUSSION

These experiments show clearly that a component or components of DSP can abrogate the normal lymphocyte response to infection with EBV and that this effect persists at very low protein concentrations. Recently, experiments showing similar effects of whole seminal plasma on the immune response to cytomegalovirus have been cited.[2] Dr A.G. Dalgleish of the Clinical Research Centre at Northwick Park Hospital has attempted on our behalf to examine the effects of DSP on human immunodeficiency virus (HIV) in a series of preliminary experiments. He has examined the effects of DSP on syncytial formation by the c8166 T lymphocyte cell line[15] and on reverse transcriptase activity in H9 cells[16] following infection with CBL-1 and RF isolates of HIV. Although some samples of seminal plasma appeared to have an inhibitory effect on syncytial formation and on reverse transcriptase these results were not consistent and further work is required. These models do not test the effect of T and B cell interactions essential in the regression assay of lymphocyte response to EBV infection.

Potential relevance to AIDS

Although it is clear that HIV is the infectious agent responsible for AIDS, a number of observations remain unexplained. Some individuals seem at greater risk of infection with HIV in spite of equivalent exposure.[17] The risk of infection does not seem to be related to the frequency of sexual exposure[17,18] and the male-to-female transmission rate seems to be approximately twice the female-to-male.[19] Heterosexual transmission of HIV is far commoner in tropical countries like Zaire and Haiti than in Europe or USA. The latent phase of HIV infection is highly variable: while some develop AIDS soon after infection, others remain asymptomatic for long periods. All these observations suggest the influence of potent co-factors affecting both the transmission of HIV and the development of disease syndromes. Because diminished immunocompetence is the hallmark of HIV infection and AIDS it seems likely that such co-factors would act by further reducing host resistance to infection and neoplasia.

Co-factors in drug users, haemophiliacs and recipients of blood

Intravenous drug abusers are an important group of HIV-infected and AIDS patients. Their susceptibility to infection is related to the direct intravenous injection of infected lymphocytes or of serum containing free virus. However, many HIV negative drug abusers have reduced numbers of T4 cells.[20] Drug abusers may also be malnourished, a further cause of immunosuppression. This may explain their reduced resistance to infections including HIV.

Haemophiliacs and blood recipients also become infected by the intravenous injection of virus. In addition, haemophiliacs without AIDS who have received multiple transfusions of Factor VIII have reduced numbers of T4 cells.[21] Patients who have received multiple blood transfusions also show evidence of impaired cellular immunity.[22]

Co-factors in tropical countries

In central Africa, the most likely co-factor is chronic viral and parasitic infection.[23] This infection results in an activation of the immune system as demonstrated by reduced T4/T8 lymphocyte ratios, increased HLA-DR and T3 lymphocytes and immune complexes (C1q binding assay). The prevalence of antibodies to cytomegalovirus (CMV), Hepatitis A and B, EBV and syphilis in African patients without AIDS is similar to that found in American homosexual males and very substantially greater than in American heterosexual men and women.[23] There are parallel differences in the immunological data. The findings in African patients might be explained by a greater exposure to other endemic infections such as malaria, trypanosomiasis and filariasis which can also affect the immune system.[24,25] Relative malnutrition and less hygienic living conditions may also play some part. However, no such factors explain the findings in homosexual American males.

Co-factors in the homosexual community

Although HIV infection is becoming more common in the heterosexual community in the United Kingdom and the USA, the majority of infected subjects have acquired the virus through homosexual practice.[26] The preponderance of homosexual or bisexual males is even greater among patients with AIDS.

Among male homosexuals, the major risk factor for transmission of HIV is receptive anogenital intercourse.[18,27-28] This seems to be independent of trauma to the anal canal.[18] Insertive anogenital, orogenital and oroanal intercourse have not been implicated in the epidemic propagation of HIV infection.[18,27] Receptive anogenital intercourse is also associated with a higher risk of the malignant complications of HIV infection.[29]

HIV negative homosexual men have a high prevalence of viral infections such as Hepatitis B, EBV and CMV. In addition, they are also at risk of developing rectal dysplasia and rectal carcinoma.[30,31] Some apparently healthy homosexuals show evidence of immunosuppression and this has been linked to receptive anogenital intercourse.[32,33] Finally, male rabbits infused with seminal plasma rectally developed evidence of systemic immunosuppression.[7]

All the above invites speculation that an immunosuppressive agent or agents in seminal plasma may play a role in the pathogenesis of some infections and of some malignancies in homosexual or bisexual males who engage in receptive anogenital intercourse. Local immunosuppression may act as a co-factor in the genesis of rectal tumours. Systemically absorbed immunosuppressive agents may make the individual more susceptible to viral infections, including HIV. Systemic immunosuppression with cyclosporine makes renal transplant patients more susceptible to lymphomas[34] and it has been suggested that this may be due to suppression of memory-T-cell proliferation.[10] A similar effect of seminal plasma immunosuppressants may explain the higher incidence of the malignant complications of HIV infection in homosexuals than in other groups of HIV patients,[35,36] although the transmission of other oncogenic viruses cannot be excluded.

Seminal plasma as a co-factor in the heterosexual community

It should also not be forgotten that "heterosexual" intercourse does not always mean vaginal penetration. Skilled, non-judgmental interviews have suggested that up to 25% of women in USA occasionally engage in anogenital intercourse and that 10% do so regularly.[37] In a study of London women, 15% reported that they had had at least occasional anal penetration and 8.2% had experienced full anal intercourse with ejaculation.[38] Two of the 3 HIV positive women in this study reported using anogenital intercourse.

However, local and systemic immunosuppression by seminal plasma is also a possibility following vaginal intercourse. Prostaglandin E is absorbed more rapidly from the vagina of Rhesus monkeys than from the rectum.[39] Even larger molecules may be absorbed vaginally. Sperm antigen is absorbed from the vagina of guinea pigs[40] and lipopolysaccharide of Salmonella typhosa from the vagina of Rhesus monkeys[41] is absorbed in sufficient amounts to stimulate the production of specific antibodies.

CONCLUSION

In the homosexual community at least it is possible that the transmission of HIV and the neoplastic complications of this infection are facilitated by the immunosuppressive effects of seminal plasma. The HIV positive homosexual should avoid not only insertive anogenital intercourse with its risk of infecting others but also should avoid receptive anogenital intercourse as this may increase his own risk of the neoplastic complications of AIDS. The same may be true for females infected with HIV.

REFERENCES
1. Stites DP, Erickson RP. Suppressive effect of seminal plasma on lymphocyte activation. *Nature* 1975; **253:** 727-729.
2. Alexander NJ, Anderson DJ. Immunology of semen. *Fertil Steril* 1987; **47:** 192-205.
3. James K, Harvey J, Bradbury AW, Hargreaves TB, Cullen RT. The effect of seminal plasma on macrophage function—a possible contributory factor in sexually transmitted disease. *AIDS Research* 1983; **1:** 45-57.
4. Rees RC, Vallely P, Clegg A, Potter CW. Suppression of natural and activated human antitumour cytotoxicity by human seminal plasma. *Clin Exp Immunol* 1986; **63:** 687-695.
5. Anderson DJ, Tarter TH. Immunosuppressive effects of mouse seminal plasma components in vivo and in vitro. *J Immunol* 1982; **128:** 535-539.
6. James K, Hargreave TB. Immunosuppression by seminal plasma and its possible clinical significance. *Immunology Today* 1984; **5:** 357-363.
7. Richards JM, Bedford JM, Witkin SS. Rectal insemination modifies immune responses in rabbits. *Science* 1984; **224:** 390-392.
8. Turner MJ, Soutter WP. The male factor in cervical neoplasia. In: *Contemporary Obstetrics and Gynaecology*. Ed. G Chamberlain. London: Butterworths; In press.
9. Turner MJ, White JO, Soutter WP. Seminal plasma and AIDS. *Immunology Today* 1987; **8:** 258.
10. Crawford DH, Sweny P, Edwards JM, Janossy G, Hoffbrand AV. Long-term T-cell-mediated immunity to Epstein-Barr virus in renal-allograft recipients receiving cyclosporin A. *Lancet* 1981; **1:** 10-12.
11. Rickinson AB, Moss DJ, Wallace LE, Rowe M, Misko IS, Epstein MA, Pope JH. Long-term T-cell-mediated immunity to Epstein-Barr virus. *Cancer Res* 1981; **41:** 4216-4221.
12. Sixbey JW, Lemon SM, Pagano JS. A second site for Epstein-Barr virus shedding: the uterine cervix. *Lancet* 1986; **2:** 1122-1124.

13. Reedman BM, Klein G. Cellular localization of an Epstein-Barr virus (EBV)-associated complement-fixing antigen in producer and non-producer lymphoblastoid cell lines. *Int J Cancer* 1973; **11**: 499-520.
14. Sternberger LA, Hardy PH, Cuculis JJ, Meyer HG. The unlabelled antibody enzyme method of immunohistochemistry preparation and properties of soluble antigen-antibody complex (horseradish peroxidase-antihorseradish peroxidase) and its use in the identification of spirochetes. *J Histochem Cytochem* 1970; **18**: 315-333.
15. Dalgleish AG, Beverly PC, Clapham PR, Crawford DH, Greaves MF, Weiss RA. The CD4 (T4) antigen is an essential component of the receptor for the AIDS retrovirus. *Nature* 1984; **312**: 763-767.
16. Hoffman AD, Banapour B, Levy JA. Characterization of the AIDS-associated retrovirus reverse transcriptase and optimal conditions for its detection in virions. *Virology* 1985; **147**: 326-335.
17. Peterman TA, Stoneburger RL, Allen JR, Jaffe HW, Curran JW. Risk of human immunodeficiency virus transmission from heterosexual adults with transfusion-associated infections. *JAMA* 1988; **259**: 55-58.
18. Evans BA, Dawson SG, McLean KA, Teece SA, Key PR, Bond RA, Macrae KD, Jesson WJ, Mortimer PP. Sexual lifestyle and clinical findings related to HTLV-III/LAV status in homosexual men. *Genitourin Med* 1986; **62**: 384-389.
19. May RM. HIV infection in heterosexuals. *Nature* 1988; **331**: 655-656.
20. Layon J, Idris A, Warzynbski M, Sherer R, Brauner D, Patch O, McCully D, Orris P. Altered T-lymphocyte subsets in hospitalized intravenous drug abusers. *Arch Intern Med* 1984; **144**: 1376-1380.
21. Carr R, Veitch SE, Edmond E, Peutherer JF, Prescott RJ, Steel CM, Ludham CA. Abnormalities of circulating lymphocyte subsets in haemophiliacs in an AIDS-free population. *Lancet* 1984; **1**: 1431-1434.
22. Gascon P, Zoumbos NC, Young NS. Immunologic abnormalities in patients receiving multiple blood transfusion. *Ann Intern Med* 1984; **100**: 173-177.
23. Quinn TC, Piot P, McCormick JB, Feinsod FM, Taelman H, Kapita B, Stevens W, Fauci AS. Serologic and immunologic studies in patients with AIDS in North America and Africa. *JAMA* 1987; **257**: 2617-2621.
24. Greenwood BM, Whittle HC, Molyneux DH. Immunosuppression in Gambian trypanosomiasis. *Trans R Soc Trop Med Hyg* 1973; **67**: 846-850.
25. Whittle HC, Brown J, Marsh K, Greenwood BM, Seidelin P, Tighe H, Wedderburn L. T-cell control of Epstein-Barr virus-infected B cells is lost during P. falciparum malaria. *Nature* 1984; **312**: 449-450.
26. Department of Health and Social Security. AIDS in the UK. *Lancet* 1988; **1**: 195.
27. Winkelstein W, Lyman DM, Padian N, Grant R, Samuel M, Wiley JA, Anderson RE, Lang W, Riggs J, Levy JA. Sexual practices and risk of infection by the human immunodeficiency virus. *JAMA* 1987; **257**: 321-325.
28. Kingsley LA, Kaslow R, Rinaldo CR, Detre K, Odaka N, Van Raden M, Detels R, Polk BF, Chmiel J, Kelsey SF, Ostrow D, Visscher B. Risk factors for seroconversion to human immunodeficiency virus among male homosexuals. *Lancet* 1987; **1**: 345-348.
29. Marmor M, Friedman-Kien A, Zolla-Pazner S, Stahl RE, Rubinstein P, Laubenstein L, William DC, Klein RJ, Spigland I. Kaposi's sarcoma in homosexual men. A sero-epidemiologic case-control study. *Ann Intern Med* 1984; **100**: 809-815.
30. Frazer IH, Medley G, Crapper M, Brown TC, Mackay IR. Association between anorectal dysplasia, human papilloma-virus, and human immunodeficiency virus infection in homosexual men. *Lancet* 1986; **2**: 657-660.
31. Gal AA, Meyer PR, Taylor CR. Papillomavirus antigens in anorectal condyloma and carcinoma in homosexual men. *JAMA* 1987; **257**: 337-340.
32. Ranki A, Valle S-L, Antonen J, Suni J, Jokipii L, Jokipii AM, Saxinger C, Krohn K. Immunosuppression in homosexual men seronegative for HTLV-III. *Cancer Res* (Suppl) 1985; **45**: 4616s-4618s.

33. Ratnam KV, Kamaruddin A, Wong TW, Sng EH, Lee J, Ong YW. Effect of ano-receptive homosexual practice on T lymphocytes and delayed hypersensitivity in transsexuals. *Aust NZ J Med* 1986; **16:** 757-760.
34. Bieber CP, Reitz BA, Jamieson SW, Oyer PE, Stinson EB. Malignant lymphoma in cyclosporin A treated allograft recipients. (Letter) *Lancet* 1980; **1:** 43.
35. Smith N, Spittle M, ABC of AIDS. Tumours. *Br Med J* 1987; **294:** 1274-1277.
36. Jaffe HW, Hardy AM, Bush TJ, Selik RM, Meade Morgan W. AIDS within population groups in the United States. *Ann Inst Pasteur Virol* 1987; **138:** 75-78.
37. Bolling DR, Voeller B. AIDS and heterosexual anal intercourse. *JAMA* 1987; **258:** 474.
38. Evans BA, McCormack SM, Bond RA, MacRae KD, Thorp RW. Human immuno-deficiency virus infection, hepatitis B virus infection, and sexual behaviour of women attending a genitourinary medicine clinic. *Br Med J* 1988; **296:** 473-475.
39. Alexander NJ, Tarter TH, Fulgham DL, Ducsay CA, Novy MJ. Rectal infusion of semen results in transient elevation of blood prostaglandins. *Am J Reprod Immunol Microbiol* 1987; **15:** 47-51.
40. Isojima S, Ashotaka Y. Absorption of sperm antigen from the vagina in guinea pigs. *Am J Obstet Gynecol* 1964; **88:** 433-438.
41. Yang S-L, Schumacher GFB. Immune response after vaginal application of antigens in the Rhesus monkey. (Abstract) *Fertil Steril* 1977; **28:** 314-315.

Discussion

Chairman: Professor C.S. Peckham

GLYNN: I would like to suggest that it is very dangerous to believe that we are underestimating the incidence of heterosexual spread. When this disease first started in the western world, it started in the heterosexual community of Latin America. There is evidence of its spreading heterosexually throughout the States and Europe, and the rate is increasing. If the rate of increase continues at that rate, and it is much lower than the rate of homosexual spread, the actual increase is still very small and very difficult to detect. But the actual rate of change may be at the very beginning of a logarithmic curve, albeit with a very flat top at the moment.

SOUTTER: It is quite clear that if you have looked at the figures that are currently available, we are not going to have large numbers of heterosexually transmitted cases of AIDS. Those of you who are involved in dealing with the media on this question need first of all to be certain of your ground. And secondly, you have to be quite clear that you do not anticipate an explosion next year. Otherwise you will end up losing the confidence of the public in your predictions. I refer you back to the question which I raised at the beginning, which was in relation to Hepatitis B. Hepatitis B spread in the same way is a more infectious organism, and it has not become a major problem in the heterosexual community. Are you really saying that HIV is going to be of the same order?

CHIN: I think that we have made it quite clear that it is a sexually transmitted disease and it moves in both directions. I think the individuals who are at risk of something like syphilis have to be concerned about HIV.

MILLS: In the United States in 1986 there was a doubling of the number of cases of AIDS in the heterosexual population in a 10-month period as well as a doubling of the incidence of AIDS in a 14-month period for homosexuals and intravenous drug abusers. So it is very difficult to think that it is an epidemic which is not going to affect the heterosexual population. We should think of means now of preventing its spread in that direction. It is very difficult to identify people's sexuality when we are talking about sexual groups. One study claimed that a third of the heterosexual men had had at least one homosexual relationship. So, we have to be very careful about these data.

SOUTTER: There is evidence that something like one-third of homosexual men will have had heterosexual relationships too, so it is not absolutely as clearcut as we would make it out.

TYLER: How did you prepare your seminal plasma?

SOUTTER: We dialysed for seminal plasma using a litre of phosphate buffer on two occasions using a filter with 25 Angstrom pore size.

TYLER: Do you also happen to know what the concentration of lymphocytes is in semen?

SOUTTER: As you probably know, lymphocytes are present in normal semen at counts of 5-10 per ml. It is entirely probable that infected lymphocytes is one of the mechanisms of transmission of HIV with sexual intercourse.

JEFFRIES: Could I just follow on this question of the immunosuppressive effect of semen? Polyamines are immunosuppressive. This has prompted the hypothesis that they may be a co-factor in HIV and the development of AIDS. I would like to know, in the culture system that you use, whether you use "neat" seminal plasma and for how long.

SOUTTER: No. We did not use "neat" seminal plasma. The seminal plasma was first dialysed and then diluted. I showed you a dose response curve which was using serial doubling dilutions of seminal plasma. We achieved 50% of the maximum finding incorporation at a protein concentration of 12.5.

JEFFRIES: So that theoretically, with the sort of dilution factor that one might expect in the genital tract or in circulation, you could imagine that immunosuppression could occur. While I agree with you that there may well be co-factors in this infection, in terms of different levels of this population who are exposed to different amounts of seminal fluid, there doesn't seem to be any influence on progression.

SOUTTER: Of course, I am aware of those data that suggest that there is no evidence of progression. There may well be some relation to transmission.

GREEN: Can I just comment on this issue of anorectal sex in heterosexuals? It has been shown that 30% of men have homosexual experiences. Very few of those actually had penetrative sex. If you look at anorectal sex none of the studies on heterosexual transmission seem to have shown this to be a factor. In areas of large scale heterosexual spread, for instance in Nairobi, the incidence of rectal sexually transmitted disease is very low, suggesting that there is a relatively low incidence of anal intercourse at least in Kenya. I would think that the prevalence of anal intercourse among heterosexuals is minimal; it is mainly vaginal transmission.

ANCELLE: I think that the situation is completely different in developing areas like Africa and the Caribbean islands from that in Europe and the United States. If anal sex counts as a factor in the European studies, I do not know exactly how. The risk factors associated with anal sex are very strong and appear in most of the studies.

GREEN: Yes, it is certainly receptive anal intercourse. I was not making that point. I was making the point that studies in heterosexual transmission show that vaginal transmission is a very viable route of transmission.

ANCELLE: Oh yes.

GREEN: One need not include anal sex among heterosexuals. The studies have not shown it to be a major factor. It is vaginal sex that is transmitting it.

CHIN: I think that sometimes we miss the forest for the trees. What we don't have are precise figures as to what the risk is per single exposure. Until someone can standardise particular sexual acts and arrive at a precise figure we have difficulties. What we do know is that receptive intercourse, whether it be anal or vaginal, is high risk. Insertive anal or vaginal intercourse is still a risk factor, but lower risk than receptive. The data are quite clear that the efficiency of transmission from male to male or male to female is quite high. The efficiency of transmission from female to male is questionable. There is clear evidence that just touching the cervix with semen from an infected donor can infect, as in the Australian study which showed that 4 out of 8 women so exposed were infected.

PECKHAM: Can I ask what population Dr Ancelle is looking at in the heterosexual European studies?

ANCELLE: We have male to female and female to male. In the female to male we have a very small population, and the females who are the index cases come from Amsterdam and are prostitutes. We cannot compare the rates of transmission as the populations are too small and they are not comparable to the population of male to female. We have a lot of intravenous drug abusers as index cases in the male to female group; we have about 150 couples. So mostly they are intravenous drug abusers, transfusion cases, bisexuals and a proportion of haemophiliacs from Germany.

PECKHAM: Are you looking at any associated infections in these groups such as CMV and hepatitis?

ANCELLE: Not CMV. Hepatitis, syphilis, yes. I would like to ask a general question regarding semen and HIV. Have there been any cultures of semen which identify exactly in which cells in the semen the virus is located?

JEFFRIES: No. I do know of studies about 2 years ago in which the virus was localised in lymphocytes, but it has not been found by virological study in spermatozoa. The problem is that in an HIV positive male the proportion of CB4 antigen-bearing lymphocytes increases in the semen quite markedly.

McMANUS: If we are trying to educate HIV patients heterosexually, we should really tell them the facts about a number of things. We run an HIV advice clinic in South London which does not have a lot of female attenders. There are about 200-300 new patients who come each month from HIV testing. This is a population of heterosexual people in whom we see a rising incidence of other sexually transmitted infections. In the period from 1983 to 1987 we have seen a rise in gonorrhoea and other sexually transmitted infections. We have no heterosexual people who are HIV positive without risk factors. There has been an increase from less than 1% of intravenous drug abusers 8 months ago who were HIV positive, to over 12%, also including partners of people who are IV drug abusers. The most worrying group is the people who are HIV positive whose partners are ex-injection users. The best we can say to those people is that if you do not know your partner's past history then you have to be careful. But if they ask, then how do you tell them that there are some heterosexual people who are HIV positive who have no contact with IV drug abusers or contacts in Africa. What we are saying to them is that we are still seeing heterosexuals who are not changing their sexual behaviour, who are still at very high risk of sexually transmitted infections. So, we may well be just about to see an HIV spread.

PECKHAM: I think that was a very good point, and one that came out very strongly in Dr Ancelle's talk, particularly the very high prevalence of IV drug abuser females in the Mediterranean countries. There is no doubt that this is coming through on European perinatal studies because these women are having babies. I think that it is just a question of time before we see an increased prevalence in this country. Some data already suggest that it is becoming an increasing problem in areas of this country, particularly Edinburgh. So I think that it is very important that we do monitor what is going on in Europe.

ANCELLE: There were data which I showed on 170 cases among 282 children with AIDS. These 170 children were contaminated by mother-to-child transmission; half of these were children whose mothers were intravenous drug users. Most of these children come from Spain, Italy and France. I think that this is an increasing problem and that it is extremely important to get the information through to the people who are abusing drugs. It is also important to tell them that they must not share needles. But you must stress the two sides. It is heterosexual transmission and needle-sharing: both equally. People will tell you that they do not share needles anymore, but that is not enough. They must also use condoms to guard against heterosexual transmission. I would stress one and then the other, because in this population it is both.

PECKHAM: I would like to sum up. There were some very provocative papers which drew attention to the desperate need for more information in order to make better predictions and in order to see how the HIV problem is growing into the heterosexual community. We have to have some idea of what is going on within a population. A lot of the information we have comes from very special groups such as people attending STD clinics, but we have very little population data. I would argue that we now need some very good population data. Obviously, there are great ethical issues and questions, which is why we haven't yet collected these data. Surveillance is very important. Some of the predictions that we saw are so close to the things that are being reported by CDSC, but we need to be able to predict further ahead and more accurately. Most of the data that Dr Chin presented actually came from the United States where there is quite a lot of population screening now, and where they are coming up with some very important information which will help to handle the problem and also evaluate some of the aspects of prevention. In this country we need to do more of the same thing.

SECTION II

NATURAL HISTORY

The impact of pregnancy on HIV-related disease

Dr E.E. Schoenbaum, Ms K. Davenny and Dr P.A. Selwyn

INTRODUCTION

The occurrence of AIDS in infants was reported soon after the recognition of the acquired immunodeficiency syndrome (AIDS) in homosexual men and intravenous drug abusers.[1-4] Case reports and the results of epidemiological surveillance of AIDS revealed that the mothers of children with AIDS were frequently intravenous drug abusers who were themselves at risk for AIDS.[2,5] This observation and the availability of assays to test for the presence of infection with human immunodeficiency virus (HIV), the newly discovered aetiological agent of AIDS, suggested that HIV was transmitted perinatally from mother to infant.[6-12] While much attention has been focused on the risks and mechanisms of perinatal transmission, there have been few studies of the natural history of HIV infection in pregnant women. Following a report in 1985 of asymptomatic mothers who had previously transmitted HIV to infants and then appeared to progress to AIDS and HIV-related illness at an accelerated rate,[13] concern was raised about the possible adverse effect of pregnancy on the course of disease in HIV-infected mothers. The known immunosuppressive effects of pregnancy and the reported increased susceptibility of pregnant women to infectious diseases provide a theoretical basis for the hypothesis that pregnancy adversely affects the course of HIV infection. Case reports of virulent presentations of AIDS in pregnant women[14-17] support this hypothesis. Few studies, however, have addressed this question, due in part to problems in assembling sufficiently large cohorts of HIV-infected pregnant women and appropriate controls. Further, much is still unknown about the natural history of HIV infection in women. Evidence that the incubation period of AIDS may be 4½ years or greater[18] suggests that studies may require many years of follow-up before the question is resolved. The increasing numbers of HIV-infected women of childbearing age[19] make resolution of questions regarding the safety of pregnancy (including early and late terminations) more urgent, and underscore the need for scientifically based counselling programmes and public health policies.

This paper will review the effects of pregnancy on the immune system and the increased susceptibility and enhanced virulence of some infectious diseases during pregnancy. Existing data on the effect of pregnancy on the natural history of HIV infection will be examined and issues related to study design and analysis of data will be discussed.

IMMUNE EFFECTS OF PREGNANCY

Investigations of the maternal immune response during pregnancy have demonstrated mild immunosuppression of predominantly cell-mediated immunity associated with a wide range of immunological mechanisms. Although much of the research in this area concerns the maternal-fetal interaction in an effort to explain why the "fetal and placental allografts" escape rejection during pregnancy,[20] the finding of physiological immunosuppression may also relate to patterns of infection observed during pregnancy.

Changes in lymphocyte number and function have been observed, including a reduced response to mitogens,[21,22] diminished cell-mediated cytotoxicity,[23] and a decrease in absolute numbers of helper T-cells.[24] Unfortunately, studies have yielded inconsistent results. For example, response to the plant mitogen PHA has been shown to occur throughout pregnancy,[22] while in other studies the depressed response was only significant in either the last 2 or only the third trimester.[25,26] In other studies no depression was noted.[21] The relative and absolute number of helper T lymphocytes has been observed to be increased,[27] decreased,[28] and unchanged.[29] Similarly, the number of suppressor T lymphocytes has been reported to be both normal[24] and increased.[30] Results of a recent study using monoclonal antibodies (OKT3, 4 and 8) to analyse lymphocyte subsets found a decrease in both relative and absolute numbers of helper T lymphocytes throughout pregnancy and noted no change in the levels of suppressor T lymphocytes.[24] These results may be inconsistent with those from prior studies in which lymphocytes were identified by different and possibly less sensitive techniques.

Studies of B lymphocytes have revealed no significant change in absolute cell number or function.[24,29] Further, quantification of immunoglobulins has shown no difference in a comparison of pregnant and non-pregnant women.[31] The fact that pregnant women have responded satisfactorily to vaccines administered during any trimester of pregnancy is further evidence of an unchanged humoral immune system.[32]

Immunosuppression has been associated with hydrocortisone and oestrogen, and somewhat less convincingly with human chorionic gonadotrophin (hCG) and alpha-fetoprotein (AFP).[33] All these hormones are markedly elevated during pregnancy. Oestradiol has been shown to inhibit graft rejection and together with hCG can cause involution of the thymus.[34] The immunosuppressive effects of corticosteroids have been well documented and include suppression of phagocytosis and lymphokine activation of the macrophages.[34] Although the hormones are increased during pregnancy, the concentration is not great enough to alter the function of previously primed maternal lymphocytes. Several *in vitro* studies have reported serum factors that are associated with reduction of maternal lymphocyte function. One study demonstrated a factor from pregnant bitches which caused functional depression of lymphocytes from non-pregnant bitches.[35] Other studies reporting suppression factors have been done with murine models.[36] However, *in vitro* effects may be significantly attenuated *in vivo*, and animal models cannot be directly extrapolated to humans.

Studies of lymphocyte function during pregnancy in response to specific antigens from pathogenic organisms have reported reduced response after stimulation with cytomegalovirus, vaccinia, herpes simplex type 1, and rubella viruses. Most studies did not relate findings to the maternal history of infection and findings have not been consistently replicated.[37]

Immune effects during pregnancy have been widely studied, and detailed reviews are available which address the maternal-fetal interaction.[23,38] Although immunosuppression occurs, data suggest a selective effect involving the cellular immune system. Overall, the effect of pregnancy on normal immune function appears to be mild. However, specific defects in response to particular organisms may be exceptional, including response to retroviruses such as HIV. In addition, the combined effects of the immunosuppression of pregnancy superimposed on a defective immune system, as occurs during HIV infection, are unknown. The interaction of the known helper T lymphocyte depletion during HIV infection with the physiological decrease which occurs during pregnancy remains speculative. If population-based studies demonstrate an accelerated course of HIV infection in pregnant women, these will be challenging and important issues to explore.

INFECTION IN PREGNANCY

It has long been observed that pregnant women fare poorly with certain infections. Those infections in which the protective effect of cell-mediated immunity predominates have been reported to cause more severe disease during pregnancy, both in reactivation of latent infection and acquisition of primary infection. Organisms observed to threaten maternal well-being to a greater degree than non-pregnant women include viruses, bacteria, fungi and parasites. Population-based studies examining the risk of viral infection among pregnant women compared with non-pregnant controls from the same community have shown increased risk to pregnant women from influenza A,[39,40] poliomyelitis,[41-43] Hepatitis A,[44-46] Hepatitis non-A non-B,[47] Hepatitis B,[48,49] Epstein-Barr,[50-53] and papillomavirus-induced genital warts.[54] Other infections for which there is evidence that pregnant women are particularly vulnerable include candida (mucocutaneous),[55] coccidioidomycosis,[56] malaria,[57] and tuberculosis.[58-61] While this list is not exhaustive it is indicative of the broad range of infections which may be more virulent during pregnancy.

Large scale studies which have investigated that course of pregnant women and non-pregnant women during epidemics have uncovered a heightened susceptibility of non-immune pregnant women to several organisms. Influenza A is associated with a lethal pneumonia in pregnant women.[39] In New York City during the 1957 influenza A epidemic 50% of women who died were pregnant, against a background pregnancy rate of 7%.[40] During polio epidemics an increased attack rate as well as a higher incidence of residual paralytic polio was noted among pregnant women in comparison with non-pregnant women.[41-43] However, conclusions of these studies may be affected by the length of time of the epidemic and the 40-week course of pregnancy. Although an increased incidence of polio during the first trimester of pregnancy has been reported,[41] the unsusceptible women who became infected in the first trimester and survived were no longer susceptible during the later trimesters, producing possible bias towards observing a worse prognosis in early pregnancy.[37]

Epidemic reports of Hepatitis A in Africa and Asia show both a greater number of cases and more frequent progression to fulminant clinical disease among pregnant women than was observed in their non-pregnant counterparts.[44-46] In these studies, pregnant women appeared to be at greater risk during the third trimester. However, these data may reflect the greater likelihood that a pregnant woman will come to medical attention and be hospitalised for illness. Similar findings have been noted for Hepatitis non-A non-B (water-borne type). For example, during an epidemic in India,[47] the incidence of infection in women aged 15-45 years was 17.3% in pregnant women and 2.1% in non-pregnant women. Fulminant hepatitis occurred in 22.2% of pregnant women and in none of the non-pregnant women. An increased incidence of Hepatitis B during pregnancy has been reported from countries with low or high prevalence, with severity of illness most marked in the third trimester.[48] It has been noted that the association of severe hepatitis and pregnancy observed in developing but not in industrialised countries may be related to nutritional status.[49] The increased nutritional demands of pregnancy in combination with the multiple infections and underlying malnutrition common in developing countries may play a role in the course of hepatitis in pregnant women.[37]

Herpesviruses have been studied in relation to pregnancy. In contrast to the studies previously mentioned, studies of herpesviruses in pregnant women have, in some instances, shown an increased rate of reactivation or more severe infection in previously infected or susceptible women.[62] The effect of primary CMV infection on infants is well known. Although studies have not shown an increase in clinical disease in mothers versus non-pregnant women, the frequency of isolation of CMV in pregnant women increases with gestation.[63] Serological detection of Epstein-Barr virus (EBV) infection is almost universal by young adulthood in developing countries and greater than 50% in population studies from industrialised countries.[50] Pregnant women have a rate of EBV reactivation which is 2.4 times greater than the rate in non-pregnant women.[51] In addition, case reports of Burkitt's lymphoma in pregnant women have described rapid and extensive progression of disease.[52,53] Susceptibility to herpes simplex virus (HSV) infections of the genitals in pregnancy has not been definitively studied. Some investigators have reported no increase in pregnant women of symptomatic genital herpes infection at the time of delivery[37] and others have reported a proclivity for pregnant women to develop genital herpes infections.[64,65] Although disseminated herpes simplex infection during pregnancy has been reported,[66] the high prevalence of herpes infection and the rarity of disseminated disease in pregnancy make the significance of the report unclear.

Studies of coccidioidomycosis are interesting in that a specific mechanism for enhancement of infection during pregnancy has been demonstrated *in vitro*. It has been demonstrated that cultures of the fungus *Coccidioides immitis* are stimulated by the addition of levels of oestradiol and progesterone in amounts comparable to those achieved in pregnant women.[56] This may explain the observed increase in disseminated *C. immitis* infection in non-immune pregnant women in areas where this fungus is endemic.

The relationship of tuberculosis and pregnancy has been controversial.[58] Prior to effective antituberculous therapy it was generally accepted that pregnancy had a deleterious effect on the course of tuberculosis. This view was so widespread that abortion was often recommended to offset the adverse effect of pregnancy. Data collected before the availability of effective therapy have not confirmed this deleterious effect[59,60] but have suggested instead that tuberculosis may flare in the post-partum period among previously infected women. Concern about enhanced tuberculosis during or after pregnancy has waned with the availability of effective therapy, and there is general agreement that the prognosis of treated tuberculosis is excellent in pregnant as well as non-pregnant women.

Some infections for which there is evidence in the medical literature that pregnancy worsens the disease prognosis have also been reported in HIV-infected individuals. Tuberculosis is frequently seen in HIV-infected individuals and is more often extrapulmonary than in individuals uninfected with HIV.[61] The presence of mucocutaneous candida (predominantly vaginal) is reported to be as high as 55% during pregnancy,[55] whereas the presence of oral candidasis in an otherwise non-immunocompromised individual meets Centers for Disease Control criteria for an advanced level of HIV infection and increases the likelihood of progression to AIDS.[67] There has been no consensus regarding the significance of oral candidiasis in pregnant HIV-infected women. Massively enlarged genital warts from papilloma virus infection have been reported during pregnancy with spontaneous regression during the postpartum period.[54] Preliminary research findings have been shown an increased prevalence of papilloma virus-associated squamous atypia on Papanicolaou smears in HIV-infected women as compared with a control group uninfected with HIV.[68] Similarly, case reports of virulent infection with *C. immitis* in AIDS patients have been linked to cellular immunosuppression due to HIV.[69] The overlap of infections seen in HIV-infected individuals and pregnant women underscores the potential for negative "side effects" from the physiological immunosuppression of pregnancy. Whether pregnancy has a negative impact on the course of HIV infection is unknown at the present time. The following section will discuss existing data which address this issue.

IMPACT OF PREGNANCY ON HIV INFECTION

The need for clearer definition of the possible deleterious interaction of the immunosuppressive effects of pregnancy with HIV infection has become increasingly compelling in view of the growing numbers of HIV-infected women of childbearing age and perinatally-infected infants. Elucidation of the risks associated with pregnancy is critical to counselling of HIV-infected women by obstetricians and midwives.

The first reported case of AIDS during pregnancy, published in 1983, described a Haitian woman who died 3½ hours post-partum at 32 weeks gestation from *Listeria monocytogenes* sepsis.[14] Although the case predated the availability of HIV antibody testing, the epidemiological data, the finding of lymphopenia and the unprecedented fatal maternal outcome from listeria infection, strongly suggested an AIDS diagnosis. The second fatal case of AIDS in a pregnant woman was reported in 1984, in a Haitian woman with *Pneumocystis carinii* pneumonia (PCP) diagnosed by bronchoscopic lung biopsy.[15] The woman died despite appropriate therapy following delivery of a preterm infant. In 1986, four additional cases of fatal PCP in pregnant women with histories of intravenous drug abuse were reported from New York City.[16,17] The cases presented between 26 and 35 weeks gestation and each resulted in death from respiratory failure.

The case reports of fatal maternal outcomes in pregnant women with AIDS caused concern that pregnancy exerts an adverse effect on the course of HIV infection. Additional evidence that pregnancy had a deleterious effect on HIV infection in pregnant women came from uncontrolled series in which high proportions of pregnant women developed HIV-related disease, and in one series with fatal outcomes. Scott *et al.*[13] identified a group of 15 asymptomatic mothers who had previously delivered infants who developed AIDS or AIDS-related complex. The women were followed for a mean of 30 months post-partum, during which time 11 of the women had subsequent pregnancies. Five (33%) developed AIDS, 7 (47%) developed AIDS-related complex and 3 (20%) remained asymptomatic. The finding that 80% of asymptomatic women developed HIV-related disease alarmed the medical community and led to the provisional recommendation by The Centers for Disease Control in Atlanta, Georgia, U.S.A., that HIV-infected women consider postponing pregnancy to avoid a worsening of their own prognosis for development of AIDS, as well as transmission of HIV to their infants.[11] In 1980 Minkoff *et al.*[70] reported related outcomes on 34 mothers selected by criteria similar to the mothers in Scott's study. All women were identified after having a child who acquired AIDS or AIDS-related disease perinatally. None of the mothers had AIDS or AIDS-related disease during pregnancy and 14 had subsequent pregnancies during prospective follow-up. Five developed AIDS and 10 developed AIDS-related complex after 27.8 mean months of follow-up. A third study from Zaire in 1986 described 5 pregnant women with HIV-related symptoms whose clinical status deteriorated from HIV-related disease and in some instances resulted in death.[71] One final uncontrolled series from Paris did not find excessive HIV-related illness after pregnancy.[72] In this study, 25 HIV-infected pregnant women were followed prospectively. Five had HIV-related disease or abnormal results on immune studies at baseline. The authors noted that pregnancy did not alter the clinical or immunological status of the women. However, 5 pregnancies were electively terminated and 1 resulted in a spontaneous abortion all at unspecified gestational age.

There are 2 ongoing prospective studies of HIV-infected pregnant women in which the course of HIV-related disease in pregnant women is compared with the course of HIV infection in women from the same population who have not become pregnant during the study. The preliminary results of these studies contrast with the uncontrolled series. In a study reported at the IIIrd AIDS International Conference in Washington, DC, Schoenbaum *et al.*[73] found no excess progression in HIV-related disease status in pregnant women as compared with non-pregnant counterparts. The women were followed for a mean 20 months and were stratified by clinical disease status at baseline. No differences in baseline status were noted. However, baseline T4 counts were lower in the women not becoming pregnant during prospective follow-up. Rates of hospitalisation for infectious diseases were lower in pregnant women. Obstetric histories were similar in both groups and the number of livebirths and pregnancies did not correlate with HIV disease progression in the pregnant women or comparison group. McCallum presented preliminary results in 1987 of a prospective study of intravenous drug abusers from Edinburgh, Scotland.[74] In this study, HIV-infected women becoming pregnant since seroconversion with HIV antibody are compared with HIV-infected women not becoming pregnant since seroconversion. All subjects were asymptomatic at baseline and had seroconverted (approximately) in 1983. No subjects in either the pregnant or non-pregnant group developed AIDS during prospective follow-up and no differences in T-cell subset analysis or immunoglobulin levels were noted between the groups.

While the case reports and uncontrolled series of HIV-infected pregnant women suggest pregnancy has an adverse effect on the course of HIV infection, there were no comparison groups against which to assess progression of HIV-related disease status. At the present time there are few other data on the natural history of HIV infection in women from which to extrapolate an adverse effect of pregnancy.

The two uncontrolled studies selected women with histories of having transmitted HIV to infants who then subsequently developed AIDS or AIDS-related complex.[13,67] Unknown factors associated with perinatal transmission of HIV to infants may also be associated with an accelerated course of HIV infection in the mothers. Factors other than pregnancy that may contribute to both poor outcome in HIV-infected women and high rates of transmission to infants include length of time of HIV infection, clinical disease or immune status at baseline, and HIV risk factor.

The two clinical studies with comparison groups failed to demonstrate an adverse effect of pregnancy on the course of HIV infection.[73,74] While these results must be considered preliminary, the inclusion of a comparison group in the study design strengthens the meaning of the results. However, it is important to identify potential selection factors in assembling a comparison group that may affect study results. For example, women with more advanced HIV infection may also be less likely to become pregnant and may be more likely to abort electively. Further, women with more advanced HIV infection are more likely to progress to AIDS or AIDS-related outcomes. A bias towards development of AIDS in the comparison group may mask important effects of pregnancy on HIV infection in the pregnant group. Ideally, a comparison group for HIV-infected asymptomatic pregnant women might include fertile HIV-infected women who for reasons unrelated to the severity of HIV infection do not become pregnant.

However, implementation of sound epidemiological methods may not always be feasible. Baseline stratification of study subjects by disease status and other factors known to affect HIV disease outcome will help to address this potential source of bias. Longer periods of follow-up may be required to resolve this issue definitively, particularly since no pregnant women developed AIDS in either of the controlled studies. Study of women with a spectrum of HIV-related disease would maximise extrapolation of results to most HIV-infected women and might uncover adverse effects of pregnancy among women with more advanced HIV-related disease not present in asymptomatic women. In addition, larger numbers of subjects should be followed to achieve sufficient statistical power for interpreting results.

In conclusion, existing data do not consistently support the hypothesis that pregnancy adversely affects the course of HIV infection, although theoretical risks, case reports and uncontrolled series describing accelerating HIV infection in pregnant women indicate a potential adverse effect. Counselling of HIV-infected pregnant women should acknowledge a potential additional risk from pregnancy but stress that preliminary results of controlled studies have not demonstrated an acceleration of HIV-related disease. Prospective study of large numbers of HIV-infected pregnant and non-pregnant women with long periods of follow-up will provide the necessary epidemiological data needed to determine the effect of pregnancy on the course of HIV infection.

ACKNOWLEDGMENTS

The authors thank Riah Ettienne for expert technical help in preparation of this manuscript.

REFERENCES
1. Centers for Disease Control. Unexplained immunodeficiency and opportunistic infections in infants—New York, New Jersey, California. *MMWR* 1983; **31**: 665-667.
2. Rubinstein A, Sicklick M, Gupta A, Bernstein L, Klein N, Rubinstein E, Spigland I, Fruchter L, Litmann M, Lee H, Hollander M. Acquired immunodeficiency with reserved T4/T8 ratios in infants born to promiscuous and drug-addicted mothers. *JAMA* 1983; **249**: 2350-2356.
3. Rubinstein A. Acquired immunodeficiency syndrome in infants. *Am J Dis Child* 1983; **137**: 825-827.
4. Thomas PA, Jaffe HW, Spira TJ, Reiss R, Guerrero IC, Auerbach D. Unexplained immunodeficiency in children. A surveillance report. *JAMA* 1984; **252**: 639-644.
5. Rogers MF. AIDS in children: a review of the clinical, epidemiological and public health aspects. *Pediatr Infect Dis* 1985; **4**: 230-236.
6. Popovic M, Sarngadharan MG, Read E, Gallo RC. Detection, isolation, and continuous production of cytotrophic retroviruses (HTLV-III) from patients with AIDS and pre-AIDS. *Science* 1984; **224**: 497-500.
7. Vilmer E, Fischer A, Griscelli C, Barré-Sinoussi F, Vie V, Chermann JC, Montagnier L, Rouzioux C, Brun-Vezinet F, Rosenbaum W. Possible transmission of a human lymphotropic retrovirus (LAV) from mother to infant with AIDS. *Lancet* 1984; **2**: 229-230.
8. Cowan MJ, Hellman D, Chudwin D, Wara DW, Chang RS, Ammann AJ. Maternal transmission of acquired immune deficiency syndrome. *Pediatrics* 1984; **73**: 382-386.
9. Lapointe N, Michaud J, Pekovic D, Chasseau JP, Dupuy JM. Transplacental transmission of HTLV-III virus. (Letter) *N Engl J Med* 1985; **312**: 1325-1326.

10. Jovaisas E, Koch MA, Schäfer A, Stauber M, Löwenthal D. LAV/HTLV-III in 20-week fetus. (Letter) *Lancet* 1985; **2**: 1129.
11. Centers for Disease Control. Recommendations for assisting in the prevention of perinatal transmission of HTLV-III/LAV and AIDS. *MMWR* 1985; **34**: 721-732.
12. Di Maria H, Courpotin C, Rouzioux C, Cohen D, Rio D, Boussin F. Transplacental transmission of human immunodeficiency virus. (Letter) *Lancet* 1986; **2**: 215-216.
13. Scott GB, Fischl MA, Klimas N, Fletcher MA, Dickinson GM, Levine RS, Parks WP. Mothers of infants with the acquired immunodeficiency syndrome. Evidence for both symptomatic and asymptomatic carriers. *JAMA* 1985; **253**: 363-366.
14. Wetli CV, Roldan EO, Fojaco RM. Listeriosis as a cause for maternal death: an obstetric complication of the acquired immunodeficiency syndrome (AIDS). *Am J Obstet Gynecol* 1983; **147**: 7-9.
15. Jensen LP, O'Sullivan MJ, Gomez-del-Rio M, Setzer ES, Gaskin C, Penso C. Acquired immunodeficiency (AIDS) in pregnancy. *Am J Obstet Gynecol* 1984; **48**: 1145-1146.
16. Minkoff H, de Regt RH, Landesman S, Schwarz R. *Pneumocystis carinii* pneumonia associated with acquired immunodeficiency syndrome: a report of three maternal deaths. *Obstet Gynecol* 1986; **67**: 284-287.
17. Antoine C, Morris M, Douglas G. Maternal and fetal mortality in AIDS. *NY State J Med* 1986; **86**: 443-445.
18. Lui KJ, Lawrence DN, Morgan WM, Peterman TA, Haverkos HW, Bregman DJ. A model-based approach for estimating the mean incubation period of transfusion-associated acquired immunodeficiency syndrome. *Proc Natl Acad Sci USA* 1986; **83**: 3051-3055.
19. Guinan ME, Hardy A. Epidemiology of AIDS in women in the United States, 1981 through 1986. *JAMA* 1987; **257**: 2039-2042.
20. Lederman MM. Cell-mediated immunity and pregnancy. *Chest* 1984; **86** (Suppl): 65-95.
21. Gehrz RC, Christianson WR, Linner KM, Conroy MM, McCue SA, Balfour HH Jr. A longitudinal analysis of lymphocyte proliferative responses to mitogens and antigens during human pregnancy. *Am J Obstet Gynecol* 1981; **140**: 665-670.
22. Purtillo DT, Hallgren HM, Yunis EJ. Depressed maternal lymphocyte response to phytohaemagglutinin in human pregnancy. *Lancet* 1972; **1**: 769-771.
23. Jacoby DR, Olding LB, Oldstone MBA. Immunologic regulation of fetal-maternal balance. *Adv Immunol* 1984; **35**: 157-208.
24. Sridama V, Pacini F, Yang SL, Moawad A, Reilly M, De Groot LJ. Decreased levels of helper T-cells—a possible cause of immunodeficiency in pregnancy. *N Engl J Med* 1982; **307**: 352-356.
25. Garewal G, Sehgal S, Aikat BK, Gupta AN. Cell-mediated immunity in pregnant patients with and without a previous history of spontaneous abortions. *Br J Obstet Gynaecol* 1978; **85**: 221-224.
26. Blecher TE, Thompson MJ. Comparison of uridine uptake at 24 hours with thymidine uptake at 72 hours in phytohaemagglutinin-stimulated cultures of pregnant and other subjects. *J Clin Pathol* 1976; **29**: 727-731.
27. Clements PJ, Yu DT, Levy J, Pearson CM. Human lymphocyte sub populations: the effect of pregnancy. *Proc Soc Exp Biol Med* 1976; **152**: 664-666.
28. Bulmer R, Hancock KW. Depletion of circulating T lymphocytes in pregnancy. *Clin Exp Immunol* 1977; **28**: 302-305.
29. Dodson MG, Kerman RH, Lange CF, Sefani SS, O'Leary JA. T and B cells in pregnancy. *Obstet Gynecol* 1977; **49**: 299-302.
30. Suzuki K, Tomasi TB Jr. Immune responses during pregnancy. *J Exp Med* 1979; **150**: 898-908.
31. Damber MG, von Schoultz B, Stigbrand T. The immunological paradox of pregnancy. *Acta Obstet Gynecol Scand* (Suppl) 1977; **66**: 39-47.

32. Amstey MS, Insel RA, Pichichero ME. Neonatal passive immunization by maternal vaccination. *Obstet Gynecol* 1984; **83**: 105-109.
33. Weinberg ED. Pregnancy-associated depression of cell-mediated immunity. *Rev Infect Dis* 1984; **6**: 814-831.
34. Rocklin RE, Kitzmiller JL, Kaye MD. Immunobiology of the maternal-fetal relationship. *Ann Rev Med* 1979; **30**: 375-404.
35. Lloyd S, Soulsby EJL. Effect of pregnancy and lactation on infection with *Toxocara canis* in dogs. *Parasitology* 1982; **85**: 39.
36. Harrison MR. Maternal immunocompetence II. Proliferative responses of maternal lymphocytes *in vitro* and inhibition by serum from pregnant rats. *Scand J Immunol* 1976; **5**: 881-889.
37. Brabin BJ. Epidemiology of infection in pregnancy. *Rev Infect Dis* 1985; **7**: 579-603.
38. Gall SA. Maternal immune system during human gestation. *Semin Perinatol* 1977; **2**: 119-131.
39. Freeman DW, Barno A. Deaths from Asian influenza associated with pregnancy. *Am J Obstet Gynecol* 1959; **78**: 1171-1175.
40. Greenberg M, Jacobziner H, Pakter J, Weisl BAG. Maternal mortality in the epidemic of Asian influenza, New York City, 1957. *Am J Obstet Gynecol* 1958; **76**: 897-902.
41. Siegel M, Greenberg M. Incidence of poliomyelitis in pregnancy. *N Engl J Med* 1955; **253**: 841-847.
42. Weinstein L, Aycoc WL, Feemster RF. The relation of sex, pregnancy and menstruation to susceptibility in poliomyelitis. *N Engl J Med* 1951; **245**: 54-58.
43. Priddle HD, Leuz WR, Young DC, Stevenson CS. Poliomyelitis in pregnancy and the puerperium. *Am J Obstet Gynecol* 1952; **63**: 408-455.
44. Morrow RH Jr, Smetana HF, Sai FT, Edgcomb JH. Unusual features of viral hepatitis in Accra, Ghana. *Ann Intern Med* 1968; **68**: 1250-1264.
45. D'Cruz I, Balani SG, Tyer LS. Infectious hepatitis and pregnancy. *Obstet Gynecol* 1968; **31**: 449-455.
46. Borhanmanesh F, Hughighi P, Hekmat K, Rezaizadeh K, Ghavami AG. Viral hepatitis during pregnancy. *Gastroenterology* 1973; **64**: 304-312.
47. Khuroo MS, Teli MR, Skidmore S, Sofi MA, Khuroo MI. Incidence and severity of viral hepatitis in pregnancy. *Am J Med* 1981; **70**: 252-225.
48. Cossart YE. The outcome of hepatitis B virus infection in pregnancy. *Postgrad Med J* 1977; **53**: 610-613.
49. Sherlock S. Jaundice in pregnancy. *Br Med Bull* 1968; **24**: 39-43..
50. Evans AS. *Viral Infections of Humans*. New York: Plenum Medical, 1984; pp.100,263.
51. Fleisher G, Bolognese R. Persistent Epstein-Barr virus infection and pregnancy. *J Infect Dis* 1983; **147**: 982-986.
52. Bammerman RHO. Burkitt's tumour in pregnancy. (Letter) *Br Med J* 1966; **2**: 1137-1138.
53. Jones DED, D'Avignon MB, Lawrence R, Latshaw RF. Burkitt's lymphoma: obstetric and gynaecological aspects. *Obstet Gynecol* 1980; **56**: 533-536.
54. Young RL, Acosta AA, Kaufman RH. The treatment of large *condylomata acuminata* complicating pregnancy. *Obstet Gynecol* 1973; **41**: 65-73.
55. Rein M, Holmes KK. Nonspecific vaginitis, vulvovaginal candidiasis and trichomas: clinical features, diagnosis and management. In: *Clinical Topics in Infectious Diseases, No. 4*. Eds. JS Remington, MN Schwartz. New York: McGraw Hill, 1986; p.294.
56. Drutz D, Huppert M. Coccidioidomycosis: factors affecting the host-parasite interaction. *J Infect Dis* 1983; **147**: 372-390.
57. Brabin BJ. An analysis of malaria in pregnancy in Africa. *Bull WHO* 1983; **61**: 1005-1016.
58. Snider D. Pregnancy and tuberculosis. *Chest* 1984; **86**: 108-138.

59. Hedvall E. Pregnancy and tuberculosis. *Acta Med Scand* (Suppl) 1953; **147**: Suppl 286: 1-101.
60. Crombie JB. Pregnancy and pulmonary tuberculosis. *Br J Tuber* 1954; **48**: 97-101.
61. Sunderam G, McDonald RJ, Maniatis T, Oleske J, Kapila R, Reichman LB.. Tuberculosis as a manifestation for the acquired immunodeficiency syndrome (AIDS). *JAMA* 1986; **256**: 362-366.
62. Agatsuma Y, Fitzpatrick P, Lee A, Kaul A, Oga PL. Cell-mediated immunity to cytomegalovirus in pregnant women. *Am J. Reprod Immunol* 1981; **1**: 74.
63. Reynolds DW, Stagno S, Hosty TS, Tiller M, Alford CA Jr. Maternal cytomegalovirus excretion and perinatal infection. *N Engl J Med* 1973; **289**: 1-5.
64. Ng ABP, Reagan JW, Yen SSC. Herpes genitalis. *Obstet Gynecol* 1970; **36**: 645-651.
65. Poste G, Hawkins DF, Thomlinson J. *Herpesvirus hominis* infection of the female genital tract. *Obstet Gynecol* 1972; **40**: 871-890.
66. Young EJ, Killam AP, Greene JF Jr. Disseminated herpes-virus infection associated with primary genital herpes in pregnancy. *JAMA* 1976; **235**: 2731-2733.
67. Klein RS, Harris CA, Small CB, Moll B, Lesser M, Friedland GH. Oral candidiasis in high-risk patients as the initial manifestation of the acquired immunodeficiency syndrome. *N Engl J Med* 1984; **311**: 354-358.
68. Schrager L, Friedland GH, Klein RS, Maude D, Schreiber K, Koss LG. Increased risk of cervical and/or vaginal squamous atypia in women infected with HIV. III International Conference on Acquired Immunodeficiency Syndrome (AIDS) June 1987, Washington; (Abstract).
69. Centers for Disease Control. Revision of the CDC Surveillance Case Definition for Acquired Immunodeficiency Syndrome. *MMWR* 1987; **36**: 35-155.
70. Minkoff HL, Nanda D, Menez R, Fikrig S. Pregnancies resulting in infants with acquired immunodeficiency syndrome or AIDS-related complex: follow-up of mothers, children, and subsequently born siblings. *Obstet Gynecol* 1987; **69**: 288-291.
71. Tshibangu K, Kayembe K, Smariuli K, Mbuyamba N. Feto-maternal risk during acquired immunodeficiency syndrome. International Conference on AIDS, Paris, France, June, 1986; (Abstract).
72. Ciraru-Vigneron N, Tan Lung RN, Brunner C, Barrier J, Wantier J, Boizard B. HIV infection among high-risk pregnant women. *Lancet* 1987; **1**: 630.
73. Schoenbaum EE, Selwyn PA, Feingold AR, Davenny K, Roberta V, Rogers M. The effect of pregnancy on progression of HIV-related disease. III International Conference on Acquired Immunodeficiency Syndrome (AIDS), Washington; June 1987; (Abstract).
74. MacCallum LI. Presentation at International Hospital Infection Society conference, 1987, London, England. Cited in *AIDS Alert* 1987; **2**: 162.

Infants born to mothers seropositive for HIV: Results from the ongoing European Collaborative Study

Professor C. S. Peckham, Dr Y. D. Senturia and Dr A. E. Ades

INTRODUCTION

As the number of human immunodeficiency virus (HIV) infections among women increases there is likely to be an increasing number of children born to seropositive mothers. Transmission rates ranging from 0-65% have been reported.[1] There are, as yet, no reliable estimates of the risk of infection in a child born to an HIV seropositive mother, but studies are in progress in several countries. At the present time our knowledge is largely based on prospective studies following children presenting with symptoms in the early months or years of life. This group does not represent the majority of HIV-infected children, and further information on the natural history of perinatally acquired infection is required.

OBSTETRIC ISSUES

By the end of 1987, 1105 adult women with AIDS had been reported to the WHO Surveillance Centre for the European region.[2] The majority were intravenous drug abusers of childbearing age. During this same period 251 children aged under 15 years with AIDS were reported, 65% of whom had acquired their infection from a mother who either had AIDS or who was at risk of AIDS (intravenous drug abuser, prostitute, a woman from a country where the prevalance of HIV infection is high or a woman whose sexual partner was in a high risk group). In the UK only 22 cases of paediatric AIDS have been confirmed; however this figure seriously underestimates the scale of the problem: children with AIDS-related complex are not included, and 173 HIV positive children have been identified by laboratory reports alone.

The justification for testing and identifying HIV positive women in early pregnancy is to offer them termination in view of the risk of intrauterine

Collaborators: C Giaquinto, University of Padua; I Grosch-Wörner, Universitätsklinikum; Rudolk Virchow, Berlin; J Mok, City Hospital, Edinburgh; F Omenca Teres, Hospital Infantil, Madrid; C Canosa, Hospital de la Seguridad Social, Valencia; H Scherpbier, Universiteit van Amsterdam; A Böhlin, Huddinge Hospital.

transmission of infection, and the possibility that pregnancy may accelerate the progression of HIV disease. It is important that all HIV seropositive pregnant women are adequately counselled so that they can make an informed choice regarding continuation of the pregnancy and be advised about the importance of reducing the chance of transmitting the infection to others by adopting safer sexual practices. A true assessment of the effect of pregnancy on the natural history of HIV infection requires comparisons between infected pregnant women and non-pregnant infected controls. Such studies are under way in the United States.[3]

Three hundred and ninety-four women had been reported as HIV seropositive by 31 December 1987 in England and Wales. At present this is estimated to represent less than 7% of HIV positive individuals, with the majority of HIV positive reports coming from high risk males. These low estimates of infection in the general population have led the Royal College of Obstetricians and Gynaecologists to recommend that antenatal screening should at present be restricted to women who are at an increased risk for HIV infection.[4]

MODES OF TRANSMISSION

There is good evidence for intrauterine transmission of HIV infection. HIV antigen has been demonstrated in amniotic fluid[5] and fetal tissue from 15 weeks gestation.[6] Virus has been isolated from a fetal sample of 20 weeks gestation with intact membranes[7] and from the thymus of an infant born by Caesarean section who died at 20 days of AIDS.[8]

We do not know whether HIV can be acquired by the infant at the time of delivery, and with current laboratory techniques it is difficult to distinguish intrauterine from intrapartum or postnatal infection. In neonates the only proven routes of transmission are intrauterine and the transfusion of blood or blood products. Although symptoms in the mother appear to influence the risk of transmission of infection, there is no evidence that Caesarean section lowers the transmission rate.[9]

The role of breast milk as a source of infection remains problematic. There is one report in the literature of extracellular virus in breast milk of 3 HIV positive mothers.[10] However, the 4 cases where breast milk was presumed to be the most likely source of infection involved transfusion of infected blood to the mother after birth.[11-13] These cases are not representative of infected mothers, and there may be a higher risk of transmission shortly after acquisition of infection when there is a peak in antigen levels.[14,15] Where safe and effective alternative methods of infant feeding are possible, such as in the United States and the United Kingdom, women who are known to be HIV positive are advised not to breastfeed. However, throughout much of the developing world breastfeeding by the biological mother continues to be the feeding method of choice irrespective of HIV antibody status, as the risk to infants of malnutrition or exposure to other infectious diseases is far greater than the possible transmission of HIV infection via the breast milk.[16]

Exposure to HIV by transfusion in the neonatal period has been shown to result in a high risk of infection, with substantial mortality and morbidity.[17,18] The screening of donated blood and plasma for antibody to HIV, and heat treatment of clotting factor concentrates, along with careful consideration of indications for use of blood products, have reduced this risk to an extremely low level.

THE EUROPEAN STUDY
Background
Much is already known about the natural history of HIV infection in haemophiliacs, but perinatal infection has not been systematically studied. In order to answer questions about the natural history of perinatally acquired HIV infection it is necessary to study the infants of a large number of women known to be seropositive. This could not be accomplished in any one European centre as numbers were too small. The European Collaborative Study was therefore designed to achieve the following objectives:

(i) to determine the prevalence of HIV infection in infants born to HIV positive mothers;

(ii) to examine risk factors influencing transmission of infection to infants, such as mode of delivery, breastfeeding, and whether the mother was symptomatic during pregnancy;

(iii) to look at the natural history of HIV infection in infants;

(iv) to identify precursors of AIDS/ARC onset in infected infants.

In order for a centre to be eligible for the study it had to ensure that HIV seropositive women are being systematically identified in the antenatal period, and that the participating paediatrician was aware of the woman's seropositive status before or at the time of birth. One paediatrician had to be available to coordinate the follow-up of the children to ensure good compliance and good laboratory procedures.

The 7 centres participating in the study are Padua, Edinburgh, Berlin, Madrid, Valencia, Amsterdam and Stockholm. New centres are still being added to the study, and it is hoped that at least 400 children will be followed.

Method of follow-up
Children are examined in the newborn period and at 3-monthly intervals using a standard protocol. Blood samples are taken at each visit for laboratory investigation.

The importance of identifying children from birth was shown clearly in the analysis of children whose data was forwarded to us in the early stages of the study, but who did not fulfil the study criteria. The majority were sick and infected, a clear illustration of how bias could be introduced.

Results (as of 31 March 1988)
By March 31 1988, 204 children had been enrolled in the study (Table 1). The majority of new cases are now coming from Spain and Italy while the numbers from Edinburgh and Berlin have declined. This may reflect differences in knowledge and attitude. In contrast to the situation in the United States, the majority of the mothers in the European Collaborative Study are white Caucasian intravenous drug abusers. Maternal characteristics are described in Table 2.

Table 1
Number of children enrolled in European Collaborative
Study
(as of 31 March 1988)

Centre	No.
Padua	64
Berlin	45
Edinburgh	31
Madrid	30
Valencia	26
Amsterdam	4
Stockholm	4
Total	204

Table 2
Maternal Characteristics

Median Age	24 years
Marital status	66% married/cohabiting
Parity	67% first born
Race	97% white Caucasian

The enrolled group comprised 103 boys and 101 girls. Their mean birthweight was 2800gm and mean gestational age 38 weeks. Drug withdrawal symptoms were present in 25% of babies but perinatal findings were otherwise unremarkable. There was a trend towards lower mean birthweight in the infants with drug withdrawal symptoms but no difference in gestational age. It is likely that the low mean birthweight for gestational age of the overall group was a result of intravenous drug abuse in the mothers rather than HIV infection.

To date, 122 children have been followed for at least 6 months, and 89 for over 1 year. The median age at last visit was 12 months. Ten children had developed AIDS or ARC (all by 9 months) and 5 of them had died, all with opportunistic infections. In addition 3 infants died in the neonatal period from problems related to prematurity. Non-specific HIV signs or symptoms were present in 13 infants; these included problems such as persistent generalised lymphadenopathy, hepatosplenomegaly, diarrhoea and failure to thrive. However, the majority of infants (178 out of 214) were clinically normal when last seen. The children with ARC all had interstitial pneumonitis, persistent oral candida or progressive encephalopathy accompanied by various nonspecific findings. All the children with AIDS fulfilled the CDC Surveillance definition.[19]There were no cases of AIDS dysmorphic syndrome.[20] The importance of not labelling children as infected when they only have non-specific signs was demonstrated by the fact that in some children these non-specific findings resolved, the child lost antibody and was clearly not infected. Children born to intravenous drug abusers are a vulnerable group in whom non-specific signs and symptoms are likely to have a multifactorial aetiology.

Transmission rate of perinatal infection

Nine of the 65 children remain antibody positive after 15 months and are therefore regarded as infected. Two have ARC or AIDS, 3 have other symptoms and 4 were clinically well when last seen. Four other children died of AIDS or ARC who would have been over 15 months had they survived. The estimated transmission rate would therefore be 19% (13/69). This is probably an underestimate as several other children known to be virus and/or antigen positive have lost antibody, and must be regarded as infected.

It is becoming increasingly clear that loss of antibody does not always infer lack of infection. More accurate information is likely to be obtained from new laboratory tests such as the *in vitro* test of antibody production[21,22] and the *in situ* hybridisation technique described by Harnish.[23] It is too early to obtain meaningful estimates of risk factors in relation to infection because numbers are still too small. However, it does not appear that vaginal delivery or breastfeeding increase the risk of infection. It is likely that clinical symptoms of HIV in the mother may be an important factor, but the increase in risk is not as clear as it appeared in the preliminary analysis.[9]

CONCLUSION

These results are only preliminary and a larger number of children born to HIV positive mothers will need to be followed-up for a much longer period before accurate information can be obtained on the natural history of perinatally acquired HIV infection. Until such information has been obtained it will be difficult to evaluate any treatment of asymptomatic children or to conduct drug trials. Because current assessments of transmission rates are less than 40%, until there is a precise way to identify infected asymptomatic infants at an early age, it would not be possible to justify the use of AZT or other toxic drugs in the first year of life.

REFERENCES

1. Friedland GH, Klein RS. Transmission of the human immunodeficiency virus. *N Engl J Med* 1987; **317:** 1125-1135.
2. World Health Organization. AIDS—Situation in the European Region as of 31 December 1987. *Weekly Epidemiological Record* 1988; **63:** 105-107.
3. Minkoff HL. Care of pregnant women infected with human immunodeficiency virus. *JAMA* 1987; **258:** 2714-2717.
4. Royal College of Obstetricians and Gynaecologists. *Report of the RCOG subcommittee on problems associated with AIDS in relation to obstetrics and gynaecology.* London: Royal College of Obstetricians and Gynaecologists, 1987.
5. Mundy D, Schinazi R, Gerber A, Nahmias A, Randall Jr H. Human Immunodeficiency Virus isolated from amniotic fluid. *Lancet* 1987; **2:** 459-460.
6. Chiodo F, Ricchi E, Costigliola P, Michelacci L, Bovicell L, Dallacas P. Vertical transmission of HTLV-III. *Lancet* 1986; **1:** 739.
7. Jovaisas E, Koch MA, Schäfer A, Stauber M, Löenthal D. LAV/HTLV-III in 20-week fetus. *Lancet* 1985; **2:** 1129.
8. Lapointe N, Michaud J, Pekovic D, Chausseau JP, Dupuy J-M,. Transplacental transmission of HTLV-III virus. *N Engl J Med* 1985; **312:** 1325-1326.

9.   Mok JQ, Giaquinto C, De Rossi A, Grosch-Wörner I, Ades AE, Peckham CS. Infants born to seropositive mothers—preliminary findings from a multi-centre European study. *Lancet* 1987; **1:** 1164-1168.

10. Thiry L, Sprecher-Goldberger S, Jonckheer T, Levy J, Van de Perre P, Henrivaux P. Isolation of AIDS virus from cell-free breast milk of three healthy virus carriers. *Lancet* 1985; **2:** 891-892.

11. Ziegler JB, Cooper DA, Johnson RO, Gold J. Postnatal transmission of AIDS-associated retrovirus from mother to infant. *Lancet* 1985; **1:** 896-899.

12. Lepage P, Van de Perre P, Carael M, Nsengumuremyi F, Njurunziza J, Butzler J, Sprecher S. Postnatal transmission of HIV from mother to child. *Lancet* 1987; **2:** 400.

13. Weinbreck P, Loustaud V, Denis F, Vidal B, Mounier M, De Lumley L. Breast-feeding in the transmission of HIV infection. *Lancet* 1988; **1:** 482.

14. Alain J, Paul D, Laurain Y, Senn D. Serological markers in early stages of human immunodeficiency virus infection in haemophiliacs. *Lancet* 1986; **2:** 1233-1236.

15. Goudsmit J, Lange JMA, Paul DA, Dawson GJ. Antigenemia and antibody titres to core and envelope antigens in AIDS, AIDS-related complex, and subclinical Human Immunodeficiency Virus infection. *J Infect Dis* 1987; **155:** 558-560.

16. World Health Organization. Breast-Feeding/Breast milk and Human Immuno-deficiency Virus (HIV). *Weekly Epidemiological Record* 1987; **33:** 245-246.

17. Pedersen C, Nielsen CM, Vestergaard BF, Gerstoft J, Krosgaard K, Nielsen JO. Temporal relation of antigenaemia and loss of antibodies to core antigens to development of clinical disease in HIV infection. *Br Med J* 1987; **295:** 567-569.

18. Saulsbury FT, Raldolph F, Wykoff MPH, Boyle RJ. Transfusion-Acquired Human Immunodeficiency Virus Infection in twelve neonates: Epidemiological, Clinical and Immunologic Features. *Paediatr Infect Dis J* 1987; **6:** 544-548.

19. Centers for Disease Control. Revision of the CDC surveillance case definition for acquired immunodeficiency syndrome. *MMWR* 1987; **36:** 3s-15s.

20. Quazi QH, Sheik TM, Fikrig S, Menikoff H. Lack of evidence for craniofacial dysmorphism in perinatal human immunodeficiency infection. *J Pediatr* 1988; **112:** 7-11.

21. Amadori A, De Rossi A, Faulkner-Valle G, Chieco-Bianchi L. Spontaneous in vitro production of virus-specific antibody by lymphocytes from HIV-infected subjects. *Clin Immunol Immunopatho* 1988; **46:** 342-351.

22. Amadori A, De Rossi A, Giaquinto C, Faulkner-Valle G, Zachello F, Chieco-Bianchi L. *In vitro* production of HIV-specific antibody in children at risk of AIDS. *Lancet* 1988; **1:** 852-854.

23   .Harnish DG, Hammerberg O, Walker IR, Rosenthall KL. Early detection of HIV infection in a newborn. *N Engl J Med* 1987; **316:** 272-273.

Paediatric AIDS in Uganda from materno-fetal infection

Dr H. Lambert and Dr H. Friesen

INTRODUCTION

Acquired immunodeficiency syndrome (AIDS) is perhaps the major new health problem faced by the world today. Nowhere is this more true than in Uganda. The country has faced repeated political and economic crises in recent years and the impact of AIDS on the country, through the loss of young working men and women, and on the already over-stretched health service, will be enormous. The first reported cases occurred in Uganda in 1982,[1,2] and the number of cases reported to the World Health Organisation (WHO) to January 1988 is 2,369. The cases show a dramatic bimodal distribution with age, AIDS being largely a disease of the over 15 year olds (the sexually active population), and the under 5 year olds, with very few cases seen in the 5 to 15 age group.

DIAGNOSIS

The diagnosis of paediatric AIDS in a developing country like Uganda, is difficult. The definitions of HIV infection and AIDS most widely used in Europe and North America, require laboratory data.[3] In 1985, at the WHO workshop in Bangui, Central African Republic, clinical case definition criteria were proposed for the diagnosis of paediatric and adult AIDS for use in countries with limited laboratory facilities. These were revised and published later that year[4] (Table 1).

Table 1   Provisional WHO clinical case definition for AIDS

Paediatric AIDS is suspected in a child presenting with at least two of the following major signs associated with at least two of the following minor signs in the absence of known causes of immuno-suppression such as cancer or severe malnutrition or other recognised aetiologies:

1. *Major signs*	i.	weight loss or abnormally slow growth;
	ii.	chronic diarrhoea of greater than one month's duration;
	iii.	prolonged fever of greater than one month's duration.
2. *Minor signs*	i.	generalised lymphadenopathy;
	ii.	oro-pharyngeal candidiasis;
	iii.	repeated common infections (otitis, pharyngitis);
	iv.	persistent cough;
	v.	generalised dermatitis;
	vi.	confirmed maternal HIV infection.

World Health Organisation. Acquired immunodeficiency syndrome (AIDS). WHO/CDC case definition for AIDS. *Weekly Epidemiological Record* 1986; **61**: 69-76.

Accurate diagnosis is of great importance, not only for the individual patient and family, but also for surveillance data.

Evaluation of the WHO criteria for adults in Zaire[5] and Tanzania[6] supported their use with some amendments. Evaluation of the WHO criteria for children, also in Zaire, concluded that they were of limited use due to their poor positive predictive value.[7] Our limited data support that view.

Over a 6-month period in 1986 we studied a group of 177 children who presented to 2 of the 4 main hospitals in Kampala, with clinical evidence of immunosuppression, including 143 who fulfilled the WHO clinical case definition criteria. Children who had another diagnosis like measles or tuberculosis which could imitate AIDS, but also of course co-exist with it, were not studied. One-third of the children had no HIV antibody detected by competitive enzyme-linked immunosorbent assay (ELISA), but did have clinical features which fulfilled the WHO case definition criteria. Thus, these children would have had a clinical diagnosis of paediatric AIDS if antibody testing facilities had not been available. The clinical features shown by this group of children were remarkably similar to the features shown by the children who both fulfilled the WHO clinical case definition criteria and had HIV antibody detected. This raises the whole question of the validity of the WHO criteria which could not, in our study, be used to differentiate between the two groups. This suggests that either the HIV antibody test used is inaccurate or the WHO criteria are not good discriminators of true cases of AIDS. To answer the former, testing for HIV antibody by ELISA carries a greater than 95% sensitivity and specificity.[8] At the time of study we were unable to retest plasma using a different technique such as Western blot assay, but data from Uganda suggest a 98% correlation between the two methods (J.W. Carswell, personal communication). This leaves us to conclude the latter.

AGE RANGE

Excluding 3 chidren aged 6, 7, and 8 years who were infected by previous blood transfusion, all the HIV antibody-positive children were aged below 5 years and 90% were aged below 2 years. Cases at both hospitals were seen again in the over-15-year-olds in a similar distribution to the country as a whole. This age distribution constitutes some evidence against suggestions that HIV infection is spread by insect vectors or social contact.[2,9,10]

Children who had HIV antibody detected but did not fulfil the WHO criteria for diagnosis of paediatric AIDS were significantly younger than the children who both fulfilled the WHO criteria and were seropositive ($p < 0.05$). This may mean that the WHO criteria are particularly unsuited to very young children, or merely that they were at an earlier stage in their disease. As facilities for virus culture or antigen testing were not available, and we do not have follow-up data, it is not possible to say how many of the children aged under 18 months were not infected but merely had prenatal transfer of maternal antibody. However, these were not asymptomatic children who were tested, but children with clinical evidence of immunosuppression.

CLINICAL FEATURES

Table 2 shows the clinical features of the children with a definite diagnosis of AIDS (seropositive and fulfilling the WHO criteria). Ninety-six percent of these children had evidence of failure to thrive as evidenced by previous clinic weight charts ("road to health charts") or by serial inpatient weights, and 30% had weight loss. It was striking that the children who subsequently were found to have HIV antibodies showed poor response to supplementary feeding (aiming for 200 kcal/kg/day) in comparison to other malnourished children fed similarly. This group of children also responded poorly to other standard treatments like antibiotic therapy for chest infections. This may be a reflection of their immunocompromised state or an indication of unusual or resistant infecting organisms. This is an area which demands further study as it may be of use in the development of improved clinical criteria.

Table 2

**Clinical features
of children seropositive and fulfilling the WHO
criteria.**

clinical feature	% with feature
failure to thrive	96%
diarrhoea > 1 month	85%
fever > 1 month	80%
cough > 1 month	68%
candidiasis	62%
rash	59%
repeated infections	45%
generalised lymphadenopathy	20%

RISK FACTORS

In Europe and North America, the majority of infected infants are born to families where one (or both) of the parents is in a high risk group such as previous recipients of blood or blood products therapy, intravenous drug users, prostitutes, homosexuals or bisexuals.[11,12,13,14] None of these parents in our study group was known to be in those risk categories.

Ninety-eight percent of the mothers of HIV positive children were seropositive, compared to 23% of mothers of seronegative children. This incidence of seropositive mothers of HIV positive children is higher than the 61% reported in Zaire,[15] and the 76% in Rwanda.[16] Eighty-three percent of the mothers were themselves well and asymptomatic.

Only 3 of the seropositive children had a previous history of blood or blood products transfusion; the remainder were presumed infected *in utero* or perinatally.

BREASTFEEDING

All the children who were being breastfed continued to be so. The evidence for the transmission of HIV infection via breast milk is at present inconclusive.[17] Current recommendations in the UK are that breastfeeding should be avoided where there is a safe and acceptable alternative.[17] Statements that breastfeeding is contraindicated, with no such qualification,[18] indicate a lack of awareness of the global impact of such advice. In most developing countries the mortality and morbidity risks associated with not breastfeeding are far higher than the small and presumptive risk of HIV transmission.

MORTALITY

Follow-up was not possible on all the children, but we know that 23% of the HIV antibody positive children died within 3 months of diagnosis. This perhaps reflects the late presentation of many of our patients, which was not confined to only those with this disease.

SUMMARY

The majority of cases of paediatric AIDS in Uganda are infected by vertical transmission of virus from mother to child, the mothers having been infected by heterosexual contact.

Paediatric AIDS in Uganda is a large problem which is showing evidence of increasing. It is an additional burden to a country where problems like respiratory tract infections, gastroenteritis and measles contribute to an already high childhood mortality and morbidity. The increase of HIV antibody in asymptomatic children is not known.

The current WHO case definition criteria are insufficient alone for the diagnosis of paediatric AIDS. This has important implications for the patients and their families, and for surveillance data. More work is urgently needed on this problem.

REFERENCES
1. Serwadda D, Mugerwa RD, Sewankambo NK, Lwegaba A, Carswell JW, Kirya GB, Bayley AC, Downing RG, Tedder RS, Weiss RA, Clayden SA, Dalgleish AG. Slim disease: a new disease in Uganda and its association with HTLV-III infection. *Lancet* 1985; **2:** 849-852.
2. Biggar RJ. The AIDS problem in Africa. *Lancet* 1986; **1:** 79-83.
3. *Morbidity and Mortality Weekly Report.* 1987; **36:** 225-230.
4. World Health Organisation. Acquired immunodeficiency syndrome (AIDS). WHO/ CDC case definition for AIDS. *Weekly Epidemiological Record* 1986; **61:** 69-76.
5. Colebunders R, Mann JM, Francis H, Bila K, Izaley L, Kakonde N, Kabaselle K, Ifoto L, Nzilambi N, Quinn TC, Van der Groen G, Curran JW, Vercauteren G, Piot P. Evaluation of a clinical case-definition of acquired immunodeficiency syndrome in Africa. *Lancet* 1987; **1:** 492-494.
6. Pallangyo KJ, Mbaga IM, Mugusi F, Mbena E, Mhalu FS, Bredberg U, Biberfeld G. Clinical case definition of AIDS in African adults. *Lancet* 1987; **2:** 972.
7. Colebunders RI, Greenberg A, Nguyen-Dinh P, Francis H, Kabote N, Izaley L, Davichi F, Quinn T, Piot P. Evaluation of a clinical case definition of AIDS in African children. *AIDS* 1987; **1:** 151-153.
8. Weiss SH, Goedert JJ, Sarngadharan MG, Bodner AJ, The AIDS Seroepidemiology Collaborative Working Group, Gallo RC, Blattner WA. Screening test for HTLV-III (AIDS agent) antibodies. *JAMA* 1985; **253:** 221-225.

9. Sewakambo NK, Carswell JW, Mugerwa RD, Lloyd G, Kataaha P, Downing RG, Lucas S. HIV infection through normal heterosexual contact in Uganda. *AIDS* 1987; **1:** 113- 116.
10. Jones P, Watson JG. AIDS. In: *Recent Advances in Paediatrics*, No.8. Ed. SR Meadow. Edinburgh: Churchill Livingstone, 1986; pp.1-20.
11. Kamani N, Krilov L. AIDS and the spectrum of human immunodeficiency virus infection in children. *Paediatric Rev Commun* 1987; **1:** 101-121.
12. Mok JQ, Giaquinto C, De Rossi A, Grosch-Wörner I, Ades AE, Peckham CS. Infants born to mothers seropositive for human immunodeficiency virus. Preliminary findings from a multicentre European study. *Lancet* 1987; **1:** 1164-1168.
13. Novick BE, Rubinstein A. Editorial Review. AIDS—The paediatric perspective. *AIDS* 1987; **1:** 3-7.
14. Rubinstein A, Bernstein L. The epidemiology of pediatric acquired immunodeficiency syndrome. *Clin Immunol Immunopathol* 1986; **40:** 115-121.
15. Mann JM, Francis H, Davachi F, Baudoux P, Quinn TC, Nzilambi N, Bosenge N, Colebunders RL, Piot P, Kabote N, Kaza Azila P, Malonga M, Curran JW. Risk factors for human immunodeficiency virus seropositivity among children 1-24 months old in Kinshasa, Zaire. *Lancet* 1986. **2:** 654-656.
16. Lepage P, Van de Perre P, Carael M, Butzler JP. Are medical injections a risk factor for HIV infection in children? (Letter) *Lancet* 1986; **2:** 1103-1104.
17. Royal College of Obstetricians and Gynaecologists. *Report of the RCOG sub-committee on problems associated with AIDS in relation to obstetrics and gynaecology.* London: Royal College of Obstetricians and Gynaecologists, 1987.

Discussion

Chairman: Professor N.F. Morris

CHIN: I should like to comment on the situation relating to the clinical definition which is currently being used in Africa. I would like to emphasise that those data are consistent findings in serological surveys which are ongoing in Uganda, but the heavy involvement is basically restricted at the present time to the urban areas. In the rural areas the preliminary data indicate that the levels of infection are much lower. In fact, only about 10% of the Ugandan population is urban at the present time—so that is one optimistic note. The figure of 25% infection is what is being claimed at the present time. With regard to the clinical definition, we will modify this with regard to adults, probably by the end of the year, and it is likely to incorporate HIV testing. If you take the clinical definition to certain parts of Africa where HIV is not present, like the Northern Sudan, it is very non-specific, and erroneously will diagnose tuberculosis and malnutrition. Where HIV is present the clinical definition has been very valuable. But the value is critical, and the clinical definition most likely will be modified to add HIV testing since it is becoming more and more available in the urban areas.

I would like to put a question to Professor Peckham. You mentioned that you believe that the preponderance of cases of infection in children is acquired *in utero*. I wonder if there are any hard data on this. If you look at Hepatitis B you know that the majority of the infections are coital rather than uterine. I am just wondering if there are any hard data on HIV to say that the preponderance of infection is uterine rather than coital.

PECKHAM: I should have said that we know that you can get intrauterine infection. We still have not proven that you cannot acquire infection by the other routes. It is not as yet possible to distinguish infection acquired early, intrapartum or through breast milk, from the intrauterine infection. Certainly in the European study women are not breastfeeding, so that obviously is not important. I think that we need to compare studies from different parts of the world.

CHIN: I am talking about intrauterine versus "at birth".

PECKHAM: But we really do not have that information, do we?

CHIN: You had made the statement that the preponderance of infections was intrauterine.

JEFFRIES: Dr Lambert in her excellent presentation made a very important point at the end, that all her babies were breastfed, and that to deprive a baby of a mother's breast milk is equivalent to signing its death certificate. We are being very careful, those of us in this country who have been discussing the implications of breastfeeding, to consider the knock-on implications in Third World countries. I have found that in certain of the Third World countries there is now a trend away from breastfeeding. Your babies may have been breastfed, but were you conscious of a move in the other direction in Uganda away from breastfeeding? LAMBERT: Certainly not in Uganda at the moment. Most of the towns didn't have any milk powder at all, let alone baby milk powder.

MORRIS: I wonder what this means in terms of bottle versus breastfeeding. If it is eventually proven, that breast milk is a factor, would this put a question mark against some of the other things that are said not to happen in the transfer of AIDS, or is it only with breast milk? Normally you would not say that any food-stuff was capable, or any bird or any insect was capable of transferring AIDS. It seems to me that in the case of breast milk you are saying this; or are you assuming that the infection is not in the milk, but is somewhere around the nipple? I am assuming that it is the milk you are talking about. If it is the milk, then you are saying that there is only one foodstuff, breast milk, which can transfer HIV infection to babies.

JEFFRIES: I think that there is little doubt that the virus is present in the milk in the lymphocytes. Dr Chin drew a parallel with Hepatitis B virus which is known to be found in milk. Hepatitis B virus has been shown to be infectious by the oral route. It is ten times higher than the minimal intradermal dose, but Hepatitis B has never been shown to be transmitted by breastfeeding. There may be other factors in terms of infection by breastfeeding—cracked nipples and so on. These are very special instances of mothers who had become infected in the postpartum period.

MOK: I would like to ask Dr Schoenbaum if, in view of her gloomy findings, she has modified her advice about pregnancy and termination for HIV positive women?

SCHOENBAUM: In almost all the preliminary studies there are women who are infected and who have become pregnant, and have multiple reasons why they consider termination aside from HIV. Their economic circumstances are often very poor and their ability to cope with the pregnancy is in question. From their point of view their concern that they may have an HIV-infected baby far outweighs their concern about their own health. I do not know whether this is typical of pregnant women, but we are seeing an increasing rate of termination in women because of the fear of vertical transmission to babies. I think that is also because they have seen so many children of their peers die of AIDS, and they have seen their colleagues die of AIDS (usually drug abusers). They do not really understand; it is almost too theoretical that they too may be at risk, in addition to what they already know to be the risk from their drug abuse. Their pregnancy may be an additional problem. We tell them that we think that there may be a theoretical risk, but we really do not know or understand at this time if it is significant or not. I must say that we see no difference at this time between the HIV positive women and the HIV negative women who are likely to opt for abortion.

HARVEY: I would like to ask Dr Lambert whether she saw any of the dysmorphic features that have been described.

LAMBERT: I was just about to ask that same question. I didn't see any of these features. However, as in many other things in medicine, if you are not looking for it you do not see it. None of the nurses I was working with commented on children looking strange.

PECKHAM: I have not seen any cases of clearcut dysmorphic syndrome in the European study. I don't know if in the States there is a difference in the different racial groups.

SCOTT: We have done a retrospective study of infants born to Haitian women, similar to your prospective study which is being done throughout Europe. In that study we are looking at dysmorphic features in those infants, taking pictures and doing measurements and recordings, but we have not really looked at it in detail. There is nothing striking in terms of differences in these infants when seen with their siblings and parents and other children. In the 200 children that we have seen there are a number of infants who do have some of the characteristics. Whether they are due to HIV or not I am not certain. We have also been doing family studies where we are looking for dysmorphic features, and looking at infected siblings and other siblings. But we do not have any definite data on that at this point.

LAMBERT: Were these dysmorphic features in children of drug abusers? We are used to seeing dysmorphia in children of alcoholics, so I have been thinking that the dysmorphia is a primary problem of the mother.

PECKHAM: These are causes which have been described as appearing in New York AIDS children. There is a recent paper where they did do a controlled study among smaller numbers of children and they did not find dysmorphia.[1]

SCHOENBAUM: I would like to add that this study came from a centre which is located on the other side of the Bronx, and we have not seen these features in our babies.

HOWIE: I would like to ask what advice should be given to women regarding termination of pregnancy simply on the grounds that they are HIV positive and their progression to clinical disease might deteriorate. There is a large number of women who are not as socially deprived as Dr Schoenbaum's population. Obstetricians still have to give an opinion of whether HIV positive status is in itself an indication for termination because of the risk of progression to disease.

SCHOENBAUM: It is a very difficult problem. We do have a number of partners of IV drug abusers in our centres that I have reported on who are not IV drug abusers any longer. We try to help them deal with the uncertainty; the fact is that we do not know if there is an adverse effect. We tell them that it is theoretically possible, but we have not observed progression during pregnancy in healthy women. We are more concerned with women who have the clinical disease. Again, it is less of an issue because they are already sick and tend to terminate on that basis. We do not know the answer. Many of these women will elect to abort because they are afraid of transmitting the infection to their children. To suggest that they abort because of progression, I think is premature, assuming that a woman is perfectly healthy at the time.

HOWIE: The evidence that pregnancy does cause acceleration of the disease is looking less and less convincing. I thought that was the message from your presentation.

SCHOENBAUM: Yes, that was why I said that we do not recommend that they terminate if they are clinically well just on the basis of their HIV positive status alone. It rarely is on that basis alone.

MOK: I am not an obstetrician, but I have been working closely with Linda McCallum whose data you have actually quoted. In women who are HIV positive in Edinburgh what we are offering is individually tailored advice where the woman is asked to undergo a full clinical evaluation to see how far along in the disease she is. In many cases where you have no evidence, no clinical evidence or any bad evidence of the women actually being ill with HIV disease, perhaps that is the best time for her to have the pregnancy. A lot of these women are desperate to have children. While they are clinically and immunologically well, that may be the best time. What do you think of that advice?

SCHOENBAUM: I have tremendous ambivalence about advising a woman that now is the time to have a pregnancy when so little is known about the risks in terms of transmission to the baby, or what will happen in the future in terms of possible treatment that may be more conducive to hazarding the advice to continue with a pregnancy. If a woman is able to postpone pregnancy, abort and then get pregnant in a few years, if age is not a major factor, and she is willing to consider that, we often encourage it.

Your suggestion is a good one. I think that each individual patient needs a good deal of counselling. It is particularly difficult in a patient at 15 or 16 weeks of pregnancy and HIV positive. You do not have time to counsel as they have to terminate before 24 weeks. But we do not tend to recommend termination purely on the basis of a possible risk to the mother.

SCRIMGEOUR: Professor Peckham, as an epidemiologist, if you are faced with a patient who is an intravenous drug abuser and who is pregnant, but has no clinical signs of the disease, what statistic would you give her as to the risk of transmission of AIDS to the baby? This is the sort of question that we clinicians are going to be faced with.

PECKHAM: This is the information that we are trying to get as quickly as possible. We cannot answer that yet. We have to wait so long before we know whether the baby is or is not infected. From the figures that I showed you we know that there is about a 25% risk of the baby being infected when born to a mother who is HIV positive. But we cannot calculate that risk in relation to whether or not she has symptoms.

SCOTT: The range is somewhere between 20-50%. In one study that we did on women who already had an infected infant it was between 50-65% for another infected infant. But that may be a very different figure for a woman who is very much further along in her illness. In general for the HIV-infected woman who has not previously had an infected infant we think somewhere between 20 and 50%.

PECKHAM: Can I raise one point? I am told that we have very stiff entry criteria, and I think that it is interesting that we had to exclude about 15 babies from Padua who were identified as HIV positive, as we did not know about the maternal status at the time of birth. We looked at those retrospectively and 90% of those babies were infected. Most of them are very sick. So even the criteria by which you select your babies will influence the risk. So it is important to start at birth; I think that is the message.

JEFFRIES: The questioner was asking about the risks of a mother having a baby with AIDS, were you not? Professor Peckham, with respect, I think what you gave the questioner was the rate of infection in those cases of babies in Europe whom we know are infected with the virus. I think that at the present time if you were to ask of the percentage who had AIDS, you have got to say that it is about 5%. So I think we have got to be careful whether we are talking about the infection or fullblown AIDS.

CHIN: That is true in terms of the mortality of infants developing AIDS in under one year. The data that are available would indicate that the progression of infants and children who are infected would probably be no less than adults. So that the information you requested might be more. So we are using, at least at the present time, a child survival rate of those infected—about 50% at 5 years.

REFERENCES
1. Quazi Q, Sheik TM, Fikrig S, Menikoff H. Lack of evidence for craniofacial dysmorphism in perinatal immunodeficiency infection. *J Pediatr* 1988; **112:** 7-11.

HIV-1 infection in infants: practical laboratory diagnosis

Dr G.B. Scott, Dr C. Hutto and Professor W.P. Parks

INTRODUCTION

As in adults, the diagnosis of human immunodeficiency virus (HIV-1) infections in most paediatric patients is dependent on the demonstration of antibodies to HIV-1-related antigens in the individual's serum. Serological assays for HIV-1 were developed within months of the identification of the virus.[1,2] The association of HIV-1 and acquired immunodeficiency syndrome (AIDS) was clearly demonstrated using these serological assays[3,4] and similar assays have been used for diagnosis of infected persons. Despite reports in the literature of the recovery of virus from seronegative individuals with AIDS,[5-7] and more recent reports of virus in macrophages of seronegatives (personal communication), the vast majority of adults and children with AIDS or HIV-related symptoms are seropositive using conventional assays.[8,9]

The use of serological assays for the identification of HIV-1 infections in infants from birth to 15 months is more problematic. Since almost 80% of paediatric HIV infections result from perinatal transmission of virus from an infected mother to her infant, the presence of transplacentally-transferred maternal IgG confuses the diagnosis of infection in this age group. The resultant delay in diagnosis of infected infants is an obstacle to understanding factors related to transmission of virus and development of disease in this age group. However, the rationale for early diagnosis of HIV-1 infection in infants relates principally to the potential for therapeutic intervention. Currently, such intervention is more relevant to the secondary complications which occur as a consequence of the HIV-1 infection, but will eventually be important for therapy of the HIV-1 infection. HIV-1-infected infants frequently develop serious and potentially fatal bacterial or other opportunistic infections within the first months of life. If infected infants can be identified early, diagnosis and therapy can be more rapidly directed towards these infants when signs of clinical disease are noted, or even earlier.

IDENTIFICATION OF HIV-1 INFECTIONS IN SERONEGATIVE INFANTS—AN ALGORITHM

Data from preliminary studies have indicated that the risk of HIV-1 transmission from an infected mother to her infant ranges from 20% to 60%.[10-12] The presence of maternal IgG in newborns of HIV-1 seropositive mothers is a limiting factor in

Figure I

Algorithm for laboratory diagnosis of HIV-1 infected infant

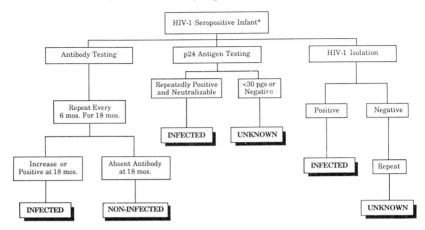

*ELISA confirmed by Western blot or other assay.

the interpretation of serological assays for HIV-1 infection and makes distinguishing infected from non-infected infants extremely difficult. For example, neither of the assays licensed in the US, the enzyme-linked immunoabsorbent assay (ELISA) or the Western blot, are quantitative. Using commonly available laboratory assays, an algorithm for distinguishing infected and uninfected infants is presented in Figure I. The most commonly used approach is the sequential measurement of HIV-1 antibody in the infant. As with other perinatal infections such as toxoplasmosis and cytomegalovirus, infection and passive antibody transfer can be distinguished by the persistence of antibody. Assays which lend themselves to objective quantitation of antibody titre, such as radioimmunoassay (RIA), provide the most efficient and accurate method for this approach. The concomitant and serial measurement and comparison of maternal and infant antibody patterns by Western blot, for example, can substantiate the persistence or loss of antibody by the infant. In the absence of stoichiometric assays, such as RIA, serial Western blots may be useful and are widely available.

Two rather technical points need to be addressed. The first is related to the relatively high total level of humoral anti-HIV-1 IgG in infected adults. Hence, very high titres of antibody may persist even in settings of passive transfer such as the newborn. Uninfected seropositive infants as measured by the highly sensitive ELISA and Western blots have been noted as late as 13 months after birth. Secondly, the assay commonly employed for diagnosis of HIV-1 infection, the whole virus ELISA, has two important characteristics, namely, great sensitivity and an inability to be used quantitatively.

The enzyme-linked antibody assays (ELISA) which measure IgG to disrupted whole HIV-1 are extremely sensitive. Because the detection systems are enzymatic, ELISA is a catalytic rather than a stoichiometric assay. Like most catalytic assays, ELISA is better suited as a qualitative measure than a quantitative one. Hence, dilutions of serum as a measure of titre of antibody levels is fraught with a number of unproven assumptions. These assumptions in whole virus assays simply do not hold, rendering comparison of sera invalid when measured by ELISA dilution. On the other hand, radioimmunoassays (RIA) for specific virion polypeptides or protein immunoblots (Western) for specific bands satisfy stoichiometric assumptions and can be employed for quantitation. With further study and careful controls ELISAs for specific viral polypeptides such as p41E may also be suitable for quantitation. Hence the dual problems of ELISA quantitation are the variable enzymatic properties of a reaction and the multivalent characteristics of the whole virus antigen mixture.

The measurement of HIV-1-specific immunoglobulin isotypes produced *de novo* by the infant and not transferred across the placenta (IgA, IgM) may also provide an earlier means of identifying infected infants. However, the immature and inconsistent neonatal immunological response to infection and the lack of a widely available assay for these immunoglobulins make this a less practical alternative for most physicians. Recent reports by Chumule *et al*[13] have also suggested establishing B-lymphocyte cultures from newborns, transforming them with Epstein-Barr virus and then attempting to measure anti-HIV-1 immunoglobulin production.

Measurement of p24 or core antigen and HIV-1 isolation when available should also be used for diagnosis of infection in infants born to infected mothers. An understanding of the limitations of the antigen assay for diagnosis is important. Experience to date indicates that antigen detection is a less sensitive measure of infection than serology. Antigen capture assays utilising the HIV-1 core protein (p24) are more widely available than virus isolation and may for some infants allow an early diagnosis. These assays, however, are positive in only approximately 20% of virus-positive asymptomatic infants. Conversely, all antigen positive infants in our experience have been positive for virus isolation. Although the p24 antigen sensitivity (approximately 30 pg of purified HIV-1 p24 per ml of serum) is extremely high, antigen is frequently not detected in the serum or plasma of many virus positive individuals.[14,15] The likelihood of detecting antigen appears to be inversely related to levels of antibody to HIV p24 protein. This probably contributes to the relatively low incidence of p24 antigen positive infants in our studies.

In our laboratory HIV-1 can be isolated from more than 80% of seropositive older children and adults, whereas, isolation in very young (less than 6 weeks) seropositive infants who are later proven to be infected has been successful in only 5/25 (20%) of patients on the initial isolation attempt. It is possible to recover virus from the majority of these infants when cultures are repeated after a few months. This suggests that virus "load" in many young infants is extremely low, further complicating interpretation of virus isolation results. Ou *et al*[16] recently reported the use of a DNA amplification technique, polymerase chain reaction, for detection of HIV in peripheral blood mononuclear cells. The technique detected proviral DNA in mononuclear cells of both seropositive culture positive and culture negative individuals and it was possible to perform the assay in less than a week. Although technically difficult to perform and available only in research laboratories at present, such assays may allow more rapid diagnosis of infection in infants.

SEROLOGICAL ASSAYS

A number of HIV-1 serological assays are currently used for diagnosis and research (Table 1). Because the accuracy of these assays for predicting infection varies, an understanding of assay parameters is relevant. The ELISA utilising disrupted whole virus as antigen is the most commonly used antibody test. This is an extremely sensitive assay and was developed for screening blood donor sera to detect infection. Because of its high sensitivity and relatively lower specificity, false positives occur frequently and its predictive value is dependent on the population screened, being most accurate when utilised in populations at high risk. If an ELISA is used for diagnostic purposes, all positive results should be confirmed with an assay with higher specificity. The Western blot is most commonly used for this purpose in the United States. The technical complexities in performing a Western blot and resultant time and economic costs, however, preclude its usefulness in screening. A number of assays utilising recombinant HIV-1 envelope or purified virion core polypeptides as antigens in ELISAs or RIA configurations are also available in many laboratories and will be more widely available in the future. These assays, though generally somewhat less sensitive than whole virus ELISAs, are highly specific and are associated with few Type I errors (false positives). Since both the quantity and presence of antibody to p24 antigen is variable among individuals, an assay for this antibody should be used in conjunction with a seroassay for *env* antibody or p41E antigen when used diagnostically to increase the predictive value. The predictive value of these assays is similar to seroassays for other organisms in that their accuracy from laboratory to laboratory is variable, and dependent on the experience of those laboratories performing the assays.

Table 1

Commonly used methods of HIV-1 antibody measurement

Method	Sensitivity*	Specificity*	Comments
Whole virus ELISA	1.0	0.5	High α error low β error
Western blot	0.9	0.9	Low α error, technically complex, stoichiometric
Specific Polypeptides			
ENV ELISA	0.5	0.75	
p24 RIA	0.7	0.9	Low α error, stoichiometric
p41E ELISA	1.0	0.9	Low α and β error

*Values are approximately relative to ideal
ELISA: enzyme-linked immunoabsorbent assay
RIA: radio-immunoassay

CORRELATION OF CLINICAL FINDINGS OF INFECTION WITH VIRAL ASSAYS

The diagnosis of paediatric HIV-1 infections, whether in infants or older children, should be made using clinical, viral and immunological data. Although some investigators have suggested that certain dysmorphic features occur in HIV-1 infected infants,[17,18] these observations have not been verified.[19] It is not known what proportion of infected infants will develop disease or laboratory abnormalities. However, markers of immunological dysfunction frequently associated with HIV-1 infection in children, elevated immunoglobulins and depleted T-lymphocyte subset numbers should be evaluated in all infants at risk of infection. Although uncommon, hypogammaglobulinaemia may be associated with HIV-1 infection in some infants. The absence or loss of HIV-1 specific antibody should be viewed very differently in these infants, since this loss may reflect inability to produce antibody rather than absence of infection. Besides immunological parameters, signs of infection may be detected with frequent and careful physical examination. Poor weight gain, developmental delay, lymphadenopathy, persistent oral thrush or hepatosplenomegaly may occur early in some infected infants and the presence of an epidemiological risk factor such as blood transfusion, absent parents, etc. should heighten one's suspicion of HIV-1 infection.

SUMMARY

The rationale for virological laboratory diagnosis of HIV-1 infected infants is based on the potential for therapeutic intervention. Using serological assays for antibodies, p24 core polypeptide antigen and virus isolation, an algorithm for virological diagnosis is presented. The most difficult diagnostic setting is in the infant born to an HIV-1 antibody positive mother since only a proportion are infected. Reliance on virological, immunological, clinical and epidemiological findings for diagnosis of paediatric AIDS is strongly recommended.

ACKNOWLEDGEMENTS
Supported by Grants AI23524 and AI20736 from the PHS, NIH, National Institute of Allergy and Infectious Diseases.

REFERENCES
1. Sarngadharan MG, Popovic M, Bruch L, Schüpbach J, Gallo RC. Antibodies reactive with human T-lymphotropic retroviruses (HTLV-III) in the serum of patients with AIDS. *Science* 1984; **224:** 506-508.
2. Weiss SH, Goedert JJ, Sarngadharan MG, Bodner AJ, Gallo RC, Blattner WA. Screening test for HTLV-III (AIDS agent) antibodies. Specificity, sensitivity and applications. *JAMA* 1985; **253:** 23-27.
3. Schüpbach J, Haller O, Vogt M, Lüthy R, Joller H, Oelz O, Popovic N, Sarngadharan MG, Gallo RC. Antibodies to HTLV-III in Swiss patients with AIDS and pre-AIDS and in groups at risk for AIDS. *N Engl J Med* 1985; **312:** 265-270.
4. Gallo RC, Salahuddin SZ, Popovic M, Shearer GM, Kaplan M, Haynes BF, Palker TJ, Redfield R, Oleske J, Safai B *et al.* Frequent detection and isolation of cytopathic retroviruses (HTLV-III) from patients with AIDS and at risk for AIDS. *Science* 1984; **224:** 500-503.
5. Pahwa S, Kaplan M, Filkrig S, Pahwa R, Sarngadharan MG, Popovic M, Gallo RC. Spectrum of human T-cell lymphotropic virus type III infection in children. Recognition of symptomatic, asymptomatic and seronegative patients. *JAMA* 1986; **255:** 2299-2305.

6.   Salahuddin SZ, Groopman JE, Markham PD, Sarngadharan MG, Redfield RR, McLane MF, Essex M, Sliski A, Gallo RC. HTLV-III in symptom-free seronegative persons. *Lancet* 1984; **2**: 1418-1420.
7.   Borkowsky W, Krasinski K, Paul D, Moore T, Bebenroth D, Chandwani S. Virus infection in infants negative for anti-HIV by enzyme-linked immunoassay. *Lancet* 1987; **1**: 1168-1170.
8.   Sarngadharan MG, Popovic M, Bruch L, Schüpbach J, Gallo RC. Antibodies reactive with human T-lymphotropic retroviruses (HTLV-III) in the serum of patients with AIDS. *Science* 1984; **224**: 506-508.
9.   Blanche S, Le Deist F, Fischer A, Veber F, Debre M, Chamaret S, Montagnier L, Griscelli C. Longitudinal study of 18 children with perinatal LAV/HTLV III infection: attempt at prognostic evaluation. *J Pediatr* 1986; **109**: 965-970.
10. Scott GB, Mastrucci MT. Mothers of infants with HIV infection: Outcome of subsequent pregnancies. (Abstract) *Third International Conference on AIDS*. Washington, D.C. June 1-5, 1987.
11. Thomas PA, Lubin K, Milberg J, Reiss R, Getchell J, Enlow R. Cohort comparison study of children whose mothers have acquired immunodeficiency syndrome and children of well inner city mothers. *Pediatr Infect Dis* 1987; **6**: 247-251.
12. Mok JQ, Giaquinto C, De Rossi A, Grosch-Wörner I, Ades AE, Peckham CS. Infants born to HIV seropositive mothers—preliminary findings from a multi-centre European study. *Lancet* 1987; **1**: 1164-1168.
13. Chumule N, Lim W *et al.* Diagnosis of perinatal transmission of HIV: Utility of *in vitro* synthesis of HIV antibodies. (Abstract) *Fourth International Conference on AIDS*. Stockholm, Sweden. June 15-16, 1988.
14. Wittek AE, Phelan M, Wells MA, Vujcic LK, Epstein JS, Lane HC, Quinnan GV Jr. Detection of human immunodeficiency virus core protein in plasma by enzyme immunoassay. Association of antigenaemia with symptomatic disease and T-helper cell depletion. *Ann Intern Med* 1987; **107**: 286-292.
15. Allain J-P, Laurian Y, Paul DA, Verroust F, Leuther M, Gazengel C, Senn D, Larrieu M-J, Bosser C. Long-term evaluation of HIV antigen and antibodies to p24 and gp41 in patients with hemophilia. Potential clinical importance. *N Engl J Med* 1987; **317**: 1114-1121.
16. Ou CY, Kwok S *et al.* DNA amplification for direct detection of HIV-1 in DNA of peripheral blood mononuclear cells. *Science* 1988; **239**: 295-297.
17. Marion R, Wiznia AA, Hutcheon RG, Rubinstein, A. Human T-cell lymphotropic virus type III (HTLV-III) embryopathy. A new dysmorphic syndrome associated with intrauterine HTLV-III infection. *Am J Dis Child* 1986; **140**: 638-640.
18. Marion RW, Wiznia AA, Hutcheon RG *et al.* Fetal AIDS syndrome score. Correlation between severity of dysmorphism and age at diagnosis of immunodeficiency. *Am J Dis Child* 1987; **141**: 429-431.
19. Qazi QH, Sheik TM, Filkrig S, Menikoff H. Lack of evidence for craniofacial dysmorphism in perinatal human immunodeficiency infection. *J Pediatr* 1988; **112**: 7-11.

Subsequent care of infants of HIV positive mothers

Dr J. Mok

INTRODUCTION

In Edinburgh, intravenous drug abusers (IVDAs) have been reported to share needles more frequently and with more people when compared to drug abusers in Glasgow or London.[1,2] Therefore, it was not surprising that when the human immunodeficiency virus (HIV) was introduced into the Edinburgh drug abusing population in 1983, the spread was rapid. With the introduction of national screening of all blood donors in October 1985, it was obvious that an alternative clinic for counselling and testing was required for this population in order to avoid drug abusers using the blood donor centre as a testing site. This alternative site was established at the City Hospital in Edinburgh in October 1985 as an open access clinic for South-East Scotland; the experience has been reported recently.[3] Three separate studies of IVDA's from South-East Scotland have reported seroprevalence rates for HIV of between 38% and 65%.[4-6]

With the setting up of the City Hospital Counselling and Screening Clinic, HIV seropositive women who had recently given birth to infants, or were in various stages of pregnancy were identified. As one third of the IVDA's attending the clinic were young sexually active women, it was anticipated that more babies would be born. Therefore, a paediatric clinic was started to coordinate the follow-up, and management of infants born to women seropositive for HIV.

PAEDIATRIC COUNSELLING AND SCREENING CLINIC

The clinic was established in January 1986, sited at the existing adult clinic. Initial referrals were from physicians who identified pregnant HIV positive women from the screening clinic, but it soon became open access with self referrals, as well as those from neonatal paediatricians, obstetricians, midwives, health visitors, general practitioners and social workers.

The clinic operates on 2 sessions a week, and is staffed by a consultant paediatrician with an interest in community child health and lately, a paediatric research registrar. During each session, a health visitor is also present, with a dental hygienist at one of the sessions. When a pregnant woman is referred, attempts are made to see her in the antenatal period, to explain the purpose and nature of the clinic as well as to seek consent for follow-up.

Although much has been written about the clinical spectrum and immunological abnormalities seen in children with HIV infection,[7-9] little is known about infected children with less severe disease. Nor is the natural history of paediatric HIV infection well understood. The paediatric counselling and screening clinic therefore aimed to quantify the risk of materno-fetal transmission of HIV; to identify factors which might contribute to this risk; to define the natural history of perinatal HIV infection as well as to treat those infants who presented with symptomatic disease.

PERINATAL CARE OF INFANTS OF HIV POSITIVE WOMEN
Delivery
The paediatrician should be alerted to an HIV positive woman in labour, and the woman informed of the various procedures necessary for herself and her infant. The use of monitoring equipment should be kept to the minimum consistent with the safety of mother and baby. Fetal blood sampling and scalp electrodes carry a risk of HIV infection to the infant, and must be avoided. A fully equipped Resuscitaire should be held in readiness, and resuscitation of the infant performed according to standard procedures. Oropharyngeal secretions should be extracted with mechanical suction, or a 60 ml syringe attached to a mucus extractor. The paediatrician should wear a plastic apron, gown and gloves while handling the infant until blood and amniotic fluid are removed during bathing. Care must be taken to keep the infant warm.

Healthy neonate
The majority of infants in the Edinburgh cohort have not required special care facilities, and have been nursed with the mother in her room without isolation. Precautions are only needed when handling blood, as in venepunctures, heel pricks and cleaning the cord, when gloves are worn. Staff should be aware of cuts or wounds in their own skin, which should be covered with waterproof dressings although gloves may be preferred where there are extensive areas of broken skin.

Intensive care
This might be required for infants born prematurely, asphyxiated because of intrauterine growth retardation or suffering from drug withdrawal symptoms. Withdrawal from methadone tends to occur later than with heroin, and staff in neonatal units should be on the alert for late signs and symptoms. The risk of horizontal transmission of HIV to other neonates or staff is extremely low, so that isolation facilities are not essential. Protective clothing should be worn during invasive procedures and when dealing with large quantities of oropharyngeal secretions, faeces or urine.

Breastfeeding
Despite reports of HIV isolation from the breast milk of infected women, and possible cases of infants being infected through breastfeeding, the risk of HIV transmission via breast milk is probably very low compared with intrauterine or perinatal infection. There are insufficient data to recommend that HIV positive

women do not breastfeed, and the European collaborative study into perinatal transmission of HIV[10,11] has shown no increased risk for infants who were breastfed. However it seems prudent to advise that breast milk from an HIV positive woman should not be used to feed another infant.

ROUTINE SURVEILLANCE IN THE COMMUNITY

The lack of sensitive tests to diagnose HIV infection in young infants means that close clinical and laboratory monitoring is the only way to ensure early detection of disease. In Edinburgh, the infant is seen at 6 weeks, 3 months and 3-monthly thereafter. The mother is given the option to attend the clinic, or be seen at home. Sixty percent of the families are seen at home, mainly due to the haphazard lifestyles of the women and the distance of the clinic, as well as the stigma some women associate with attending an "AIDS clinic". At each visit, the paediatrician elicits a clinical history and conducts an examination of the infant while the health visitor performs developmental screening. The height, weight and head circumference are carefully documented and blood taken for virological tests (HIV antibody, antigen and virus cultures), immunological and haematological monitoring (IgG, A, M; full blood count with differential white cell count, T lymphocyte subsets and platelet count).

Most of the mothers do not attend local child welfare clinics, although encouraged to do so. This means that our health visitor has to discuss normal child care issues and immunisation procedures (see below). The majority of infants are immunised at the screening and counselling clinic. The mothers are also asked about their own health, and given the option to be seen by an adult physician.

PROGRESS OF THE EDINBURGH COHORT

From 1 January 1986 to 31 December 1987, 40 infants born to 37 HIV seropositive women have been followed up at 165 attendances. Figure I shows the age distribution of the cohort at the last attendance. Clinical data of the infants and mothers are presented in Table 1. All are white Caucasian.

Table 1

Clinical data of 40 infants of 37 HIV positive women

Boys (n)	19	
Girls (n)	21	
Gestation (wks)	29-42	($\bar{x} = 38.2$)
Birth weight (g)	930-4000	($\bar{x} = 2822$)
Spontaneous vaginal delivery (n)	39	
Neonatal special care (n)	7	
Mother's age at delivery (yrs)	17-33	($\bar{x} = 23.6$)
First born (n)	19	
IV drug use during pregnancy (n)	11	
Risk activity—IVDA	32	
Heterosexual contact	5	

Figure I

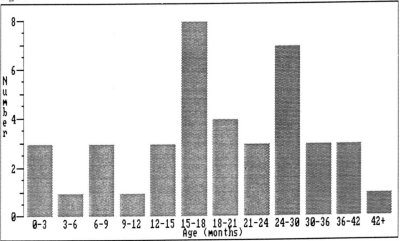

Age distribution of Edinburgh cohort on 31 December 1987.

After a median follow-up period of 15 months, 4 children have shown clinical evidence of HIV infection. Signs and symptoms were non-specific, and appeared at 6-9 months. This consisted of significant lymphadenopathy (nodes > 0.5cm in > 2 non-contiguous sites) in 4 children, hepatosplenomegaly in 3 children, recurrent respiratory infections in 4 children, eczematous eruption in 4 children and failure to thrive in 1 child. The enlarged lymph nodes as well as liver and spleen were noted to fluctuate in size over time, being most pronounced when the children were first suspected to be infected. The remaining 36 children were clinically well when last seen. Neurological abnormality (ataxic diplegia) was seen only in 1 infant who was delivered at 31 weeks gestation and had neonatal meningitis followed by hydrocephalus. The developmental progress of the rest of the cohort has been within normal limits. One other child has also been diagnosed as having cystic fibrosis. Abnormal laboratory tests were noted as follows: hypergammaglobulinaemia (in the 4 HIV-infected children as well as the child with cystic fibrosis), thrombocytopaenia in 3 children, with T4 lymphopaenia (<1000) seen in only one child although T4/T8 was > 1.5 in 5 children. Maternal HIV antibody has persisted in 6 of 29 infants over 15 months old, 4 of whom are symptomatic. Figure II shows the numbers of children tested at each follow-up interval together with the numbers who were HIV negative. Antibody loss occurred from 6-18 months (median 12 months). HIV antigen tests have recently been performed in 16 children, and none found to be positive. Positive HIV culture results have been obtained in the 4 symptomatic children.

CLINICAL MANAGEMENT

While a diagnosis of AIDS usually results in a high mortality, many children will present with less severe illnesses which nonetheless require therapy. In the absence of an effective anti-viral drug, current treatment is supportive and directed at the symptoms of HIV infection.

Figure II

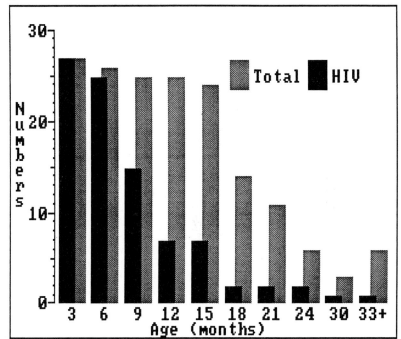

Loss of maternal HIV antibody. The histograms depict total numbers of children tested at each follow-up period, and the numbers found to be HIV positive.

Recurrent infections

Defective humoral immunity has been reported, and affected children present with recurrent bacterial infections despite persistently raised serum immunoglobulin levels.[9] Empirical treatment has been instituted with regular infusions of intravenous gammaglobulin. In Edinburgh, the regime used is 200 mg/kg on a 3-weekly basis. Although the humoral defect is not reversed, there has been a decrease in the number of infections and a significant fall in the days of hospitalisation.[12] Oral candidiasis can result in feeding difficulties and be resistant to topical therapy. Systemic drugs, i.e., Ketoconazole, may have to be used. Pneumocystis carinii pneumonia (PCP) can be treated with high-dose Cotrimoxazole or Pentamidine. Following a diagnosis of PCP, prophylaxis is recommended with Cotrimoxazole.

Lymphocytic interstitial pneumonitis

Although the mortality with lymphocytic interstitial pneumonitis is lower than that seen with PCP, the morbidity can be significant. Affected children show varying degrees of hypoxaemia which might necessitate supplemental oxygen therapy. Parents can be taught the use of this at home. Some children also respond to steroid therapy.

Nutrition

A combination of anorexia and oral candidiasis will lead to an inadequate caloric intake. The advice of a paediatric dietitian should be sought, although it may be necessary to resort to nasogastric or parenteral feeding. Recurrent or protracted diarrhoea will result in dehydration and electrolyte imbalance, requiring close hospital monitoring.

HIV encephalopathy

This presents with delayed milestones or developmental regression, and is usually progressive.[8,13,14] Seizures can be controlled with conventional anticonvulsants. Progressive motor and intellectual dysfunction result in a multiply handicapped child who will require the services of physiotherapists, occupational therapists and social workers, as well as special educational facilities. The encephalopathy reported in adults with AIDS responds favourably to treatment with Zidovudine,[15] and similar trials in children also need to be conducted.

IMMUNISATION

Concerns have been raised regarding the safety and efficacy of childhood immunisations for HIV-infected children, and guidelines have been devised for immunisation of children who are at risk of HIV infection.[16] In general, live vaccines are contraindicated in children with compromised immune systems, because of the potential for disseminated infection with the viral or bacterial vaccine strain. Any immunisation could accelerate the disease by providing antigenic stimulation.

When immunising children at risk of HIV infection, it is not always known whether the child has normal immune function. Of the 40 children in the Edinburgh cohort, 36 received diphtheria/tetanus or diphtheria/tetanus/pertussis immunisation; 32 inactivated polio vaccine, 4 oral polio vaccine, while measles vaccine was given to 13 children over 15 months of age who were HIV antibody negative, clinically well and had normal tests of immune function. No adverse reaction was reported in any child, nor was vaccine-related poliomyelitis seen in any household member who was HIV-infected.

Recent evidence indicates that live vaccines (polio, measles and BCG) can be given safely to symptomatic HIV antibody positive children, especially in areas where the infections are prevalent and life-threatening.[17,18,19] The practice in Edinburgh tends to be rather more cautious and considers the fact that other household members might be immunocompromised. (See Table 2)

Table 2

Immunisation of children at risk of HIV infection (Edinburgh perinatal transmission study)

---

1 *Children with normal clinical and immune status*
   Diphtheria, tetanus, pertussis (unless other contra-indications exist to pertussis vaccine)
   Inactivated polio vaccine (oral polio if no other family member immune compromised)
   Measles vaccine

2 *Children with HIV disease*
   Diphtheria, tetanus, pertussis (as above)
   Inactivated polio vaccine
   No measles vaccine—hyperimmune gammaglobulin is offered following significant exposure
   All mothers also have their Hepatitis B status checked, and the infant immunised if appropriate

DAY CARE AND SUBSTITUTE PARENT CARE

In Edinburgh, women who are HIV seropositive come from areas of the city with multiple deprivation. Therefore, the problems of drug abuse, unemployment, imprisonment and single parent families only compound the diagnosis of HIV infection. Parenting skills are limited, and while many mothers manage to care for their infants with support from health care and social work staff, some have continued to abuse drugs following the birth of their infants.

The Lothian Region Social Work Department has pioneered training programmes in the care of infants at risk of HIV infection for their own staff as well as foster families.[20] As a result, staff in Children's Centres (Day Nurseries) have been able to integrate such children into normal facilities. Close liaison with the paediatrician has meant that advice on specific health issues is readily available. Children with symptomatic HIV infection, or those with anti-social behaviour, i.e. biting, obviously need closer supervision, and this has been made possible by increasing the staff:child ratio.

While 3 infants have been placed in the care of grandparents, 8 have been successfully looked after by foster families. Initially, seminars were held for all foster families, where basic facts were given on AIDS, transmission of the virus and the low risk of infection during casual contact. Good hygiene practices were emphasised. Specific issues addressed were the uncertain outlook for the child and the need to assume HIV infection with an immune system that could be depressed. Good back-up facilities for respite care were made available, and mutual support amongst the foster families has proved invaluable. At the time of writing, 1 child has been adopted by his foster family, while 3 other children in foster care are going through the legal procedures for adoption.

HIV ANTIBODY TESTING AND ALTERNATIVE CARE

While a positive antibody test in an adult is a sensitive indicator of HIV infection, the presence of passively transferred maternal antibody limits the usefulness of this test in young infants. Foster parents must be assured that there are no risks of HIV transmission during normal household contact, as long as good standards of hygiene are maintained. It is therefore not necessary for them to know the HIV status of children placed in their care. Indeed, emergency foster placements usually mean that arrangements for testing are not feasible. Prospective adopters are seeking reassurances that an HIV-infected child is not placed with them. Many adoption agencies are now screening women who wish to offer their baby for adoption. Screening should begin with a careful history to elicit risk activities, in keeping with current practice where a detailed family and social history is obtained from the mother. Identification of any risk factor should then lead to counselling the woman regarding HIV testing. Where the woman's test is positive, there will still be difficulties in placing her infant due to the present lack of sensitive tests to identify HIV infection in young children. Routine testing of all infants placed for adoption is not recommended.

EDUCATION

Current recommendations are that the number of people aware of the child's HIV status be kept to the minimum necessary to assure proper care of the child, and to detect situations in which the potential for transmission may increase.[21,22] Parents may choose not to disclose their child's infection to any child care staff. It is therefore imperative that staff in all establishments dealing with children (nurseries, playgroups, schools, day care facilities) should adopt routine procedures for handling blood and secretions (including sanitary towels) regardless of whether children with HIV infection are known to be in attendance.

A child with symptomatic HIV disease runs a greater risk of infection in an unrestricted school setting, and special educational provisions may be required. HIV encephalopathy resulting in developmental delay will also mean the child will need special educational facilities, which could range from special classes to tuition at home. Close liaison between education and paediatric staff will ensure the best possible provision for each child.

FUTURE PROVISIONS

Because 80% of children are infected as a result of materno-fetal transmission, it is important to consider the mother's health at all times. Concomitant illness in mother and child is not uncommon, and intravenous drug abusers may not have an extended family available for support. In Edinburgh we are looking towards a supported accommodation unit, where the ill mother can be helped to look after her child. Intensive care facilities for children will have to be developed as more children become ill. It is conceivable that less severely affected children will survive into adolescence, and there could also be asymptomatic carriers of HIV in their teens. Such adolescents need to be counselled on the implications of their disease, starting with healthy living and avoidance of risk activities which will contribute to disease progression. Safer sexual practices have to be instituted. The adolescent will also need help to come to terms with anger towards his parents, fear about his own future and guilt that he might infect his sexual partner and offspring.

CONCLUSIONS

The need for prospective studies to determine the prevalence of perinatal transmission, as well as define the natural history of HIV disease in infants born to seropositive women has been highlighted.[10] In setting up such a study in Edinburgh, the paediatric counselling and screening clinic has been recognised as the centre in the United Kingdom with the largest cohort of infants of HIV positive mothers. The experience gained in the clinical are has been invaluable, and close liaison with the Social Work Department as well as voluntary agencies mean that social, family and other factors are identified and guidelines developed for the subsequent care of infants born to HIV positive women.

REFERENCES
1. Robertson JR, Bucknall ABV, Wiggins P. Regional variations in HIV antibody sero-positivity in British intravenous drug users. (Letter) *Lancet* 1986; **1:** 1435-1436.
2. Brettle RP. Epidemic of AIDS related virus infection among intravenous drug abusers. (Letter) Br Med J 1986; **292:** 1671.
3. Brettle RP, Bisset K, Burns S *et al.* Human immunodeficiency virus and drug misusers; the Edinburgh experience. *Br Med J* 1987; **295:** 421-424.

4. Peutherer JF, Edmond E, Simmonds P, Dickson JD, Bath GE. HTLV-III antibody in Edinburgh drug addicts. (Letter) *Lancet* 1985; **2**: 1129-1130.
5. Robertson JR, Bucknall ABV, Welsby PD, Roberts JJK, Inglis JM, Peutherer JF, Brettle RP. Epidemic of AIDS related virus (HTLV-III/LAV) infection among intravenous drug abusers. *Br Med J* 1986; **292**: 527-530.
6. Brettle RP, Davidson J, Davidson S, Gray JMN, Inglis JM, Conn JS, Bath GE, Gillon J, McClelland DBI. HTLV-III antibodies in an Edinburgh clinic. (Letter) *Lancet* 1986; **1**: 1099.
7. Rubinstein A. Paediatric AIDS. *Curr Probl Paediatr* 1986; **16**: 365-409.
8. Belman AL, Ultmann MH, Horoupian D, Novick B, Spiro AJ, Rubinstein A, Kurtzberg D, Cone-Wesson B. Neurological complications in infants and children with acquired immune deficiency syndrome. *Ann Neurol* 1985; **18**: 560-566.
9. Bernstein LJ, Krieger BZ, Novick B, Sicklick MJ, Rubinstein A. Bacterial infection in the acquired immunodeficiency syndrome of children. *Paediatr Infect Dis* 1985; **4**: 472-475.
10. Mok JQ, Giaquinto C, De Rossi, A, Grosch-Wörner I, Ades AE, Peckham CS. Infants born to mothers seropositive for human immundeficiency virus. *Lancet* 1987; **1**: 1164-1168.
11. Senturia YD, Ades AE, Peckham CS, Giaquinto C. Breast feeding and HIV infection. *Lancet* 1987; **2**: 400-401.
12. Williams PE, Yap PL, Mok JQ, Bingham J, Brettle RP. Treatment of HIV antibody positive infants with intravenous immunoglobulin. *Communicable Disease Surveillance* 1987; **33**: 7-9.
13. Epstein LG, Sharer LR, Oleske JM, Connor EM, Goudsmit J, Cook S, Dowling P. Neurologic manifestations of human immunodeficiency virus infection in children. *Pediatrics* 1986; **78**: 678-687.
14. Belman AL, Diamond G, Dickson D *et al.* Pediatric Acquired Immunodeficiency syndrome. Neurologic syndromes. *Am J Dis Child* 1988; **142**: 29-35.
15. Yarchoan R, Brouwers P, Spitzer AR, Grafman J, Safai B, Larson SM, Berg G, Fischl A, Wichman A, Thomas RV, Brunetti A, Schmidt PJ, Myers CE, Broder S. Response of human-immunodeficiency-virus-associated neurological disease to 3'-azido-3'-deoxythymidine. *Lancet* 1987; **1**: 132-135.
16. ACIP. Immunisation of children infected with human T lymphotrophic virus type III/lymphadenopathy associated virus. *MMWR* 1986; **35**: 595-606.
17. Krasinski K, Borkowski W. Response to polio vaccination in children infected with human immunodeficiency virus. Presented at 1987 meeting of the Society for Pediatric Research. Albuquerque: Society for Pediatric Research 925, 1987.
18. Sension MG, Nzila N, Duma M *et al.* Does concomitant HIV infection and measles infection in African children lead to increased morbidity and mortality? *IIIrd International Conference on AIDS*, Washington DC, 1987.
19. Carswell M. BCG immunisation in the children of HIV positive mothers. *AIDS* 1987; **1**: 258.
20. Black A, Skinner K. Placement of children at risk of HIV infection. In: *The implications of AIDS for children in care.* Ed. D Batty. London: British Agencies for Adoption and Fostering, 1987; pp.36-47.
21. *AIDS. Guidance for educational establishments in Scotland.* HMSO, January 1987.
22. American Academy of Pediatrics, Committee on School Health, Committee on Infectious Diseases. School attendance of children and adolescents with human T lymphotrophic virus III/lymphadenopathy associated virus infection. *Pediatrics* 1986; **77**:430-431.

Discussion

Chairman: Professor N.F. Morris

WHITELAW: I would like to ask Dr Scott two questions. In a child with chronic pneumonitis is it obligatory to have a lumbar series to distinguish pneumocystis from the lymphoid interstitial variety, and what do you see in the encephalopathy when examined neuropathologically?

SCOTT: In general, we have initially done a lumbar series on our children with chronic lung disease, although we do not know at that point what we are looking at. The majority of those have lymphoid interstitial pneumonitis or pneumocystic disease, and some have CMV in addition to one or both of these. At the present time we no longer do biopsies. We do aspirates for the diagnosis of PCP and tuberculosis since we have a high incidence of tuberculosis in our area. We watch it over a period of time but we do not necessarily biopsy it to find out the pathology. That rules out CMV, pneumocystis, TB and routine bacterial infections. In terms of the encephalopathy, virologically we have been able to identify the organism in the brain. Histologically I think they have found some multinucleated giant cells.

WHITELAW: So lymphoid pneumocystis is really a diagnosis of exclusion, a diagnosis without effective treatment?

SCOTT: The only way you could make the diagnosis is by biopsy, but you can make a presumptive diagnosis by bronchoscopy and by ruling out other causes. And also by having a typical clinical picture.

GREEN: Could I ask you about this issue of encephalopathy in children. There does seem to have been some degree of over-diagnosis of encephalopathy in adults with HIV infections. I wonder how accurate the assessment is. On the other hand, you do not want to underestimate, because it is notoriously difficult to know all about the brain function of an infant of 15 months. The other thing was a question of whether you think that encephalopathy is a sole problem in children in the absence of opportunistic difficulties.

SCOTT: There is a typical picture of encephalopathy that does occur in a child who presents initially with delayed milestones and progressive regression, who has usually a very normal immunoglobulin level, or they may be hypo-gammaglobulin anaemic. They are typical of a "failure to thrive" picture. They have fairly low T4 counts. So it seems that very early on in life for one reason or another they start out not doing well, and then progress. That is one picture. Most children progress to becoming very stiff and lose their muscle control totally, very much like cerebral palsy. There is another group who seem to have some cell development delays, but may catch up either with an improvement of their infection status or an improvement in their nutrition. Some of these children catch up totally; others do not. That is the group that we cannot identify as definitely HIV-infected. I think that in prospective studies like Dr Mok is doing and the European Collaborative Study, it would be a very nice group to look at using developmental testing. We are doing that in our retrospective study, and we test them every 3 months. If they are HIV positive we look at HIV antibody synthesis in the brain or in the spinal fluid. We are looking at CT scans as well in these infants. At least we are going to find out more information about what the long term picture is going to be in terms of development. When we try to culture HIV from spinal fluid even in children with severe encephalopathy it is not 100% positive. Yet we have seen some positive viral cultures in spinal fluid of children who are asymptomatic. So the CSF may act as a reservoir for the infection, and something may happen to allow progression of the infection into the central nervous system.

GREEN: What about much older children? Can we verify this problem in children who may have no other problems?

SCOTT: It is unpredictable. We had a 5-year-old who had a blood transfusion at age 2, who at age 5 started out with some ataxia; nobody knew what he had while he was regressing until someone remembered the fact that he had had an earlier blood transfusion. They tested him, and he was HIV positive. But he presented solely with the little bit of ataxia, a little bit of speech difficulty, and started to do poorly in school. He had nothing else for a long period of time. We really do not understand why some children present with only encephalopathy.

I would like to ask Dr Mok a question. When you identify an HIV positive child in a family, do you look at the siblings?

MOK: I think it depends very much on the ages of the siblings. We know for a fact that HIV arrived in Edinburgh at the end of 1983. So when there are 10-year-olds and 11-year-olds in a family you obviously do not look at them. But when there is a child born after 1983, yes, we certainly do look at them.

WOOD: Thinking of some of the cases which Dr Scott described, it is so like cases of severe combined immune deficiency disease that the person who is looking for that sort of thing is now going to have HIV at the top of the list of diagnostic possibilities. One is going to have to address the question of the selection of cases for HIV testing in paediatric outpatients, irrespective of knowing whether the families are high risk or not.

MOK: It depends very much on your own clinical practice as to how much you explain your investigations to the parents. I would hate to have to deal with a positive result having not got the consent of the parents for testing for HIV.

SCOTT: It would be a lot easier to deal with if you told the mother that this is included in a differential diagnosis and that you are going to do all the different tests.

LAMBERT: Of the children that you deal with who have recurrent bacterial infections, can you tell us what sort of bacterial infections they have, and were they unusual infections? Secondly, could I ask if you see any cases of Kaposi's sarcoma?

MOK: The children that I see have predominantly respiratory infections—the "snotty nosed child"—who probably would have gone to the general practitioner or the paediatrician. They would never have considered HIV as a diagnosis. I have not seen the more severe infections like pneumonia or meningitis.

SCOTT: It is very interesting that out of our prospective study, and our children are not that far along in terms of age—perhaps reaching 12-15 months—those that have been identified are all clinically symptomatic. In fact, 2 of them have already died, one from pneumocystis and the other from severe encephalopathy. So, at least in our prospective infants, all of those who are HIV positive or culture positive, have severe systemic disease. I refer to those who are HIV positive or culture positive, which is much different from what Dr Mok described. I do not know whether it is a difference in the virus load or the climate, or what. The kind of bacterial infections which are the commonest are pneumococcus, streptococcus Type B, some salmonella and occasional staph. And many times they do not deal with the organism in the order that we anticipate that they should. For instance, I saw a throat infection and treated for that, and the patient developed meningitis a few days later. Many of the children have otitis media on a recurrent basis, but that is not very specific. But meningitis and other such infections are very aggressive.

MOK: I would like to ask if anyone could offer an explanation as to why 2 prospective studies should have such different results. Is is because in Miami they have seen HIV for much longer than we have in Edinburgh? Is it racial? Biochemical?

MORRIS: May I ask the epidemiologists that question. Do they have figures as to why the 2 studies do not necessarily correspond?

PECKHAM: I think that a lot depends on whether the child is infected or not. We have not yet been able to look at the group who were infected in relation to symptoms, and those who were not infected in relation to symptoms. Some of the symptoms might be related to the type of children. Secondly, we have had some very sick children in the multicentre study; we have had children with neurological problems, one with acquired macrocephaly, and quite severe neurological problems and encephalopathy. I think that we have not yet gone on long enough to really know what we are going to find.

SCOTT: Some of our babies may still be too early to be easily identified.

MOK: It cannot be just the length of follow-up because Dr Scott has been doing a follow-up to 15 months or even a shorter length of time, and yet she is seeing children with all these problems.

PECKHAM: But they do not know how many are infected yet. We have to wait until they are all over 15 months before we can say that they are or not infected. Perhaps there are many more infected because there may be other risk factors that will influence the rate of transmission. I think that we do not know yet. We must be very cautious.

SCHOENBAUM: It is also quite possible that there is a significant difference in length of infection in the mothers. You say that you know that the mothers are infected; you actually know that they seroconverted. Your information dates from 1983. In the United States we have information since 1978, so potentially many of the mothers are at a different point of their disease.

ANCELLE: I wonder also if in heterosexual studies there was a link between the clinical status of the mother and the child. I had the impression that the mothers were clinically more advanced than in the infant studies.

SCOTT: We are a little early in our study to have that kind of data. I think that 2, or maybe 3 of those infants came from mothers who had already delivered an infected infant. So that may be a slightly different situation. The other 2 that I recall had asymptomatic mothers. But there may very well be a common denominator.

SCHOENBAUM: Just to make it more complicated I would like to mention that of the 23 seropositive mothers that I have quoted, we have studied their babies prospectively and have found results very similar to those of Dr Mok in Edinburgh, with only 2 having CDC classification AIDS, and almost all losing antibody. Some of them had nonspecific symptoms and underwent diagnostic tests, but they are not really sick.

SCOTT: We do not really know exactly what our seronegative rate is.

JOHNSTONE: Referring to the 10 babies whom you diagnosed as having AIDS in 1982, of whom 5 are still alive, after the 6 intervening years, is it possible to assess the quality of life of those surviving children?

SCOTT: It is easier for me to do it from date of birth, because then I know who they are. We have some children who were born in 1979 at least 2 of whom are asymptomatic, except for some odd lymphadenopathy. But other than that, I could not pick them out of a group. They are quite healthy with normal development and a very mild degree of symptoms, and have remained so over a long period of time. So there are children who are going to do well. The prospective study will give us a lot more information about the children.

JOHNSTON: These were children who had been diagnosed as having AIDS?

SCOTT: Yes. It is interesting if you look at survival, we have a large group of children from 1979, 1980, 1981 who are still living. Then when you look at our survival rate from later on—from the last 2 years—it looks worse. But I think that this is due to the fact that we have not yet seen the long term outcome from those children who were born in 1986 and 1987. What we are seeing in those 1979-1980 groups are a number of children who died early but in the long term could have done well. I know that there are series of children who are in school and clinically well. So there is a subgroup—we do not know how many of them there are, not a majority—but they are certainly there. The other thing that I think is important is the impact on obstetrics. I think that from a paediatric point of view, we want to prevent disease. One way that we can think about preventing disease is early diagnosis of the mother and possibly treatment of infants at the time of birth if they are HIV positive or at risk, or certainly if they are infected. You can see from the statistics that the majority of these children, at least those we know now, have caught the disease in the first few weeks of life. The majority are going to die in that time period. So we have a very small window of time to deal with these children. If we know that they are HIV positive at birth because you have tested the mother or you have done some evaluation of the mother, that helps us a great deal. I cannot tell you that today I can go out and treat every HIV positive infant born to an HIV positive mother. But in the future that should be possible, and I think that it is going to be very important to be able to make those identifications early. From my point of view and those of my colleagues in the field, early therapy is the best way to deal with this. Also, if it is transmitted around the time of delivery, possibly early therapy may even prevent the disease.

STEELE: May I ask Dr Mok if she has anything to tell us about children of HIV positive fathers?

MOK: HIV positive fathers when the mother is negative? I have about 20 of these children in my cohort. The reason for enrolling them in the study was just in case the mother seroconverted. But the mothers have all stayed negative and the children have remained well. Even when you look at the nonspecific findings which my paediatric colleagues tell me are very common in the selection of converts, they are not as frequently seen in the children of HIV positive fathers when the mother is negative. All of them remain well; their functions are completely normal.

WHITELAW: If your study is epidemiologically designed to look at the natural history, what is the influence of the use of immunoglobulin infusions? Is this standardised into the whole of the European study? Could you tell us what are the grounds on which you start infusion, and how long do you go on?

MOK: The criterion used for starting is recurrent infection, such as diarrhoea, and that is about it. Children do seem to have an improved quality of life in that if they do have infections, they are shorter lived and there is a significant reduction in their stays in hospital.

HARVEY: I would like to ask Dr Mok about immunisation, particularly the BCG. From what you said from the WHO recommendations, quite a lot of these might have been candidates for the BCG. Quite often in London we have to use the BCG.

MOK: It is just not common practice.

HOWIE: You do not have a prejudice against it?

MOK: It is not something we do routinely in Edinburgh.

SCOTT: I think the other piece of information about immunisation is that there are a certain number of deaths from measles in HIV-infected children who acquire the natural infection but who have not been immunised. I think that this information will probably lead to liberalisation of immunisation.

THOMPSON: Could I return to the question of the baby whose father is positive and the mother negative? Would you please comment on the management of this family?

MOK: We treat the child normally with the whole immunisation procedure. They attend local clinics and there are no special precautions.

TYLER: Were the fathers using protective measures before they attempted pregnancy, or were they on a protective course before pregnancy occurred?

MOK: Actually some of them have continued to have unprotected intercourse. It is quite amazing what some of the mothers put themselves through. We do discuss issues of safe sex with them because of the danger of transmission. But the sort of excuses that we get for not using condoms are sometimes quite incredible. They just do not use condoms.

SCRIMGEOUR: What were the chances of the subsequent sibling being HIV positive?

SCOTT: We have done that on an expanded number. We had 25 mothers who had subsequent infants. It ended up being a 50% transmission rate in that group— for a woman who had an HIV positive infant and then went on to have subsequent pregnancies. In the first study we did the rate was 65%.

JEFFRIES: You seemed to be impressed with the use of zidovudine in neonates. Some of us have also experienced the use of this drug in adults. Could you give us a thumbnail sketch as to what your impressions are at the present time of the use of this drug, in terms of its virological effect possibly on antigen and in terms of toxicity in children?

SCOTT: I think we have had less experience in the United States than they have in some parts of Europe. We have done a case study on about 30 children in the United States. In general the drug appears to be well tolerated and the side effects are similar in terms of having to watch the white count and the platelet count. But those problems seem to be easily overcome and we have not seen any severe unremitting anaemias or children who have stopped growing.

MOK: I recall the experience that Graham Watson has had in Newcastle where he has used a portion of zidovudine in 3 haemophiliacs and one with vertical transmission. The children were started very early on in the disease based on T4 counts. They were impressed on how minimal the side effects were (personal communication).

SCOTT: I think that Pizzot in Washington has had some problems with zidovudine in children but has found some reversal of neurological symptoms.

HUDSON: We have heard that the incidence of Caesarean sections is extremely low in this sort of series. Can we collect any information from the United States or Europe which would give us any guidance at this stage on the relevance of Caesarean sections in terms of the status of the babies? My impression is that we just do not know the answer.

SCOTT: The answer is that we do not know. In our prospective studies some of them have Caesarean section while others have had natural delivery, and we have not followed them long enough to know whether there is any effect. In our other series less than 10% have had Caesarean sections that were infected.

HUDSON: That would be less than the Caesarean section rate for the United States.

MORRIS: What was the theory behind the Caesarean section? Was it that there was less risk of transference?

HUDSON: I believe that viral transmission through an infected genital tract to a fetus in transit could introduce infection which perhaps had not gone across transplacentally earlier.

PECKHAM: From the evidence we have so far there is no difference at all between the infection rates in those that deliver vaginally and those who have Caesarean sections. There is no suggestion that Caesarean section reduces the infection rate.

MOK: In Berlin where all the babies are delivered electively by Caesarean section they are still seeing infected babies.

SHARP: This is what you would expect, is it not? The only reason that I can see for avoiding a vaginal delivery would be the potential trauma to the baby, and therefore the greater likelihood of blood getting through a non-intact integument. That would be equally operative in Caesarean section as far as the exposure to blood is concerned. The only difference is maybe that minor trauma is more likely to the baby coming through the vaginal canal naturally.

SCOTT: What has worked out very nicely in our hospitals is that we have a clinic one afternoon as a combined Ob/Gyn clinic and there is a specialist there so that when parents come to us if the mother needs to see an Ob/Gyn specialist she can go to him while we see her child. This has worked out very well in terms of sharing information as well as making the parents happy when they come in and have the two people to see at the same time. I think that it has improved the clinical care of the family unit.

JOHNSTONE: The patients that we have seen tend to go into labour somewhat prematurely. Fifty percent of them deliver within 2 hours of admission to the labour ward. So they tend to admit themselves late, sometimes in the second stage, sometimes in the third stage!

MORRIS: One of the issues that has been pressed into the background is whether all women having babies should be tested. From your experience have you seen many babies who have escaped the net, so to speak? In other words, have you picked them up as being HIV positive, even though they have not gone through your high risk group? Obviously, there are some mothers who have had infected babies who have not been picked up by the present methods of scrutiny because they do not necessarily fall in the high risk groups, and therefore would not have been screened.

SCOTT: You miss about 50% of them through that mechanism. Right now in our hospital we are not doing maternal screening. The only way that we have of identifying people is through our own prospective study or through the development of symptoms in the children.

MORRIS: Do you think that there is a lot to be said for knowing as shortly after birth as possible so that we can instigate treatment which at the moment can be somewhat primitive, but hopefully will become more sophisticated later on?

SCOTT: I think that it is important to identify the child because you are going to teach that mother when she should bring the child into the clinic.

MOK: I certainly have been referred at least 5 children where the mothers have gone through the normal procedures of going to an antenatal clinic, and have been delivered of a child, where they have not been picked up as being seropositive. Dr Johnstone will tell the story of the one and only emergency Caesarean section that we had of a woman who did not think that she belonged to a risk group. It was only when the anaesthetist thought that she had puncture marks and decided that she should be tested when she was being anaesthetised. But that is not normal. Usually we do this. But there is certainly a case for identifying women and babies early. If they had not been closely followed up the symptoms will be missed as will the progressive T4 counts.

HUDSON: This surely brings us back to the ethics of antenatal testing. There would be different constraints on that to the voluntary consent and full knowledge which is obviously required in the antenatal scene. The welfare of the infant will depend on that knowledge.

SCRIMGEOUR: In your series in which those patients presented to you with no warning and were found to be HIV positive, when you went back to the mother were the clues there and had they been missed?

SCOTT: A large number of our infants were born to mothers who had emigrated from Haiti. The mothers were not symptomatic when they delivered their infants; they themselves were perfectly well and unaware that they were threatened. In the majority of these cases the father has been the index case in the family and has served as the sentinel case for recognition of the infection in the mother. These would never have been self-identified cases.

SCRIMGEOUR: Except for the country of origin. Is it possible for you in Miami to say that all those girls who come over from Haiti should be screened?

SCOTT: We could not do that. The Haitian population was identified by the CDC as a high risk group, for reasons that were not very clear, and that has caused a great number of problems in the community. Other women who also have the infection because of heterosexual spread are no different, and so you cannot choose one group to screen. I think that if you are going to do screening you have to offer it to everyone.

LUCAS: Can I take up the point made about postnatal screening? It does raise an interesting ethico-legal problem that we are going to have to face sooner or later. If we are going to screen neonates because of this "window", then ultimately we will find parents who do not want their children screened because their own HIV status will be discovered as a result. How is that going to resolve?

SCOTT: I do not think that you should be screening the neonate. I think you should be screening the mother. Or if you are going to do anonymous screening like they have done in Boston and, I think, in New York, they used the Guthrie neonatal test where no one knows who the patients are. That just gives you prevalence data. I think that you should screen the mother, counsel the mother, and then test the infant. I do not think that the infant should be screened first unless there is a medical reason to do so.

MOK: I think it goes back to the issue of why you are screening. If you are only screening because you would like to know what the HIV prevalence is amongst the antenatal population, then anonymous screening using the Guthrie test would seem to be a good idea. But if you are screening to identify infants that you might do something about, then you are going to need consent.

LUCAS: That is the situation that I was talking about. I agree that if you screen the mothers first, then that solves the problem, but if you cannot do that does the parent have the right to refuse consent for his child to be screened? Is that ethically acceptable?

SCOTT: I would not like to have to make that decision.

HARVEY: I think that the parent does have the right.

LUCAS: I agree with you, but the point of issue here is that, as Dr Scott has pointed out to us, it is important to diagnose the condition as soon as possible in neonates.

HARVEY: I agree totally with Dr Scott that one needs to test the mother.

RAFFLES: I think certainly that paediatricians would go along with Dr Harvey in agreeing that the mother is the person that you really ought to be testing. In our hospital we know that there are undiagnosed HIV positive infants in the community from a screening programme that was carried out. We have now been given today a whole list of symptoms. I think that it is going to expose paediatricians' inaction to an even greater difficulty as from today. That is to take back this list of symptoms and ask themselves whom they are going to treat. It is good that this point has been raised now, and that there are going to be many years of discussion before it is resolved fully.

MOK: I agree that for a symptomatic child you have no option but to test. But we are talking about presymptomatic diagnosis. Do you go along with testing every child who walks into a paediatric clinic?.

RAFFLES: At present the answer would be no, unless we had grounds to request permission from the mother. There would be nothing against a study using the correct ethical channels that involve requesting permission from the mother to screen the child for HIV, on the grounds that they are involved in a clinical study from which they can opt out. I think, though, that at the moment clinics do not have the time, nor the training to be AIDS counsellors or HIV testing counsellors. But given the facilities, we could do that. I think that one place that would be important would be in our drug dependency clinic. Fewer than 30% of the women who eventually become pregnant who attend our drug dependency clinic actually attend the antenatal clinic at less than 30 weeks. They literally come in and out of the park. Our last patient was found unconscious in the park at 32 weeks.

SCOTT: The other important aspect that you pointed out is that if you are going to do voluntary testing or screening with permission you have to have the mechanism in place to do the rest of the follow-up, the referrals, the testing of parents and the counselling and education. If you do not have those facilities then you really should not go into screening.

RAFFLES: If I could just draw a parallel—in the area where I work we all do sickle cell screening. We have great difficulties from angry parents who say that they did not know we were screening for sickle cell. We have one set of parents who have threatened to sue us. In fact, the information was given to the parents, but nobody sat down and actually read it out to them. That is an easier disease to deal with, but the same ethical considerations are there.

MOK: Could we take it one step further? Having identified an infant of an HIV positive woman, where do we stand if the mother refuses follow-up? Does the baby have to be seen?

HARVEY: I do have some anxieties that about 75% of the babies are going to lose their antibodies and are not infected. If an HIV positive mother had said to me that, because of identifying the baby, she felt it would cause problems for her family, and that she could not talk about it because she could not live with the consequences, I do wonder whether it was worthwhile identifying the baby in that case. It depends critically on whether it is advantageous for the children who are infected to be identified early. If it improves the prognosis then it is worthwhile doing it. If not, then it might very well cause more anxiety problems than the identification would actually solve.

SCOTT: It may give the woman an option.

LAMBERT: I think we must realise the immense moral and ethical arguments. There are also legal arguments. As far as I know the medical defence unions have not made a statement on the testing of babies. But also, as far as I know, in the strict legal sense, parents do not have the right to allow their children to be entered into any kind of clinical trial, although it does happen all the time.

SCOTT: The other issue is the HIV positive infant who ultimately becomes negative. Once that baby is identified as negative, normal, and noninfected, how do you put that into the chart to ensure that the baby is not in future identified as being HIV positive?

JOHNSTONE: It always seems to me when we talk about testing, that the paediatricians, for example, feel that they really cannot do this, and that we should be talking to the mother. They say that their paediatric clinic is busy, and that therefore we should spend our time at the antenatal clinic counselling mothers and explaining the problem. Our clinics are busy as well, and it is a huge exercise to counsel a large number of women. Surely the logical thing is for each area to establish the prevalence and decide whether or not they have got a problem. If they do a large screen periodically and they do not have a problem, then that is fine; they can carry on. Six months or a year later they can look at it again. When they have defined a problem that is the time to look at it and see what it takes: how many counsellors they are going to need, exactly what they are going to do, set up the follow-up services, and really do it in a responsible way. I am sure that even now there are areas that do not realise they have a problem. They should be doing this systematically, and intermittently. As soon as they think they have a problem then they need a full attributable screen. But it seems silly to set up a huge screening programme if you do not know what you are going to turn up; it is expensive and it is upsetting to everyone.

THOMPSON: I accept the fact that we should identify high risk areas and low risk areas. We are a low risk area, and we would screen, say 500-1000 of our population. Is that what you are suggesting?

JOHNSTONE: Yes, you take a month, and you screen everyone during that time.

THOMPSON: But the question is, if you are doing this anonymously, do you tell the patients that you are screening that month?

JOHNSTONE: You would have to tell the population that it is going on.

THOMPSON: You are going to have patients who will refuse to be screened, and they may represent high risk cases. So you are not going to get ideal screening.

JOHNSTONE: I think that whatever screening system you have, there are going to be some patients who are not going to be tested unless you test them without telling them. And I do not think that is a possibility.

SCOTT: This is another question for Professor Peckham since she raised the issue—and for Dr Mok as well. I was recently asked if an HIV positive woman might breastfeed her infant knowing that she was HIV positive, with its probable small risk. What would your response be to that?

MOK: I had a recent case just like that, and I said "Yes". She very successfully breastfed her infant.

PECKHAM: I think that sometimes we do not think enough about the advantages of breastfeeding. We are looking at the equation in an unbalanced way. It could be beneficial to breastfeed even though there might be a small increased, unquantifiable risk. So I would agree with that.

LUCAS: In theory, it is an unquantifiable risk, but there is some perhaps not particularly convincing evidence for infection via breastfeeding. But you might be more convinced by the very sizeable literature on the transfer of HTLV-I via breastfeeding, and prophylactic effect of bottlefeeding and also the beginning of the literature on direct experimental work in primates showing that retroviruses of other sorts can in fact be acquired during breastfeeding. When you take that into consideration, the risk is a little bit greater. Also, in the West one really would be very hard pressed to find hard data against bottlefeeding in morbidity terms. I think that one has to be realistic. There are really very little data.

McELWEE: Do we mean to give control over making decisions to the people who use our services? We need to be very clear about that. We need to make clear statements to the people who are using our services if that is our intention.

MORRIS: The most important thing that has emerged from our discussions is that although we have some excellent data, it has demonstrated that what we need is much more solid information so that we can guide our colleagues. I do not know of many obstetricians in this country who are aware of some of this information, even in some of the units where it happens. If obstetricians are going to take sensible decisions on the management of mothers they will need to have this information. I think that this applies not only to this country, but also abroad. I was in Asia where I met people who denied the presence of AIDS in the East. I think that they too need to hear more from us. Otherwise they are going to let it drift on, and they will be in a worse position. Maybe it is true, as was suggested in some of the papers, that so far the East has not become infected, but I think that one of the problems is that they are not looking for it. It is true that they do not have many advanced cases yet, but in a city like Seoul there are 750,000 prostitutes. So once the prostitutes become infected, they could create an alarming source of heterosexual transfer. We must emphasise the need for expanding the amount of support for research studies both in this country and others

SECTION III

OBSTETRIC MANAGEMENT PROBLEMS

Methods and reliability of antenatal diagnosis (including the effect of passive immunisation)

Professor W.P. Parks

(This paper was presented to the Study Group by Dr G.B. Scott on behalf of Professor Parks, but the author was unable to submit a manuscript for publication.)

Antenatal HIV screening—ethical considerations

Professor P. W. Howie

INTRODUCTION

Antenatal HIV screening has roused much controversy in the medical press. Discussion has centred round whether screening should be offered to all pregnant women or only to those in high risk groups, whether samples sent to the laboratories should be anonymous or identifiable and, most importantly, whether prior consent from the mother is required. It is easy to understand the basis for this controversy because, although antenatal HIV screening has advantages it also creates several problems.

CASE FOR ANTENATAL HIV SCREENING

Three reasons can be advanced in favour of antenatal HIV screening. The first is that screening identifies an HIV seropositive mother so that, after appropriate counselling, she can be offered termination of pregnancy. The second, argued by Sir Richard Doll in January 1987[1] and re-stated with several distinguished colleagues[2] is that HIV screening of pregnant women, by providing epidemiological data on prevalence, would help to fight the disease within the community. The third reason, which is less commonly stated, is that antenatal screening would help to prevent cross-infection, however small that risk might be, to other patients and staff.

It should be noted that only the first of these three reasons offers direct benefit to the mother and depends upon the assumption that pregnancy accelerates HIV seropositive women to clinical disease. It also assumes that seropositive mothers would opt for termination of pregnancy, so that to be sure of benefit it would be necessary to have prior knowledge of the mother's views about termination, in a manner similar to that required for consent for alphafetoprotein screening.

PROBLEMS OF ANTENATAL HIV SCREENING

While antenatal HIV screening offers benefits it also creates serious problems. The main problem relates to the consequences of a positive HIV result for the infected individual and her family. It is the understandable desire to avoid these severe personal and social consequences that gives rise to considering strategies which involve anonymous screening without consent. Other problems relating to antenatal HIV screening are more practical, such as finding resources for sample collection, laboratory testing and above all, for counselling, which may be very time consuming. There is also the problem of false positive results which require verification by Western blotting in order to avoid incorrect individual diagnosis and the rendering of prevalence studies as invalid.

DEFINITION OF TERMS

Discussions in the medical press have sometimes been confused because separate questions have become intertwined and because terms, especially "anonymous screening", have meant different things. It is therefore necessary to define the questions that need to be asked and the terms which are being used.

Three separate issues can be identified:
(i)   Should screening be elective or selective?
(ii) Should sample containers be anonymous or identifiable?
(iii) Should screening be done with consent (voluntary) or without consent?

These 3 questions, although interrelated, raise different ethical issues and require separate discussion.

SHOULD ANTENATAL HIV SCREENING BE ELECTIVE OR SELECTIVE?

Elective screening refers to an offer of HIV screening to all mothers; in contrast, selective screening is an offer of HIV screening to pregnant mothers in defined "high risk" groups. This question, although highly relevant to practising obstetricians, does not pose any specific ethical dilemmas. The answer to this issue revolves around the availability of resources and whether elective screening would give value for money. Thus, this question raises issues of management and of clinical judgement rather than any particular ethical problem. The Royal College of Obstetricians and Gynaecologists through its Report of the sub-committee on problems associated with AIDS in relation to obstetrics and gynae-cology (see Appendix), does not recommend routine HIV testing for all pregnant women at the present time. Should the prevalence of the disease increase rapidly in women of childbearing age this policy may have to be reconsidered and changed in the future.

SHOULD HIV SAMPLES BE ANONYMOUS OR IDENTIFIABLE?

The term "anonymous screening" has often been used as interchangeable with "unconsented" or "involuntary screening" and this has created confusion. For this paper, "anonymous screening" refers to the testing of an unlabelled untraceable sample in the laboratory. An identifiable sample is one which is labelled with the name or number of an identified subject. Anonymous testing used in this sense may be done with or without the mother's consent.

Defined in this way anonymous testing does not raise severe ethical problems but 3 possible objections to anonymous testing could be made. Firstly, the quality of prevalence studies will be reduced if anonymous testing is used because it will be more difficult to identify high and low risk individuals with confidence. In some cases it will not be possible to eliminate false positive results with confidence as testing on a further sample would be required. Some ethical objections can be raised against any research which is clearly sub-standard and may lead to false conclusions. Secondly, breaches of anonymity, although unlikely, are possible. For example, a new nurse to the antenatal clinic might write the name on a sample which is meant to be anonymous and which turns out to be HIV seropositive. Although such an event may be unlikely, any system which depends upon humans is liable to error. Should a patient who wished to remain anonymous be identified, such an event would create severe problems. Thirdly, should a prevalance study show that say 10 out of 3,000 patients were HIV seropositive this might create anxiety amongst the individuals who knew that they were part of that population, lest they were one of the 10 seropositive individuals, Furthermore, suspicion might be created amongst the staff dealing with that population knowing that they would have to deliver some individuals who were HIV positive. This latter objection could only be overcome if the results of prevalence studies were also kept confidential so that no hospital or area could be identified.

Despite these points, anonymous testing does not create major ethical difficulties provided the system is run efficiently and the prevalence results are handled with the necessary degree of confidentiality.

IS CONSENT FOR ANTENATAL HIV TESTING NECESSARY?

The major ethical dilemma concerns the question of consent. Screening "with consent" means that maternal permission for the test is obtained before the blood sample is drawn. Screening "without consent" involves HIV testing on part of a blood sample, drawn for other purposes, without the prior permission of the mother. This latter practice raises the ethical issue of informed consent. The case for testing without consent was put by Sir Richard Doll in 1987[1] and supported by Sir Douglas Black[2] and others in December of the same year. The main arguments in support of such a policy are that prevalence data will benefit the whole community, that testing without consent can do no harm to individuals and that testing without consent is already carried out for other conditions.

The validity of HIV screening without consent was questioned by Gillon in an article to the British Medical Journal in March, 1987.[3] In that article, Gillon points out that carrying out HIV testing without consent on antenatal mothers for the purpose of prevalence studies falls into the category of non-therapeutic medical research. The Declaration of Helsinki of 1983, states that in non-therapeutic medical research, the subjects should be volunteers who have the opportunity to abstain from participation after adequate information has been given. The Declaration goes on to state that the interests of science and society should never have precedence over the interests of individuals.[4] Thus, it is clear that any policy which involves HIV testing without consent challenges the established ethical principle of informed consent.

IS ANTENATAL HIV TESTING WITHOUT CONSENT REALLY NECESSARY?

In his analysis of HIV testing without permission, Gillon[3] goes on to ask whether testing without consent is really necessary. He examines some of the arguments which have been advanced in favour of HIV testing without consent. These were that:

(i)   It would be too cumbersome to obtain consent;
(ii) Prevalence studies would be inaccurate if withdrawal was allowed;
(iii) Testing without consent was already practised in other circumstances;
(iv) Consent was not legally necessary;
(v)   Consent was already implied;
(vi) Testing without consent could do no possible harm.

These different arguments will now be examined in turn.

Obtaining consent is too cumbersome

Gillon argues that signed witnessed consent is not required and all that is necessary is a general understanding on the part of the patient about what is involved. Information could be appropriately given in an explanatory leaflet sent to the mother before her first visit to the antenatal clinic giving any mother who did not wish to have antenatal HIV screening the opportunity to opt out. In this way, many of the practical difficulties would be overcome and detailed individual explanations would not be required.

Prevalence studies will be too inaccurate if withdrawal is permitted

It is certainly true that if there were large numbers of individuals who declined to participate in prevalence studies the value of the results would be seriously undermined. However, it appears that acceptance rates have been high in most studies that have been undertaken, particularly if the obstetricians in charge pursue the policy with enthusiasm.[5] When prevalence studies are done with consent, it provides the opportunity to identify high and low risk mothers with greater accuracy and there is also an opportunity to confirm the result on a second sample. Thus, prevalence studies with consent and without consent are evenly balanced as far as advantages and disadvantages are concerned.

Testing without consent is already practised

Because it has been common practice to carry out tests for conditions such as syphilis without specific consent from pregnant mothers does not necessarily justify the practice. Two wrongs do not make a right. A major difference between syphilis and HIV testing is that testing for syphilis confers an advantage upon the patient in a way that HIV testing does not. If it is argued that an offer of pregnancy termination to an HIV seropositive mother is an advantage to her, this will only be true if it is known that the mother would agree to a pregnancy termination. To justify such a claim of benefit it would be necessary to seek the mother's views about termination before the test were carried out and this is equivalent to obtaining consent for the test. It is not possible, therefore, to mount a satisfactory defence for HIV testing without consent on the grounds that testing without consent is carried out for other conditions. Indeed, it may be necessary for obstetricians to re-examine their practices and to consider giving all antenatal mothers a pamphlet with a list of all conditions which will be routinely tested on the blood samples withdrawn at the antenatal clinic.

Is consent for antenatal HIV screening legally necessary?

At its annual representative meeting in 1987 the British Medical Association passed a resolution "that testing for HIV antibodies should be at the discretion of the patient's doctor and not necessarily require the consent of the patient". In response to that resolution the BMA Council obtained a legal opinion from Mr Michael Sherrard, QC who said that in his view if a patient was tested for HIV without giving consent, the doctor would be at risk of being charged with assault. In an article summarising the position in the British Medical Journal it was stated that the GMSC endorsed the decision of the BMA Council not to implement the decision of the annual representatives meeting.[6] Although the resolution of the BMA had not been specifically referring to antenatal HIV testing, it is nevertheless clear that it may well be legally necessary to obtain consent to be sure of avoiding prosecution.

Is consent for HIV testing already implied?
In his article, Gillon[3] argues that any assumption that consent is implied by the patient allowing blood to be taken is undeniably false. It would certainly be unjustified to assume that consent was implied if no patient benefit could be demonstrated as a result of taking blood for the test. If in any circumstance there is any doubt about "implied consent" then there is an obligation upon the doctor to acquire specific permission.

Is it true that HIV testing without permission can do no possible harm?
Gillon's view[3] is that this is a doubtful ethical argument because there are some forms of behaviour which are wrong even if the consequences are likely to be good and no one will be harmed. Apart from the general ethical arguments, there are some practical reasons why testing without consent may cause some harm. One possible adverse effect is that if patients suspected that HIV testing was being carried out without consent they might stay away from such clinics. This might be especially true of high risk mothers who knew that they might have a chance of being HIV seropositive and also be in need of the antenatal care offered at the clinic. Earlier in this paper, mention has been made of the adverse consequences should any breach of anonymity occur by accident, and of the anxiety that might develop in patients who knew that they were part of a population in whom HIV seropositive mothers had been identified. These specific points are part of the more general argument that mistrust may develop between patients and medical staff if it becomes known that any procedures are being carried out on patients without their consent. The ethical principle of informed consent has been developed over many generations, and it would be most unwise to set it aside for any reason without serious consideration of the adverse consequences.

Antenatal HIV testing and the rights of staff and other patients
In discussions on antenatal HIV testing it is usually assumed that the rights of the individual patient are paramount. While the statement is undoubtedly true it does not mean that the rights of the staff and other patients to protect themselves deserve no consideration of any kind. If patients are identified as HIV seropositive, it is unreasonable to expect staff to expose themselves to potential risk during delivery, however small that risk might be, without giving them the

opportunity to take the necessary precautions to protect themselves. The same argument applies to other patients who will share the hospital facilities with the HIV positive mothers. This issue is not the paramount consideration in the debate concerning consent for antenatal HIV testing, but it serves to reinforce the view that prior consent should be obtained before HIV testing is carried out.

CONCLUSIONS

From this paper, it is argued that there is a strong case for antenatal HIV testing, especially in mothers who are in high risk groups. Whether HIV testing is extended to all pregnant mothers will depend partly upon available resources and partly upon the anticipated prevalence of the disease in any specific population. HIV testing in antenatal patients provides an opportunity for much needed prevalence studies, but there are dangers in carrying out such studies without the prior consent of mothers both from the ethical and legal standpoint. Existing experience suggests that most antenatal mothers will give their consent for antenatal HIV testing. Whether HIV testing should be carried out on anonymous or identified blood samples does not raise major ethical issues, but it appears that most mothers would prefer to know the result of their own sample, and the arguments for and against anonymous testing are evenly balanced. At present, it would appear that the preferred policy for antenatal HIV testing should be identified samples after prior consent.

REFERENCES
1. Doll R. A proposal for doing prevalence studies of AIDS. *Br Med J* 1987; **294:** 244.
2. Bodmer W, Cox D, Doll R, Durbin J, Hoffenberg R, Kingman J, Pefo J, Weiss R, Black D. HIV testing on all pregnant women (Letter). *Lancet* 1987, **2:** 1277.
3. Gillon R. Testing for HIV without permission. *Br Med J* 1987; **294:** 821-823.
4. Declaration of Helsinki. In: *The Handbook of Medical Ethics*. London: British Medical Association, 1984; pp.73-76.
5. AIDS and the Newborn. Report on a WHO Consultation. Copenhagen, 9-10th April, 1987.
6. Beecham J. Support for BMA council's decision on AIDS. (Editorial report). *Br Med J* 1987; **295:** 1428-1429.

Discussion

Chairman: Dr J. W. G. Smith

SMITH: In terms of practical clinical care, you said that that it is your practice to assume that babies born of infected mothers are infected themselves, until proven otherwise.

SCOTT: Unfortunately, the nurseries that we have only permit a "form" of isolation, which involves placing the infants in a particular.part of the nursery and using gown and gloves when handling them.

MOK: In your prospective studies how many negative virus cultures would you accept before you declare an infant free of infection?

SCOTT: I would have to put that into context with the clinical status of the infant. If there are any clinical signs or symptoms of HIV infection and the antibodies and the virus cultures are negative, we would still continue to follow that baby very vigourously. In cases of lymphadenopathy or hepatosplenomegaly we continue attempts to isolate the virus in that infant. In the infant who is clinically well, and the antibody is declining and the first 1 or 2 viral cultures are negative, we would probably not do a viral culture on every visit. However, we would continue to do cultures every 6 months to a year during our follow-up.

MOK: To what age?

SCOTT: In general, at the moment up to 15 months of age. With some of the newer data one could perhaps make a case for 18-24 months of age.

LUCAS: Professor Howie, you introduced 3 pairs of terms to clarify the situation in this ethical field. May I introduce another which I think might be helpful — the difference between research and audit. It is very revelant to the Helsinki Declaration that a patient has the right to know that they are having research done on them. Could I give you a couple of examples of what I would see as audit to see if you think that the anonymous screening for HIV could fall under this umbrella? Firstly, if you were to present the number of Caesarean sections that you performed last year, that would involve the presentation of patient data obtained anonymously, probably without consent, and you would not regard that in any way upsetting. You would not feel that you would need to approach the patient in that case. To give you a slightly more relevant example, we recently approached our ethical committee in Cambridge because we were worried about the high aluminium content of artificial intravenous feeds for premature babies. We asked if we could look at throwaway samples of blood and urine for aluminium. We were told by the ethics committee that this was not research; it was in fact, audit. Therefore, we did not require the patient's consent. I know that this does not resolve the issue of whether one should go for consent or non-consent, but it does tackle one important part of it. Do you think that the anonymous screening for HIV could be regarded as audit rather than research?

HOWIE: I do not think that you can justify it in that way. I do not think that it takes away from the fundamental issue of the need to do it with consent. In the case of the Caesarean sections, the patient knows that she has had a Caesarean section, so I do not think that is relevant. I do take your point though about the powdered milk and the aluminium. I think that in that case it is a balanced argument, but I do not think that the aluminium content in powdered milk has anything like the same level of implication for the patients. Obviously, it is a contentious issue, but I am not sure that the examples which you put overcome the difficulties.

LUCAS: Aluminium toxicity is damaging to brain, bone and blood. So we are talking abut the diagnosis of a potentially very serious problem.

HOWIE: But if there is aluminium in the milk it does not carry the social stigma of an HIV positive result.

GLYNN: I would like to make some points which I think are important. One which we keep forgetting is the problem of false positives. However, the HIV antibody tests are far more accurate than any other serological tests. Samples do get mixed up, but not very often. But no one is ever reported as positive until at least 3 or 4 tests have been done. The only way you can verify your results is by doing some anonymous testing.

I would entirely agree, in view of the Helsinki Agreement, that you should do no harm to the patient or anybody else on the basis of doing good to society. But there are degrees of harm. When you suggested that looking for aluminium cannot be compared to looking for HIV you said implicitly that it is not an absolute judgement. Assuming that there are no risks, then you can do no harm to the individual. I am not sure that I am too impressed by the arguments about the anxiety to staff and the patients that are being tested. Also, any doctor treating patients is benefitting from the research that has been done over the past years, with or without consent. Much of the research has been done on doctors themselves and by themselves. I should think that they would be happy to support future research.

HOWIE: I accept your point that the false positive issue is not a particular problem. Other doctors have given a slightly different view. Pregnancy may have more complications with false positives, but that is another issue.

SIMMONS: The argument has been put very clearly by Professor Howie. Dr Glynn says that ethics are not absolute, which is debatable. It was interesting that when this particular subject was debated in the Ethics Committee in this College, when some 2 to 3 years ago we tried to make a case for anonymous testing, the Committee, which is composed equally of lay and professional representatives, gave an absolutely unanimous answer. Anonymous testing for AIDS, without consent, was regarded in this particular debate as unethical. When that was taken to Council again it was absolutely unanimous.

McELWEE: The reality sometimes is that in a clinical situation with anonymous testing we are hoping that everyone that we test will be negative. The trouble starts when we get a positive result in an inappropriate place such as in an ordinary outpatient clinic or in an out-of-London antenatal clinic. I know of one woman last year who was told she had 3 days over Christmas to consider a termination of pregnancy because that was the only option open to her. We have to be very careful about what happens. Here it might be a debate, but out there people are practising testing without consent and then acting on it, not keeping it totally anonymous.

HOWIE: If it was intended to be anonymous, then the result should not have been divulged.

McELWEE: The intention was that it was to be anonymous. They just wanted to see if they had HIV in the area. But the consultant pathologist who had the name of the person sent it back to the consultant who felt that he had to tell the woman.

PATEL: I would support Professor Howie. I think that in Dundee and Edinburgh we have the two areas where the incidence of HIV positives in the population is quite high because of drug abuse. We also have this dilemma about deciding whether there should be anonymous testing with or without consent. If we opt for testing with consent, then a significant minority will opt out. In reality it does appear that the population would be very happy to be tested. If they do not wish to know the result they will say so. In a proper epidemiological study that would give us far more information, identifying not only the prevalence of HIV positives in the population, but also yielding epidemiological evidence that would come from high risk, and other groups in the population. In a pilot study both in Edinburgh and Dundee patients wanted to be tested with consent.

MILLS: I would like to extend the debate to HIV prevalence after screening the population with consent. We are dealing with a disease which we cannot cure. The only weapon that we have against it is prevention of spread. We are dealing also with a disease where there is a long latent period between infection with HIV and the development of AIDS. If we wait until we have the data on registered cases of AIDS we are going to have a higher prevalence of infection in the population. We have already debated whether we really do have the risk of HIV infection and AIDS in the heterosexual population. I think that without anonymous HIV screening in the population with consent we are going to have to wait far too long to get this sort of data to make our aims effective in the prevention of the spread of this disease.

JEFFRIES: I have little conflict with Professor Howie's conclusions. One has to to remember that we are dealing with a potentially very serious situation, and a changing situation. I accept that the College made a policy decision 2 years ago, but I think that things have changed since then. I would be very much against anything that affected the individual patient, but I think that we must bring 2 other factors into this equation. One is that it is looking now as though we can do something for these children who are HIV positive. Also, there are benefits in identifying positives, such as the effects of counselling on the family. Consent to testing comes down to good medical practice. When it comes to anonymous screening, there is information from London which indicates that the rate of positives is a lot higher than some people suspect. The first piece of information relates to one survey of the previous year's antenatal bloods where about 1% of the tests were positive, indicating a 0.3% prevalence in the antenatal population. In another study where patients in the antenatal clinic had been tested with their consent, the uptake was 68%. Of that group of 1000 sera 13 were found to be positive. Of these 13 positives the hospital believed that 12 would have been identified as having been exposed to a risk group or activity. One was picked up from someone who was not obviously in a risk group. One wonders what the rate would have been in the 32% of women who declined to be tested. So I would not be too influenced by decisions made 2 years ago; there are signs in this community, certainly in London, that the situation is changing very rapidly with the increasing prevalence of intravenous drug users. There is a strong case now for anonymous testing. In those regions with a high prevalence they may wish to select the point where testing will become routine in the antenatal clinic. Others may hold off for months or even years.

GLYNN: It is very important to distinguish between the tests that you do as a part of good clinical practice to help a particular patient as opposed to epidemiological surveillance where you want to get general information for the benefit of everyone. It is essential that the patient knows what is happening.

SCHOENBAUM: In New York City we have decided on anonymous testing, and we have learned a lot from anonymous testing. In the Bronx 2% of babies are infected. Anonymous testing has been carried out throughout the city in clinics devoted to prenatal care and abortion and found also that about 2% of the babies were infected. At our hospital we administer extensive counselling as well as screening to all prenatal patients. In addition, anyone who wants to be tested can order HIV testing on a confidential basis — what we call anonymous link study. The lab does not know who the patient is, but the patient is told the result and the doctor knows and may or may not put it in the chart depending on the agreement that he has with the patient. In addition to the anonymous link, patients can go to anonymous centres where they are the only person who knows the result.

There was obvious concern from the midwives and obstetricians that perhaps mandatory antenatal testing should be instituted, or certainly aggressively offered in a prenatal clinic. What we found was that less than 1% of the bloods from the prenatal clinic were positive for HIV antibody. In cord blood it was about 2%, but in the emergency room the prevalence was 8% of women who suspected that they were pregnant and had pregnancy tests done. Over 10% of general visitors who came to the emergency room were positive. Extensive education was necessary, but there were extremely limited funds. The state has now mandated that anyone who offers prenatal care should offer testing, but no money has been forthcoming to pay for the counselling and other follow-up services. So we have decided to concentrate our efforts on the emergency room and attempt to reach those women who are not getting prenatal care. It would not have been obvious to us if we had not done the anonymous testing. If we just focussed on the prenatal clinic we would not reach the large population of positives.

HOWIE: May I ask how you define anonymous testing?

SCHOENBAUM: It is largely a collaboration between the laboratory and the researcher. When the blood comes to the reseacher he is getting sera with no identification from the laboratory. The HIV testing is then done by a second laboratory or it could be done by the same laboratory as long as the blood was returned with no identification.

HOWIE: So that would limit your ability to know whether you were penetrating into the low risk or the high risk population.

SCHOENBAUM: Actually we refined the anonymous testing to an advanced degree. Depending on the level of collaboration with the laboratory we have been able to link the blood to gender, to race, to insurance type, to what clinic is sending the blood. These are very large numbers of bloods, so it would be impossible to go back and say who had a very low prevalance. It would be very dangerous to do this in small clinics where one could possibly guess who was positive.

There have been studies where the anonymous blood comes to the researcher unlinked to name, date of birth or anything which would allow you to identify the patient, but the chart is actually written to the researcher. So he knows the diagnosis and he knows that there has been a suspicion of a risk factor.

Others have suggested testing blood for drugs anonymously to see if there is a positive suspicion of drug use. It has evolved to a very detailed level of data collection, but it is still anonymous. Anyone who has ever been involved in anonymous testing knows that if it is not done absolutely correctly and carefully it is possible for the anonymity to break down.

HUDSON: The investigation mentioned by Dr Jeffries was approved by a human ethics committee which has legal and lay representation on it. This is examination of historical stored serum which has been taken for other investigations. There are no names or details attached. Obviously, the results cannot be verified in any way because there is no way of getting confirmatory specimens. The investigation can make a great deal of difference to the local plans for care, and I do not think that there would be any legal implications.

SMITH: I have the impression that there is strong support for Professor Howie's views, both scientifically and ethically, that voluntary named screening programmes are greatly preferable. But he did say that it has not been tried on a scale yet to find out if people do take part. Dr Jeffries' observations suggest that over 30% of people in the London area would not be prepared to take part in a voluntary programme.

JEFFRIES: That was in one particular hospital. But the acceptance rate depends very much on whether the women in the antenatal clinic are informed. I know a number of places in Europe where testing is being done on a routine basis with informed consent where nobody refuses. I take the point that has been made that if it is known that testing is going on in a particular clinic, then one may well be driving people out of hospital. It is a difficult decision.

SCOTT: Just recently in the New England Journal of Medicine[1] they published the results of a very large series of testing that was done in Boston and the surrounding area. They took neonatal blood that was designated for PKU testing. The eluted the blood and did serial HIV testing on it. From that very small amount of blood they were able to do the testing on several thousand patients. From that they were able to arrive at a prevalence rate for various hospitals in that area. The results will be used very much as those in New York have been used, to plan for health care programmes in those areas. Certainly, in that article it was felt this was a very reasonable way to do the testing. It was an unlinked type of testing, and considered ethical.

HEDGE: A large number of women have such an implicit trust in the medical profession that even if you tell them that this is an anonymous test, and so nobody will know the result, they actually believe that if anything is wrong the doctor will not let them slip through the net. The doctor will actually see them "okay". So if anyone is doing a study like that you have to go overboard to spell out that even if they are positive they cannot be told.

SIMMONS: I would just like to comment on what Dr Jeffries said about changing position. It seems to me that, despite that, the ethics of anonymous testing is unaltered. Essentially what he has said is that this is "my blood". If you do an investigation then he is entitled to know the results and act upon them. Although historically one has done that sort of investigation without consent, this is an error. People's expectations in relation to the profession have altered also. They expect to be informed now in a way which they did not formerly. We cannot go back to what was done 50 years ago, ethically, in the context of society as it is today. It seems to me, on the evidence of what the Ethics Committee here would say, that if you can conduct this within accepted guidelines and get the information, then that should at least be the initial approach. If at the end of that investigation it is found that the information cannot be obtained within accepted ethical guidelines of the system, then there may be a case. It may be a government decision. Where there is a national emergency that requires dispensation outside normal behaviour that is a government decision through the Department of Health as it would be in the case of war. We are talking about a national emergency which requires behaviour outside normal standards. That is something that needs to be decided by the administration. That is not something that a medical ethical body could decide.

GREEN: One of the issues here is that you do not need to have an "either/or" situation. Either you are going to have anonymous testing or many women are going to have the test and find out what their test results are. We intend to carry out some anonymous testing with consent. With intravenous drug abusers it is a slightly different population. At the same time we are going to test them, and should they wish to have HIV tests, they are available. We talk to them about that. We never push the test on them. We try to make it clear what the advantage of being tested is. One of the issues about informed consent is that very often people are not informed very well, and the consent that they give is sometimes under some degree of duress. If you are approached by someone who is an eminent medical figure, and who tells you that the test is available, who tells you that "you can refuse to have it but . . .", then very often it is very difficult for a woman under those circumstances to refuse.

JOHNSTONE: It is unhelpful for us to muddy the situation by confusing or not telling the patient. I do not think we should be discussing testing secretly or without consent. I am sure there would be a broad level of agreement from all of us that that should not happen. To confuse anonymous with secret is just unhelpful.

For us to carry on year after year talking about and remaining in ignorance of the prevalence has an ethical dimension in itself. We have not talked much about the expense of counselling, for example 10,000 women a year. Either you pretend to counsel them, or else you do it properly. And that is very expensive. It is perfectly reasonable to carry out anonymous testing with the population knowing what is going on. We have to say to everyone, as we did in Lothian, that we will test them but they have to attend a counselling session which is held in each hospital once each week. In this way they can have the implications of testing explained to them. It is possible to have prevalence screening, and yet allow people to opt out and opt in by going along to the counsellor. That is cheap; it is much cheaper than approaching every woman in the clinic.

HARE: I come from East Anglia where the incidence of AIDS is the second lowest in the country. I have the results of testing for two series last year. Of 4,400 specimens 63 were positives. A number of those were duplicates and a number of people have been diagnosed later to East Anglia. Are you really suggesting that the ethical situation has changed over the past 2 years because of the increase in prevalence in parts of the country? In that case, where does that leave us in East Anglia? From the kind of incidence that we presume from those figures that I have quoted, does Dr Glynn still say that false positives are not a significant factor in areas like East Anglia? Perhaps someone could tell me how much it costs?

GREENWOOD: I work with the DHSS but I do not know the answer to that question. If a woman consents now to give an antenatal sample then we could go on and test it. If, as I understand it, it is being suggested that this sample of blood be kept for a number of years in the laboratory, who then does that blood belong to—to the woman? or to the health authority?

SMITH: I have discussed this question with legal people, and I do not think that there is a correct answer. Probably the legal bottom line is that it is the property of the person who donated the blood. As to the cost, I think that when everything is taken into account it is about £3.00 per test.

GLYNN: If you are concerned with the individual patient, then the chance of a false positive being false because of a laboratory error is extremely low, and prevalence does not come into it. There is a very low possibility indeed that this matters. If you do the test with a 99.5% specificity you have a 1 in 200 chance of a false positive. If you get a positive, you will do 2 or 3 tests which means that your chances of eventual positive is rather less than one in a million. Your prevalence is higher than that. I should like to comment on Mr Simmons' point. He said that ethics do not change, but they do. We do not think the same way about things as we did 20 years ago. I would be very worried if, because of what we see as a dire emergency, we were to change our ethics. If we cannot find the information we need ethically, then I am afraid that I would just not seek it, even if a government were to give me a dispensation on ethics. I have no great faith in the ethics of government.

HOWIE: I understood that the results of the anonymous testing showed a surprisingly high incidence of positive results. Does that not now indicate that the real investigation should be by consent so that you can identify whether there are high risk or low risk parts of the population. From a practical point of view that is what it is important to know.

JEFFRIES: I think that there is probably a need for a number of different studies in terms of different sectors of the population. Coming to Mr Hare's point, the kind of occasional sampling he described is of considerable use and would be done on a geographical basis. One can go for a truly guaranteed anonymous screening based on Guthrie testing, for example. This may suggest the desirability or otherwise of going ahead with a more aggressive programme of testing with informed consent. What is the situation with regard to risk activity as opposed to other possibilities in the community? What is the geographical distribution? We know that Edinburgh has a problem and Dundee has a problem, and London's problem is increasing. There may be other pockets of drug users that we are not aware of. I wonder whether Mr Simmons would rule out the possibility of something more centralised which cannot possibly get back to the individual patient, along the lines of Guthrie testing.

SIMMONS: If things have changed, and you feel that there is a need to review the situation, the College would do so on the advice of this Study Group. Having looked at the question once, the College would look again. The ethical dimension would go to its Ethics Committee, and that would advise the Council. They would certainly agree to the need to look at this problem again in the light of the information which has been provided.

SCRIMGEOUR: Several times it has been mentioned that Edinburgh has a problem. We know that we have a problem amongst intravenous drug abusers; we know that we have certain high risk patients. What we do not know either in Edinburgh or Dundee is what the rest of the community is doing. This is essential information. What we have done in our pilot studies is to ask the patients, both in terms of a written form given to them before they come to the clinic, and a verbal enquiry at the antenatal clinic as to whether they would prefer to know that they were being tested, and whether they would prefer to know the result having been tested. I think that what is going to happen if we drag our feet much longer is that the patients are going to tell us what to do. They are certainly going to tell us that they want to know that they are being tested. They want to know the result of the test and the implications. Otherwise we are going to land in that situation that was described so eloquently.

REFERENCE
1. Hoff R, Berardi VP, Weiblen BJ, Mahoney-Trout L, Mitchell MJ, Grady GF. Seroprevalence of human immunodeficiency virus among childbearing women: estimation by testing samples of blood from newborns. *N Engl J Med* 1988; **318**: 525-530.

Counselling the HIV positive pregnant woman

Dr B. Hedge

INTRODUCTION

In Europe and America today most women infected with human immuno-deficiency virus (HIV) are found to belong to groups at high risk for HIV infection. That is, they or their sexual partners have been injecting drug users,[1] or they are the partners of bisexual men or haemophiliacs,[2, 3] or they or their partners have had sexual contact with people from the Caribbean or Central Africa.[4] However, there is increasing evidence that HIV infection now extends to heterosexually active young people with none of these traditional risk factors. Hoff *et al*[5] found a 0.2% prevalence rate for HIV infection in women giving birth in hospitals in Massachusetts, but noted that the infection rate varied within the geographical area sampled, being highest (0.8%) in inner city hospitals and lowest in suburban and rural hospitals (0.09%). Tempelis *et al*[6] noted cases of HIV infection in serum samples from blood collected in sexually transmitted disease (STD) clinics and premarital testing sites in the San Francisco Bay area which indicate that HIV is present in heterosexuals with no other risk factors than unprotected sexual intercourse.

Although the spread of HIV within the heterosexual population in the UK lags behind the spread in North America,[7] there is no reason to suppose that it will not follow the same trend. Indeed the number of cases of AIDS in the United Kingdom reported to the Communicable Disease Surveillence Centre and the Communicable Diseases (Scotland) Unit indicates a similar but delayed trend in this country with 47 adult heterosexuals (non-injecting drug users) and 13 children reported by the end of February 1988. Of these adults 9 are presumed to have been infected in the United Kingdom. As the number infected with HIV is many times greater than the number presenting with AIDS it seems likely that the number of HIV seropositive women currently conceiving will increase markedly over the next few years.

If a woman knows she is HIV seropositive then she can be alerted to the issues concerning pregnancy and childbearing before conception,[8] but a number of women will discover their HIV status when already pregnant and some will fail to prevent conception although they are aware of their seropositivity.[9] The report of the RCOG sub-committee on problems associated with AIDS in relation to obstetrics and gynaecology[10] recognises that the seriousness of the consequences of intrauterine transmission of HIV is sufficient to comply with the requirements of the 1967 Abortion Act. The first decision to be made by a seropositive woman is whether to continue with the pregnancy or to seek termination. A major difficulty encountered by the HIV positive woman when deciding whether to continue with a pregnancy is the uncertainty attached to the outcome of the event. Not only is the rate of transmission of HIV uncertain but it is also not clear what the effects are of HIV on the pregnancy or of pregnancy on the mother's health.

This paper argues that counselling should be made available to these women and suggests the issues which should be addressed, the problems encountered when a counselling service is not available and factors which are likely to make counselling effective.

HIV AND PREGNANCY

There are a number of reports addressing the issues relating to pregnancy in the HIV positive woman[11,12] so only a brief summary of the problems is given here.

Intrauterine transmission of HIV

Mok[13] suggests that not all mothers infected with HIV transmit the virus to the fetus. A working estimate is that at least 50% of the infected infants will develop AIDS.

Perinatal infection

There are reports of HIV infection from cervical secretions,[14,15] which suggest that infants could be infected during vaginal delivery.

Post-natal infection

Zeigler et al[16] report transmission of HIV from mother to baby via breast milk. Although this is supported by Thiry's report of the isolation of HIV from breast milk,[17] there are a number of reports of babies breastfed by seropositive mothers who have not contracted the infection.[18]

The effect of the virus on pregnancy

There are few reports of the effect of HIV on the outcome of pregnancy. Johnstone et al[19] compared the outcome of pregnancies in HIV positive and HIV negative but well women who had a history of injecting drug use or who had HIV positive partners. They found adverse outcomes equally in the two groups but more spontaneous abortions in the seropositive group. However, they suggest that the abortion rate in the HIV positive group seemed low and so there is little evidence that HIV adversely affected the outcome of pregnancy in well women. It is not clear whether these findings would remain the same in women who were already symptomatic or whether they should be generalised to a non drug abusing population.

The effect of pregnancy on a woman's health

There have been suggestions[11,12] that pregnancy might accelerate the progress of HIV disease. Some cases have been reported where the health of the mothers did deteriorate during pregnancy,[13,19] but once again there is little substantial evidence. Mayer *et al*[20] report a case of T-cell activation being increased during pregnancy which could suggest that the mother's health was at risk. However whether this would hold true for women at different stages of infection is not known.

Summary

It is then not possible to tell a pregnant woman what the outlook is for her or her baby's health, or the likely outcome of her pregnancy. The information only gives estimates of outcomes and it is not clear that the information available now will apply to all HIV women, or to groups with different lifestyles or at all stages of infection. Nor is it possible to suggest any option, either to terminate the pregnancy or to continue with it, that will guarantee that the mother remains healthy. The decision of whether to continue with the pregnancy may well be hard to make, but can also be hard to live with. Psychological difficulties may well be seen in those attempting to make or live with such decisions.

PSYCHOLOGICAL PROBLEMS ASSOCIATED WITH HIV

When counselling is not encouraged or not readily available a wide range of psychological problems have been seen in those who are HIV positive. These are described in detail by Miller *et al*[21] and Coates *et al.*[22] A number of psychological problems are encountered by most HIV positive women when pregnant, but Shaw and Palev[23] note the particular impact that HIV may have on those women who see their primary role to be that of mother and caretaker. Although the difficulties encountered will be specific to each particular case generalisations can be made, and the following reactions are commonly seen.

Shock

A frequent reaction to the discovery of pregnancy is shock. Shock is often most easily dealt with by denial of the event which caused it. In this situation denial of pregnancy can lead to the pregnancy being continued without reasoned consideration of possible outcomes. Not only may the option of termination not be considered, or only considered in the later stages of pregnancy, but denial of the pregnancy may result in the woman not receiving adequate antenatal care.

Anxiety

The number of uncertainties to be considered can generate excessive anxiety in an HIV positive woman. There is some suggestion that stress itself is immunosuppressive,[22] and so should be minimised in those who are HIV positive. A further complication is that stress also makes rational thought more difficult and decisions become harder to take.

Depression

Even when the decision of whether to continue with the pregnancy has been made depression is often seen. Whatever the decision, there is no positive message that by acting this way the woman will remain well, and little possibility that pregnancy will be an option at a later date. If a spontaneous miscarriage occurs the desire to become pregnant again can be increased, and it is suggested that if further pregnancies are prevented depression and anger may well be seen.

Anger and frustration

When pregnancy occurs in women who have, or whose partners have stopped using drugs anger and frustration are frequently encountered. Although these women have effected a major change in their lifestyle, towards a pattern of greater social "acceptability" these changes have come too late to prevent infection with HIV. The anger generated is often directed towards those medical and associated professionals who helped with their change in lifestyle, and further advice and help from these authorities may well be rejected, and with it necessary antenatal care and support.

Loss of control

The loss of control over such a natural event as having a child can lower a woman's self-esteem, especially in those for whom childbearing is of primary importance. Women who have been drug abusers or see themselves as having been excessively sexually active often already have a low self image and so a further inadequacy can accelerate depression and may have a detrimental effect on current relationships or on the care of existing children. Self-esteem can also be undermined when women with HIV are perceived as being drug users or prostitutes simply because they are infected with the virus, irrespective of the veracity of such perceptions. This may result in withdrawal and self-imposed isolation from society and medical services.

Obsessional behaviour

When a woman decides to continue with a pregnancy having been informed of the risks, every different bodily sensation can be interpreted as a sign that HIV disease is progressing, rather than as a sign of pregnancy or as a symptom of anxiety. Involuntary thoughts of progressive illness and compulsive activities such as body checking can take up considerable periods of time and can lead to work deteriorating and relationships falling apart.[24]

Guilt

Pregnancy can also increase feelings of guilt especially if one partner feels responsible for aquiring the infection (eg. the drug using partner). Such feelings can be intensified if the baby is born sick or dies and may lead to suicidal thinking and even to the rejection of those one has infected in order to spare them pain.

THE CHARACTERISTICS OF EFFECTIVE COUNSELLING

Miller *et al*[25] suggests that the efficacy of counselling does not seem to be primarily dependent on the counselling style used or the particular caring profession of the counsellor. What is important is that counselling is readily available and that certain basic principles are maintained.

It has been observed that in medical consultations few facts are retained especially in times of stress.[26] This suggests that when counselling an HIV positive pregnant woman important information should be repeated several times in simple language and in concrete terms.[27] This can most easily be done by the counsellor translating general statements (eg. the likely risk of an HIV positive baby becoming ill and dying) into specific scenarios with the parts being "played" by the woman's family and friends.

It can be useful to encourage the woman to consider the best possible and the worst possible outcomes for the baby, for herself and for others involved. This approach is less traumatic than simply discussing the possible negative consequences. It also illustrates well the range of dilemmas which may have to be faced if the pregnancy is continued. It can also be helpful to elicit emotions which the woman would expect to feel for each considered outcome and to discuss how she might cope with such feelings.

It can be seen then that a necessary requisite of good counselling is sufficient time for adequate discussion. It is also important that counsellors are familiar with the latest medical evidence relating to HIV and the pregnant woman, so that accurate, up to date information is available.

When counselling about any aspect of HIV great emphasis must be placed on the need for confidentiality. This is a matter of routine in STD clinics but needs to be built into counselling centres everywhere. The more people involved with a woman the easier it becomes for accidental breaches of confidence to occur. This may suggest changes in obstetric practice to a system where women are allocated one or two key workers who, except for emergencies, will see them through their pregnancies.

The qualities of a counsellor which have generally been found to enhance therapy are warmth, empathy and genuineness.[28] This suggests that to counsel HIV positive patients a counsellor should be able to accept, understand and feel comfortable discussing various sexual and social lifestyles. It does not imply that good counselling can only be given by those of a particular sex or sexual orientation, or by those with a lifestyle similar to the patient.

While HIV infection has been seen mainly in homosexual men and injecting drug users, counselling has generally been made available in STD clinics and Drug Dependency Units. However, most women are more frequent users of antenatal and gynaecological out-patient facilities and so the finding[29] that women were less likely to accept counselling sessions held in a STD clinic comes as no surprise. Rather it does suggest that as HIV is increasingly seen in the traditionally "low risk" groups counselling should be made available in those places which are already acceptable to women such as Family Planning Clinics, antenatal clinics and gynaecological out-patient clinics.

Who needs counselling?

The HIV seropositive woman may or may not have a stable partner who may or may not be the father of the child she is carrying. There will be some women whose partner is already sick, dying or dead. This means that it is important that counselling be directed at the pregnant woman together with any others who are significant in her life. This could be a partner, friends or relatives. Future care of the woman if she becomes ill and of the baby, if the mother is unable or unwilling to look after the child, are matters to be discussed. Therefore the involvement of all concerned as early as possible ensures that relevant information reaches those who need to know. Decisions and joint decision-making can then be encouraged. Partners who are involved can be very supportive and lessen the need for professional help at a later date.[24] However, as experience has shown, the decision to involve "significant others", particularly on a longer-term basis, must rest with the patient herself.[24]

When should counselling be given?
Counselling should be made available as early as possible during pregnancy so there is time for issues to be discussed and for the woman to arrive at an informed decision as to whether to continue with the pregnancy or to request a termination. Women for whom the discovery of their HIV positive status coincides with the onset of pregnancy will be under acute stress and may well take time to report the pregnancy. These women have little time to consider a termination. It is, therefore, of vital importance that a support service which has provision for immediate counselling is available.

The aims of counselling
The primary aim of counselling is to provide the necessary medical and social information for informed decisions to be made. However, as Miller[21] notes, one of the psychological effects of being HIV positive is a feeling of loss of control over the future. In the HIV positive pregnant woman this perceived loss of control can easily manifest itself as a failure to make any decision regarding the continuation of the pregnancy and so allow the pregnancy to continue by default.

A second important aim is therefore to ensure that some decision is made. Although the woman should be encouraged to take time and consider the alternatives, some time limit will usually be necessary. It is beneficial to agree during the first counselling session on a specific date by which the decision of whether to continue with the pregnancy will be taken. It is important that this choice is made by the woman, and that she is clear that it is her decision, not that of the counsellor or of any member of the medical profession. It is not the role of a counsellor to make the decision for her. The pregnancy remains the responsibility of the woman and the right to continue with it hers. Often by recognising and respecting a woman's responsibilities and choices a counsellor can restore a sense of control and increase self-esteem. The decision of whether to continue with the pregnancy is then more likely to be made rationally than emotively. Counselling should also provide ongoing support, as and when necessary to assist the woman to live with her decision whatever the outcome.

Psychological intervention
As noted earlier some women will experience quite marked psychological trauma when faced with both HIV infection and pregnancy. For those women there should be access to psychological or psychiatric expertise as necessary.

Psychological intervention may be necessary when a woman is severely distressed. Although the cause of this distress is novel, its manifestations are classic and there are many well established treatment programmes available. An approach which focusses on enhancing the woman's coping abilities and her self-esteem has been found effective.[30] Specifically, such intervention can provide the woman with techniques to manage excessive anxiety and stress, skills to aid decision-making, ways of coping with depressed and suicidal thoughts and with obsessional behaviour and ruminations.[31-34] Self-esteem can also be boosted by recognising the woman's right to control the pregnancy and respecting her decision.

The uncertainty of a baby's HIV status for some time after birth and of the child's continuing good health if seropositive means that the psychological problems encountered during pregnancy do not remit at birth. If support is not available increased difficulties with any existing family and with ongoing relationships may occur. It is important to recognise that the tensions associated with HIV are always dynamic, and many issues in counselling recur as new crises emerge over time.

As HIV has such a stigma attached, many seropositive people are counselled to tell as few people as possible of their status. A repercussion of this can be that only a limited number of people are available to give support over these difficult periods. It would seem essential that counselling be available to minimise trauma and to maximise quality of life.

CONCLUSIONS

As well as providing HIV positive pregnant women with the necessary information for an informed decision to be made concerning the continuation of the pregnancy, effective counselling helps women make and then live with their decisions. It also provides continuing tailor-made support as and when necessary, whether the pregnancy has been terminated or continued. Counselling also aims to provide access to other relevant professionals in order to maintain the woman's mental and physical health.

If the necessary counselling facilities are to be available for HIV positive pregnant women then an effective liaison must be established between the obstetricians, counsellors and supporting services such as social and community workers, psychologists and psychiatrists.

Although the number of women currently requiring these services is small, there are indications that the numbers are increasing and will continue to do so for some years. It is therefore suggested that obstetricians and gynaecologists address the issue of counselling HIV positive women now, so that facilities are available when needed.

REFERENCES
1. France AJ, Skidmore CA, Robertson JR, Brettle RP, Roberts JJK, Burns SM, Foster CA, Inglis JM, Galloway WBF, Davidson SJ. Heterosexual spread of human immunodeficiency virus in Edinburgh. *Br Med J* 1988; **296:** 526-529.
2. Allain JP. Prevalence of HTLV-III/LAV antibodies in patients with haemophillia and their sexual partners in France. *N Engl J Med* 1986; **315:** 517-518.
3. Guinan ME, Hardy A. Epidemiology of AIDS in women in the United States 1981 through 1986. *JAMA* 1987; **257:** 2039-2042..

4. Fischl MA, Dickson GM, Scott GB, Klimas N, Fletcher MA, Parks W. Evaluation of heterosexual partners, children and household contacts of adults with AIDS. *JAMA* 197; **257:** 640-644.

5. Hoff R, Berari VP, Weiblen BJ, Mahoney-Trout L, Mitchell ML, Grady GF. Seroprevalence of human immunodeficiency virus among child bearing women. *N Engl J Med* 1988; **318:** 525-530.

6. Tempelis CD, Shell G, Hoffman M, Benjamin RA, Chandler A, Francis DP. Human immunodeficiency virus infection in women in the San Fransisco Bay area. *JAMA* 1987; **258:** 474-275.

7. Evans BA, McCormack SM, Bond RA, MacRae KD, Thorp RW. Human immunodeficiency virus infection, hepatitis B virus infection, and sexual behaviour of women attending a genitourinary medicine clinic. *Br Med J* 1988; **296:** 473-475.

8. Steele SJ. Pre-conceptual counselling. In: *AIDS and obstetrics and gynaecology*. Eds. R Hudson, F Sharp. London: Royal College of Obstetricians and Gynaecologists/Springer-Verlag, 1988; pp.317-319.

9. Scott GB, Fischl MA, Klimas N, Fletcher MA, Dickinson GM, Levine RS, Parks WP. Mothers of infants with the acquired immunodeficiency syndrome. Evidence for both symptomatic and asymptomatic carriers. *JAMA* 1985;**253:** 363-366.

10. Royal College of Obstetricians and Gynaecologists. *Report of the RCOG Subcommittee on problems associated with AIDS in relation to obstetrics and gynaecology*. London: Royal College of Obstetricians and Gynaecologists, 1987.

11. Pinching AJ, Jeffries DJ. Aids and HTLV-III/LAV infection: consequences for obstetrics and perinatal medicine. *Br J Obstet Gynaecol* 1985; **92:** 1211-1217.

12. Peckham CS, Senturia YD, Ades AE. Obstetric and perinatal consequences of human immunodeficiency virus (HIV) infection: a review. *Br J Obstet Gynaecol* 1987; **94:** 403-407.

13. Mok JQ, Giaquinto C, De Rossi A, Grosch-Wörner I, Ades AE, Peckham CS. Infants born to mothers seropositive for human immunodeficiency virus. Preliminary findings from a multicentre European study. *Lancet* 1987; **1:** 1164-1168.

14. Vogt MW, Witt DJ, Craven DE, Byington R, Crawford DF, Schooly RT, Hirsch MS. Isolation of HTLV-III/LAV from cervical secretions of women at risk for AIDS. *Lancet* 1986; **1:** 525-527.

15. Wofsy CB, Cohen JB, Hauer LB, Padian NS, Michaelis BA, Evans LA, Levy JA. Isolation of AIDS-associated retrovirus from genital secretions of women with antibodies to the virus. *Lancet* 1986; **1:** 527-529.

16. Ziegler JB, Cooper DA, Johnson RO, Gold J. Postnatal transmission of AIDS-associated retrovirus from mother to infant. *Lancet* 1985; **1:** 896-898.

17. Thiry L, Sprecher-Goldberger S, Jonckheer T, Levy J, Van de Perre P, Henrivaux P, Cogniaux-Le-Clerc J, Clumeck N. Isolation of AIDS virus from cell-free breast milk of three healthy virus carriers. *Lancet* 1985; **2:** 891-892.

18. Senturia YD, Ades AE, Peckham CS, Giaquinto C. Breast-feeding and HIV infection *Lancet* 1987; **2:** 400-401.

19. Johnstone FD, Maccallum L, Brettle R, Inglis JM, Peutherer JF. Does infection with HIV affect the outcome of pregnancy? *Br Med J* 1988; **296:** 467.

20. Mayr P, Fuchs D, Fuith L, Hausen A, Reibnegger G, Werner ER, Watcher H. Allogeneic activation is increased during pregnancy. A risk factor in HIV infection? *Br J Obstet Gynaecol* 1987; **94:** 1000-1002.

21. Miller D. Psychology, AIDS, ARC and PGL. In: *The management of AIDS patients*. Eds. D Miller, J Weber, J Green. Basingstoke: Macmillan, 1986; pp 131-149.

22. Coates TJ, Temoshock L, Mandel JS. Psychosocial research is essential to understanding and treating AIDS. *Am Psychol* 1984; **39:** 1309-1314.

23. Shaw N, Palev L. Women and AIDS. In: *What to do about AIDS*. Ed. L McKusick. Berkeley: University of California Press, 1986; pp 142-154.

24. Miller D. *Living with AIDS*. Basingstoke: Macmillan, 1987.

25. Miller D, Green J, McCreaner A. Organising a counselling service for problems related to the acquired immune deficiency syndrome (AIDS). *Genitourin Med* 1986; **62:** 116-122.
26. Ley P, Spelman MS. *Communicating with the patient*. London: Staples, 1967.
27. Bradshaw PW, Ley P, Kincey JA, Bradshaw J. Recall of medical advice: comprehensibility and specificity. *Br J Soc Clin Psychol* 1975; **14:** 55-62.
28. Rogers CR. The necessary and sufficient conditions of therapeutic personality change. *J Cons Psychol* 1957; **21:** 95.
29. Anonymous. Fewer pregnant women agree to to the test. *New Scientist* 1988; **117, 1602:** 35.
30. Namir S. Treatment issues concerning persons with AIDS In: *What to do about AIDS*. Ed. L McKusick. Berkeley: University of California Press, 1986; pp 86-94.
31. Nicholls KA. Psychological care in general hospitals. *Bull Br Psychol Soc* 1981; **34:** 90-94.
32. Walker CE, Hedberg A, Clement PW, Wright L. *Clinical procedures for behaviour therapy*. Englewood Cliffs: Prentice-Hall, 1981.
33. Beck AT. *Cognitive therapy and the emotional disorders*. New York: International University, 1976.
34. Beech HR, Vaughan M. *Behavioural treatment of obsessional states*. Chichester: Wiley, 1978.

Termination of pregnancy

Dr F.D. Johnstone

BACKGROUND

Whereas in England and Wales it is still predominantly homosexual men who are infected with human immunodeficiency virus (HIV), HIV seropositivity in Scotland occurs largely in intravenous drug users (60% of all HIV seropositivity) and 60% of those infected in this way live in Edinburgh. This situation arose because of an epidemic of intravenous drug abuse (IVDA) in the early 1980s, documented by the rise in drug-related morbidity during that time, together with widespread sharing of equipment. The introduction of HIV, probably from a single source in mid-1983, meant that the infection swept through the drug-using community.[1] A third of IVDA are women, and others are becoming infected from HIV positive partners. Edinburgh therefore has a serious local problem with HIV infection and pregnancy.

KNOWN PREVALENCE OF HIV IN PREGNANCY

Testing for HIV in pregnancy in Edinburgh has been by case finding rather than screening, and plans to carry out a total prevalence study in early 1987 were stopped to allow a large attributable screening programme, though this has not yet started. Therefore the prevalence of HIV infection in pregnancy is still unknown. Of over 300 pregnant women whose HIV status is known, the only seropositives were found in those who had injected drugs themselves (50% of whom were seropositive), or those whose partner was known to be seropositive through drug use. Table 1 shows that no seropositives were found in the remaining categories of risk activity.

Table 1

Women with known HIV status during pregnancy—Edinburgh 31 December 1987

Risk Factor	Number of individuals tested (including retrospectively)	HIV positive No.	%
IVDA	120	61	50
Partner IVDA and HIV +ve	34	6	18
Partner IVDA (HIV status unknown)	48	0	—
Other drug used by patient	15	0	—
Other indication	98	0	—

IVDA = intravenous drug abuser

If we consider pregnancies in Edinburgh City residents only, which terminated between October 1985 and December 1987, and extrapolate total city figures from the 1985 data (the most recent year for which figures are available), we find that in approximately 1.5% of pregnancies the mother was screened for HIV by the Maternity Service. The known prevalence of HIV, and this is certainly an underestimate of the true figure, is approximately 0.4%. However, this varies according to the outcome of the pregnancy, with a known prevalence of approximately 0.3% in term deliveries, but 0.7% in induced abortions. There is also variation between hospitals, and in 1.1% of terminations carried out at Edinburgh Royal Infirmary/Simpson Memorial Maternity Pavilion the woman was known to be HIV positive.

USE OF INDUCED ABORTION BY HIV POSITIVE WOMEN

Pregnancy outcome in HIV positive women (up to December 1987) is shown in Table 2. Out of 79 pregnancies, 30% were terminated. Though this is a high proportion it cannot be assumed that HIV status was the sole indication. The pregnancy outcome in seronegative women who were tested for the same indications (ie. intravenous drug abuse or a partner known to be seropositive) is shown in the same table. Out of 101 pregnancies there were 20 induced abortions, not significantly different from the seropositive women. Similarly, in pregnancies occuring before HIV, those women who were seropositive had had 22% of their 97 pregnancies terminated. This therefore is a population whose use of induced abortion is likely to be above average even without the additional problem of HIV infection.

In several of the pregnancies the diagnosis of HIV infection was made only retrospectively or late in pregnancy. In others the woman attended too late for termination of pregnancy to be considered. Of women who have attended recently who were less than 20 weeks when first seen, and who had detailed

Table 2

Pregnancy outcome in women who are HIV seropositive,
and also women who are HIV seronegative but were tested for the same indications.

	HIV +ve	HIV +ve (same indication)	Total
Number of women	65	91	156
Number of pregnancies	79 (100%)	101 (100%)	180 (100%)
Delivered	38 (48%)	68 (68%)	106 (59%)
Pregnant	6 (8%)	6 (6%)	12 (7%)
Spontaneous abortion	11 (14%)	7 (7%)	18 (10%)
Termination	24 (30%)	20 (20%)	44 (24%)

counselling, 50% opted for termination of pregnancy and this may be more representative of future trends. Several had termination predominantly because of social factors, but at least 5 women had wanted pregnancies which were terminated purely because of HIV infection or medical advice; 2 women had AIDS and 1 had chronic liver disease and ARC.

ASSESSMENT OF THE HIV POSITIVE PATIENT IN PREGNANCY
Two of the critical factors in advising about pregnancy are the risk of the fetus becoming infected and the likely state of the mother's health over the subsequent few years. To a certain extent, assessment of the mother may help in defining both these risks.

There is a widely held belief, not yet adequately substantiated by data, that the risk of the fetus becoming infected *in utero* is related to the mother's immune status; that is, transplacental infection is most likely when the immune system becomes compromised and viraemia increases. Certainly the European Collaborative Study[2] has shown that infection is 9 times more common in babies whose mother had symptomatic HIV infection during pregnancy.

As far as the mother is concerned, there are a large number of data, mainly from homosexual men, highlighting markers for imminent progression to AIDS. Clinical markers include persistent oral candidal infections, weight loss, fever, diarrhoea, seborrhoeic dermatitis and hairy cell leukoplakia of the tongue. A simple but highly predicitive investigation is a full blood count, where leucopaenia, a low platelet count or a normochromic anaemia are good predictors of the later development of AIDS.[3] Less generally available investigations which should nevertheless be used in assessment are T4 lymphocyte count, presence of HIV antigenaemia and antibody to the major HIV core protein p24. The development of AIDS over a 2-year period in one study was 20 times higher among men who were HIV antigen positive than among those who were HIV antigen negative,[4] while another study suggested that 49% of patients might develop AIDS within 2 years from the reappearance of antigenaemia.[5] Decline in anti-p24 may parallel increase in antigenaemia, and be associated with disease progression[4-6] or may precede antigenaemia as a correlate of prognosis.[7]

It is therefore essential to assess symptoms carefully and to examine the patient for the signs mentioned above. In addition, increasingly it will be appropriate to carry out the investigations listed above. Some women who are prepared to accept the general risks described in continuing pregnancy may nevertheless opt for termination if they are shown to have unfavourable immunological or virological features. Advice which is based on accurate assessment of the individual is more likely to be accepted than blanket statements of risk.

INITIAL COUNSELLING ABOUT PREGNANCY
Some of the points which must be covered are shown in Table 3. The mother's attitude to the pregnancy and to abortion is clearly of major importance. Social factors are important, because 37% of the previous children of HIV positive women have been cared for by others (though not necessarily in an official care arrangement), and some women still abusing drugs have major social difficulties.

Table 3

Initial counselling about pregnancy

Mother's attitude to pregnancy and abortion.
Social factors.
Risk of baby acquiring HIV infection and AIDS.
Risk of maternal progression to AIDS.
Life expectancy and health of the mother.

HIV seropositive pregnant women in Edinburgh have tended to be young, unemployed, to come from areas of the city with multiple deprivation and many of the women have severed family ties. The risk of the baby acquiring HIV infection, and the risk of maternal progression to AIDS have been dealt with elsewhere in this volume. Suffice it to say that in Edinburgh, in a cohort of HIV positive women, no deterioration in clinical or immune status was found in the women who had had pregnancies since seroconversion compared with the women who had not (L MacCallum, personal communication). As far as the mother's health and life expectancy are concerned, rates of progression to AIDS of 8-10% per year after 3 years of HIV infection, and continuing for an unknown number of years, are widely accepted. The effect that early treatment with anti-viral drugs will have on this is uncertain.

Where the woman is less than 22 weeks pregnant and presents seeking termination of pregnancy without consideration of HIV problems, this is clearly justified under the 1967 Abortion Act because of the risk of fetal infection and the possibility that the woman's health and life expectancy may be limited. Where the pregnancy is wanted, there should be detailed counselling about the risks of pregnancy. Some women will elect to have an abortion on these grounds. Should the woman still wish to continue the pregnancy, she must be fully investigated and assessed as described above. If she shows markers of imminent illness, then the rather stronger risks should be discussed with her again. Where her immune status is satisfactory, or where she decides against termination despite ominous investigations, or if she is more than 22 weeks gestation, the pregnancy should continue. Even with a poor outlook for themselves and the child, some women will choose to continue with the pregnancy, as do some women with other life threatening conditions.

It is of the greatest importance during this process to avoid seeming to force the woman to a particular conclusion. It is she who must make the decision, and we can only offer general guidance and some idea of the risks involved. More than most groups of women, drug users may be resentful of authority and it is important that they regard their medical advisors as sympathetic and likely to help and support them, rather than as remote and dictatorial figures.

WHEN IS THE RIGHT TIME FOR PREGNANCY?

The mean age of onset of intravenous drug use was only 17.5 years and drug use was sometimes a transitory or occasional activity. Many infected ex-users are in their early twenties and now leading a stable lifestyle and looking forward eagerly to starting a family. Motivation to have a baby may in some cases be increased by the desire to succeed at something and to integrate into a society where success in material, educational or employment terms may have eluded them. In these circumstances, to have to cope with the implications of HIV infection for their own health, and also accept advice that that they should never have children may be unacceptable. If they are to have a child sometime, when should this be? Advice about this has importance not just for the individual patient, but also for the wider drug-using community where this information spreads. In the past we have advised that pregnancy should be postponed for as long as possible, and the argument we have put to patients is that in a few years more will be understood about the disease and the risks of pregnancy and we will be clearer about the long term outlook for the woman herself with the availability of new anti-viral drugs. This had the advantage of getting the patient's cooperation in preventing pregnancy, but without closing the possibility of pregnancy for the future. Whether this advice is correct is arguable. There is another school of thought that postponement will simply mean that pregnancy occurs at a later stage in the progress of the disease; there may be more chance of immune compromise and viraemia, and hence probably more risk of fetal infection and maternal progression to AIDS. In the absence of more definite information about the effects of pregnancy, there is no alternative at present to assessing each woman individually and in the light of all available information trying to offer her advice directly relating to her situation. Blanket policies are inappropriate.

PRECAUTIONS TO BE TAKEN DURING TERMINATION OF PREGNANCY

As with all procedures on HIV positive patients, care has to be taken to eliminate risks of infecting other patients or staff. These risks are currently seen as being remote,[8-10] but nevertheless precautions have to be scrupulous in view of the high exposure to blood in our speciality and the catastrophic consequences of infection. Only 9 of 24 HIV positive patients who had terminations first presented before 12 weeks, and altogether half had suction termination and half had prostaglandin termination of pregnancy. Many other patients having termination have been treated as a high infective risk because of continued HIV exposure, even though HIV negative.

For suction termination of pregnancy, the case is done last on the list and the theatre is stripped, leaving only the operating table covered in polythene sheets, a very simple anaesthetic machine using halothane (with N_2O and oxygen mixture from the piped supply), a disposable suction apparatus and a disposable suction collection bag for the products of conception. The operator and anaesthetist wear waterproof gowns, goggles and double gloves, and all drapes are disposable. The volsellum is the only instrument likely to cause a perforating injury to the operator. After the operation all disposable equipment is removed in marked, double bags. Although interpretation of local guidelines varies, all that is considered to be required thereafter is to clean any obvious blood spillage with hypochlorite or gluteraldehyde, and to clean the theatre. The theatre should be ready for use within an hour.

Prostaglandin termination is carried out using Cervagem pessaries. Ureaphil is no longer available for more advanced pregnancies. The only major risk of exposure to blood is at manual removal of placenta, especially as elbow-length removal gloves are no longer available. A waterproof gown should therefore be used. This procedure is carried out in a special "high infective risk" room in our labour ward.

There can be particular problems with venous access in current or ex-drug users and occasionally anaesthesia has to be given by an inhalation. There can be concern about giving large doses of narcotics during second trimester abortion to a woman who has recently stopped using drugs, in case this reawakens the desire.

This is a possibility, but intramuscular narcotics for pain probably have limited potential to do this, and adequate analgesia should certainly not be withheld on this account. Epidural anaesthesia is an alternative and the risks in each individual case have to be balanced. We routinely check these patients for chlamydia trachomatis and other sexually transmitted infection, and have treated women with depressed immunity with prophylactic antibiotics.

FUTURE CONTRACEPTION
Although there have been suggestions that the oral contraceptive pill could be a co-factor for transmission of the virus,[11] in the absence of any clear evidence that it influences progression of disease we have continued to advise its use for some women. At the same time, however, the couple should continue to use the sheath as a barrier.

CONCLUSION
Termination of pregnancy in women infected with HIV will continue to be important. It should be clear that there are many uncertainties regarding the outlook for mother and baby if pregnancy continues. Advice and management should depend on careful assessment, and consideration of the individual.

REFERENCES
1. Robertson JR, Bucknall ABV, Welsby PD, Roberts JJK, Inglis JM, Pewtherer JF, Brettle RP. Epidemic of AIDS related virus (HTLV III/LAV) infection among intravenous drug abusers. *Br Med J* 1986; **292:** 527-529.
2. Mok JQ, Giaquinto C, DeRossi A, Grosch-Wörner I, Ades AE, Peckham CS. Infants born to mothers seropositive for human immunodeficiency virus. Preliminary findings from a multicentre European study. *Lancet* 1987; **1:** 1164-1168.
3. Carne CA, Weller IVD, Loveday C, Adler MW. From persistent generalised lymphadenopathy to AIDS: who will progress? *Br Med J* 1987; **294:** 868-869.
4. De Wolf F, Goudsmit J, Paul DA, Lange JMA, Hooijkaas C, Coutinho RA, van der Noordaa J. Risk of AIDS related complex and AIDS in homosexual men with persistent HIV antigenaemia. *Br Med J* 1987; **295:** 569-572.
5. Pederson C, Nielson CM, Vestergaard BF, Gerstoft J, Krogsgaard K, Nielsen JO. Temporal relations of antigenaemia and loss of antibodies to core antigens to development of clinical disease in HIV infection. *Br Med J* 1987; **295:** 567-569.
6. Weber JN, Wedworth J, Rogers LA. Three-year prospective study of HTLV-III/LAV infection in homosexual men. *Lancet* 1986; **1:** 1179-1182.
7. Forster SM, Osborne CM, Cheingson-Popor R. Decline of anti-p24 antibody precedes antigenaemia as correlate of prognosis in HIV-1 infection. *AIDS* 1987; **1:** 235-240.
8. McCray E. Occupational risk of the acquired immunodeficiency syndrome among health care workers. *N Engl J Med* 1986; **314:** 1127-1132.
9. Henderson DK, Saah AJ, Zak BJ, Kaslow RA, Lane HC, Folks T, Blackwelder WC, Schmitt J, LaCamera DJ, Masur H, *et al.* Risk of nosocomial infection with human T-cell lymphotropic virus type III/lymphadenopathy-associated virus in a large cohort of intensively exposed health care workers. *Ann Intern Med* 1986; **104:** 644-647.
10. McEvoy M, Porter K, Mortimer P, Simmons N, Shanson D. Prospective study of clinical, laboratory and ancillary staff with accidental exposures to blood or body fluids from patients infected with HIV. *Br Med J* 1987; **294:** 1595-1597.
11. Piot P, Kreiss JK, Ndinya-Achola JO, Ngugi EN, Simonsen JN, Cameron DW, Taelman H, Plummer FA. Heterosexual transmission of HIV. *AIDS* 1987; **1:** 199-206.

Discussion

Dr J.W.G. Smith

GREEN: Counselling covers several quite separate issues, such as helping the woman to come to a decision as to whether or not she is going to terminate. The difficulty is that there is no consensus about what the advice should be. Some months ago we were providing women with information, biased toward termination, far more than it would be today. These changes are making things very difficult. We do not know what changes there are going to be in the next year or so. We still do not know what the real risk is to the child in terms of the infection rate, progression to AIDS, or what the risk is to the mother given all the complexities of her status etc. That makes it difficult to give a clear explanation to a woman, and therefore it is difficult for her to decide.

The second issue she must decide is whether she is ever to become pregnant again. If she is going to terminate, then you are not only terminating her pregnancy but you are also saying to her that it is probably going to be unwise for her to become pregnant again. So you are going to have to deal with those issues because her health is probably going to get worse. If she decides to continue then surely the largest issue in terms of counselling is going to be helping the woman to prepare for what comes after the birth, because she is going to have a lot of problems. She is going to have social difficulties. She is going to have problems of child care if she should be hospitalised. Is she going to tell the child minder that the child may be infected, when we will not know whether the child is infected for perhaps 15 months after birth. She is going to have to live with those sort of problems. Preparation for what could happen after the birth is going to be a fairly important issue in counselling these women.

HEDGE: If she does not have a termination, we take the woman through "what if she becomes sick", "what if she and her partner die" . . . every single eventuality on that level. Then she can make the best decision. We never try to say that we know the answers to any of the risk factors, although women and their partners press us all the time. They want a simple yes or no, but we cannot give them that.

It may be that you have a healthy woman in front of you who says that all she ever wanted out of life is to have children. If you advise this woman to terminate then she will become pregnant at a later stage in the disease which will be more hazardous. There may be other reasons why she wants to become pregnant. So you may have this termination only to find that she is pregnant again. The whole

157

issue is very complex, and we try to take up as much of this as possible before the decision is made. Obviously, if she decides to go on with the pregnancy we go on with the counselling.

GREEN: If these issues are fully examined before the decision is taken, then the woman may feel that the pressures are on her to terminate. Therefore it becomes even more difficult to deal with her if she does intend to continue the pregnancy. Some drug abusers become very resistant to the idea of being terminated. Often pregnancy is the only thing in a woman's life that gives her any status or any point to life, so she simply is not going to terminate. She may have bad housing, bad social conditions, cannot look after a child. It is all too easy under those circumstances to go overboard and offer biased advice. But it has to be the woman's decision.

SMITH: I was very struck by the amount of time spent, both by the obstetrician and counsellor. In places like East Anglia who does this job? Is it your job, or do you have counsellors?

HARE: I have not been faced with specific termination because of HIV, nor have most of my colleagues. We obviously have a pool of counsellors within each health authority who theoretically could be drawn in. We presume that they would be. A lot was said about counselling about termination. It needs to be done anyway about *all* terminations. It would be a shame if termination counselling for HIV cases was put in the limelight, and termination counselling for others was to suffer.

STEELE: The borderline between giving factual information and factual advice about something and pressuring someone is very grey. We all know the operations, but if you are asked to spell out the probabilities, we tend to spell them out in such a way that most people would not go ahead, just the same as most of us would not wish to take off in an airplane if the pilot did the same thing on the tarmac at Heathrow. If we are looking at people who are abusing drugs, the social implications of pregnancy may actually be quite intimidating if one looks at them honestly. I do not know the answer to this. It is very difficult to spell these out without biasing it one way or the other. Speaking to colleagues before coming to this meeting, the reaction of very many obstetricians and midwives, and most other people is that if pregnancy occurs in the presence of infection then termination is the obvious answer.

Consumers' concerns about AIDS

Mrs A. Spiro and Dr R. J. D. George

INTRODUCTION

The consumers to be considered are women of childbearing age. Their concerns are based primarily around the wellbeing of themselves, their children and their partners. To date no studies were found that considered *well women* in the community or addressed their attitudes or concerns to HIV. It was felt that a study investigating issues concerning HIV in this group was required. After considerable consultation, it was decided that pregnant or immediately post-partum women would be a difficult group to study. Any form of interview or questionnaire directed at this group could involve unnecessary anxiety. It was therefore felt to be more appropriate to study a group of women of similar age who were not considering pregnancy in the immediate future.

Women attending family planning and *well-women* clinics in Harrow, Middlesex were chosen. The clinics were evenly spread across the borough to achieve a broad mix of cultures and socio-economic groups. A questionnaire was drawn up to cover issues of HIV that were related to the consumer and about which they might be concerned (See Appendix). It was hoped that by exploring their knowledge of HIV a picture of the areas of uncertainty would arise. Future health education programmes could be aimed at filling these gaps in knowledge. Questions were also asked about their sexual practices and whether these had changed. General attitudes about the transmission of HIV and anxieties about mixing socially with HIV carriers were explored.

METHOD

Women attending the family planning clinics and *well-women* clinics were interviewed by a nurse. They were asked whether they would be willing to complete a questionnaire while they waited for their consultation. Only one woman refused to complete the questionnaire and a total of 364 women responded. When they had completed the questionnaire they were asked to post it into a box, so that their answers remained entirely confidential and anonymous. The nurse then handed each woman a leaflet on HIV and AIDS, that had been produced by the Health Authority. A large number of women attend family planning clinics in Harrow, and this group was easily accessible and appropriate to study. Larger numbers could have been studied but numbers had to be restricted because of time constraints.

RESULTS

As Figure Ia shows, 55% of the women in the group were between 20 years and 29 years of age, although 13% were between 15 years and 19 years. Fifty-seven percent were single, 35% were married and 8% did not answer this question (Figure Ib). Fifty-nine percent of the group did not have children, 31% had at least one child and 10% did not answer (Figure Ic).

Figure Ia

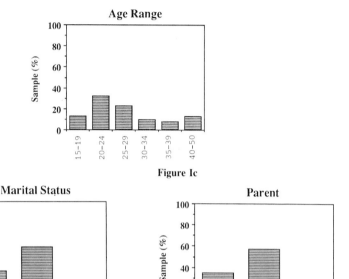

Figure Ib   **Figure Ic**

When asked whether they had read the Government literature last year, 73% said they had. Thirty-eight percent felt there was not enough information on HIV in their area and 35% thought there was sufficient information. However, 20% did not know and 7% did not respond.

Seventy-nine percent felt that there was not too much money being spent on AIDS and HIV and 54% thought more money should be spent.

The answers the women gave showed a good basic knowledge and that much of the message of the Government's campaign had been assimilated (Figure II). Ninety-nine percent knew they could catch HIV from an infected sexual partner and 94% thought they stood a greater risk of catching it if they had many different sexual partners. Ninety-seven percent thought that sharing needles for intravenous drugs was a way of becoming infected with HIV. Only a small percentage of women were worried about touching, coughing, clothing, utensils and shopping. Eighty-one percent thought condoms reduced the risk of spread of HIV.

Figure II

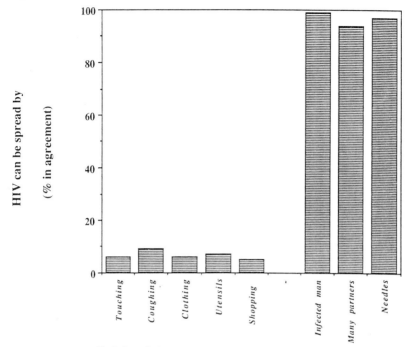

Basic knowledge: possible methods of spread of HIV.

There emerged several areas of doubt where knowldege was poor (Figure III). Several of these were associated with medical investigation or treatment. Twenty-two percent of the women were concerned that they might be infected with HIV if they had an internal examination. Fifty percent thought they could still be infected through blood transfusions in Britain today. Thirty-five percent were concerned about contracting HIV infection after a blood test. Eleven percent indicated that they felt there might be a risk in attending clinics. Doubt was also expressed about transmission of HIV to the baby during pregnancy, as 14% were not certain that this could happen. Forty-two percent were uncertain about a baby catching HIV during Caesarean section. Sixty-one percent were not sure whether HIV could be transmitted through breast milk. Twenty-six percent thought that there was no risk in a baby receiving untreated, donated breast milk, and 50% thought pasteurised breast milk was safe. As far as their own sexual habits were concerned, 46% felt there was still a risk of HIV infection if they kept to one partner and 24% were worried that kissing on the mouth might be a way of becoming infected with HIV.

A positive response was received in their personal attitudes towards screening (Figure IV). Seventy-five percent of women thought all couples planning to have a baby should be screened for HIV antibodies. Seventy-eight percent thought all

Figure III

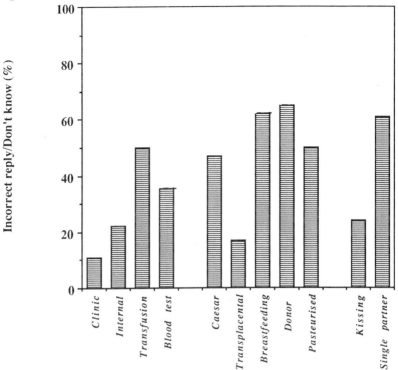

Areas of doubt—incorrect reply or uncertainty as to risk of contracting HIV.

pregnant women should be screened, and 71% thought doctors should seek permission first (Figure V). Sixty-one percent thought everyone should be tested, and 70% thought all doctors and nurses should be tested. Eighty-four percent answered that they would agree to having a blood test for HIV (Figure IV). If they were found to be infected, 60% would want to be sterilised. Forty-nine percent of women would like their own blood stored in case they needed a blood transfusion. Six percent of women knew someone who was HIV positive.

The women were asked how many sexual partners they had at present (Figure VI). Only 4% did not answer this question and 2% had no present sexual partner. Seventy-six percent answered that they had 1 partner, 10% that they had less than 5, 4% less than 10 and 4% more than 10. When asked how many partners they had had in their lifetime 36% answered 1, 43% less than 5, 8% less than 10 and 8% more than 10. Five percent did not respond to the number of lifetime partners question (Figure VII). Seventy-two percent said they had not changed their sexual habits since the AIDS publicity (Figure VIII). However, 26% said they were keeping to 1 partner and 16% said they had reduced the number of partners. Thirteen percent replied that they were using a condom.

Figure IV

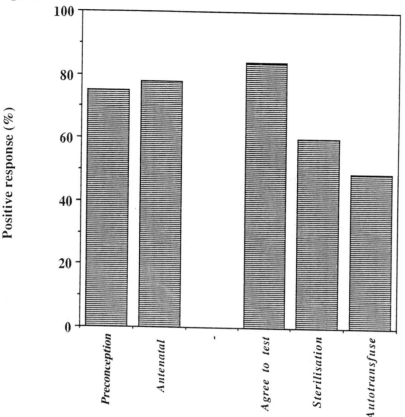

Personal attitudes: showing percentage of sample in agreement with screening preconceptually and antenatally; percentage agreeing to an HIV blood test; percentage wishing for sterilisation if positive; percentage who would prefer autotransfusion if possible.

Considerable concern was expressed over their children mixing socially with people known to be HIV positive. Only 32% were happy for their children to visit a friend they knew was infected. Forty percent were happy about their child attending a school where the teacher was known to be carrying HIV. Thirty percent were happy about their child staying the night in the same house as someone with HIV. However, only 12% felt people with the virus should be isolated.

The women were asked which groups in society were responsible for the spread of HIV. Eighty-one percent thought drug addicts, 72% thought homosexuals and 59% thought promiscuous people. Thirty-eight percent felt the permissive society was responsible for spread.

Figure V

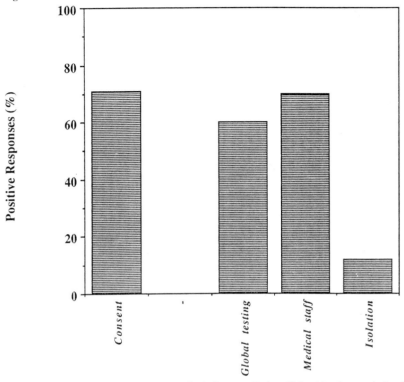

General attitiudes showing: percentage who believe medical staff should gain permission for HIV test; percentage wishing whole population to be tested; percentage that think medical/nursing staff should be tested; and the number who consider HIV positive individuals should be isolated.

When asked which groups were responsible for the prevention of HIV spread, most women thought it was primarily up to each individual. However, 59% thought the Government had a role and 50% thought that parents, individuals, NHS and schools all had an equal role in prevention. Also, 38% felt religious teachers had a role to play in education.

DISCUSSION

This study was carried out exactly a year after the Government's campaign on AIDS. It showed that the group studied had an excellent basic knowledge of the sexual transmission of HIV. This reflected the emphasis of the campaign and demonstrated that the information had been retained.

In the area of numbers of sexual partners this study confirms a previous study[1] that most women have one sexual partner at one time and most have less than 5 sexual partners in a lifetime.

Figure VI

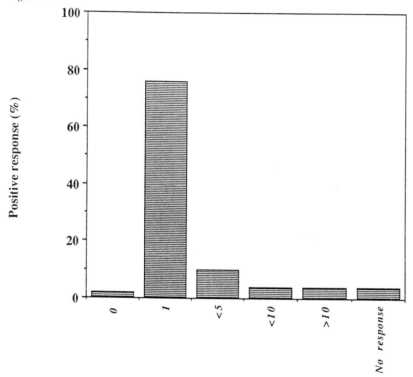

Number of current partners: distribution.

The replies were positive in their personal attitudes towards screening. Most women thought that antenatal mothers and couples thinking of having a baby should be offered screening. Most thought permission for screening should be sought.

This attitude is also held by another consumer group, the National Childbirth Trust. It believes that antenatal screening for AIDS should be available, nationwide, to all pregnant women who request it. This will enable those who are HIV positive to choose whether to continue with the pregnancy or to have a termination. The National Childbirth Trust believes that screening should be done only with the woman's permission, and women should be able to make their own informed choices. Counselling should be available both before and after tests are done and results are treated with the utmost confidentiality.

This study highlighted several areas of consumer concern. The first being those surrounding medical examination, blood tests and blood transfusions. There was some uncertainty over transplacental transmission, and transmission through breastfeeding and donated breast milk. Many women were also concerned about Caesarean sections.

Figure VII

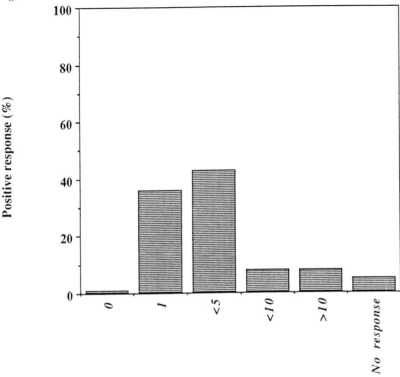

Number of lifetime partners: distribution.

There appears to be a need for a further health education campaign to reassure women that medical investigations, operations or, indeed, attendance at clinics are not activities that present risks of contracting HIV.

Women are concerned about their children mixing socially with individuals with HIV. Although most of them were happy that HIV was not transmitted through plates, cutlery, touching, coughing or meeting people in crowded places, they were unhappy about their children making friends with families where there was HIV infection. This attitude can lead to discrimination against children who have HIV or individuals who work with children. Perhaps this attitude will change with time, as it becomes more obvious to the general public that transmission does not occur in normal social contact.

Drug addiction was seen as being most responsible for the spread of HIV in Britain with homosexuality coming a close second. Interestingly, promiscuity was not seen to be as important in its spread. This group sees HIV as a disease primarily of drug addicts and homosexuals. These women thought the government should lead the way in prevention, closely followed by parents, individuals, NHS and schools.

Figure VIII

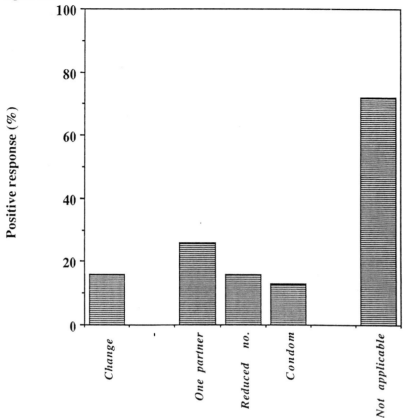

Change in sexual behaviour: showing percentage of women who have changed, and methods by which they have changed.

There appear to be two main areas that need to be targeted in health education campaigns: first the safety of mother and child by reassuring women that medical examinations, blood tests, Caesarean sections and clinic attendances are not activities that present risks; and second, helping society change its attitudes to HIV so that it corresponds with the available knowledge.

REFERENCES
1. Evans BA, McCormack SM, Bond RA, MacRao KD, Thorp RW. Human immunodeficiency virus infection, hepatitis B virus infection, and sexual behaviour of women attending a genitourinary medicine clinic. *Br Med J* 1988; **296**: 473-475.

Appendix:
Questionnaire used in the study

We would be grateful if you could complete the following questionnaire. Your answers will help us in the future planning of services for women of childbearing age. We do not require your name and your answers will remain entirely anonymous. Many of the questions are about AIDS, but not all refer to behaviour or situations that are high-risk.

You are asked to tick Yes/No/Don't know. Several responses may be appropriate for some questions. If you do not understand a question, just leave it blank.

Thank you for your co-operation and help.

Questionnaire

Age:...................years   Married/Single

	Yes	No	Don't know
KNOWLEDGE			
I have children	☐	☐	☐
I have read the Government Literature sent through the door on AIDS, in January 1987.	☐	☐	☐
CAN THE AIDS VIRUS BE SPREAD BY:			
Touching?	☐	☐	☐
Coughing?	☐	☐	☐
On clothing?	☐	☐	☐
Cutlery?	☐	☐	☐
Plates?	☐	☐	☐
Meeting people in crowded places — shops?	☐	☐	☐
— clinics?	☐	☐	☐
Having a blood test?	☐	☐	☐
Having an internal examination?	☐	☐	☐
Having sexual intercourse with an infected man?	☐	☐	☐
Having sexual intercourse with many different partners?	☐	☐	☐
Having sexual intercourse with one partner?	☐	☐	☐
By kissing on the mouth?	☐	☐	☐
Sharing needles for intravenous drugs?	☐	☐	☐
Having blood transfusions in U.K. today?	☐	☐	☐

	Yes	No	Don't know
Can people of all races catch the virus that causes AIDS?	☐	☐	☐
Can a person catch the virus and not know for months?	☐	☐	☐
or years?	☐	☐	☐

CAN A BABY CATCH THE VIRUS THAT CAUSES AIDS:

in the womb?	☐	☐	☐
by being breastfed?	☐	☐	☐
during a Caesarean section?	☐	☐	☐
from being fed untreated, donated breast milk?	☐	☐	☐
from being fed pasteurised, donated breast milk?	☐	☐	☐

ATTITUDES/PRACTICE	Yes	No	Don't know
Do you think that all people should be tested for the AIDS virus?	☐	☐	☐
Do you think all couples planning to have a baby should be tested for AIDS antibodies?	☐	☐	☐
Do you think all doctors and nurses should be tested for evidence of infection by the AIDS virus?	☐	☐	☐
Do you think all pregnant women should be tested for evidence of infection by the AIDS virus?	☐	☐	☐
If you had evidence of infection by the AIDS virus would you be sterilised?	☐	☐	☐
Do you think doctors should ask permission before testing for the virus?	☐	☐	☐
Would you agree to having a blood test for the AIDS virus?	☐	☐	☐
Would you like to have your own blood stored in case you need a blood transfusion?	☐	☐	☐
Have you changed your sexual habits since the AIDS publicity?	☐	☐	☐
If so, how? — By using a condom?	☐	☐	☐
— Keeping to one partner?	☐	☐	☐
— Reducing your number of partners?	☐	☐	☐

	Yes	No	Don't know
How many sexual partners do you have now? (Please tick)			1
			less than 5
			less than 10
			more than 10
How many sexual partners have you had in your life? (Please tick)			1
			less than 5
			less than 10
			more than 10
Do condoms prevent the spread of the AIDS virus?	☐	☐	☐
Do condoms reduce the risk of speading the AIDS virus?	☐	☐	☐
Are you happy with the Government's advertising campaign?	☐	☐	☐
Do you know anyone with AIDS or the AIDS virus?	☐	☐	☐

WOULD YOU LIKE YOUR CHILD TO:	Yes	No	Don't know
Visit a friend you know is infected with AIDS?	☐	☐	☐
Go to a school where a teacher or pupil has the AIDS virus?	☐	☐	☐
Have tea with a friend who has the AIDS virus?	☐	☐	☐
Stay in the same house as a friend who has the AIDS virus?	☐	☐	☐
Should all people with the AIDS virus be isolated?	☐	☐	☐
Is enough information on AIDS available in your area?	☐	☐	☐
Is too much money already being spent on AIDS?	☐	☐	☐
Is too little money being spent on AIDS?	☐	☐	☐

What, in your opinion, has been responsible for spreading AIDS in this country?
Please tick one or more of the following:

Air Travel

Unemployment

Poor discipline

The permissive society

Promiscuity

Homosexuality

Drug addiction

The Church

Society's attitudes

Scientific research

Nothing

Who should be trying to prevent the spread of AIDS?
Please tick

Parents

Government

N.H.S

Schools

Religious teachers

Individuals

Each individual

SECTION IV

OBSTETRIC CARE

Changes in routine antenatal and postnatal inpatient practice

Miss J. Brierley and Miss C. Roth

The advent of human immunodeficiency virus (HIV) and the anticipated increase of infection in our population, has presented those giving care during pregnancy and childbirth with a challenge to our current practices which requires a reasoned and practical response. This presentation will examine some of the issues surrounding current practice and research findings which may provide a basis for further change.

INTRODUCTION

Many maternity units have begun to respond by designing an infection control policy to be implemented when a woman has been identified to be HIV antibody positive thus creating a two-tier infection control system.[1] There are several limitations to this approach. Firstly, it presumes that all women at risk of HIV infection can be identified. However, since medical and social history with medical examination cannot reliably identify all women infected with HIV, it is highly unlikely that all those infected will be identified. Furthermore, even in areas of "high risk" population groups, voluntary testing, based on active case-finding and self-identification, failed to detect 86% of HIV infected women.[2] Secondly, even if routine universal testing were carried out, some women found to be antibody negative may nonetheless be infected, because of the period (sometimes prolonged) before seroconversion.[3] Thirdly, a problem in using selective precautions lies in the fact that, because of their elaborate nature, their implementation results in breach of confidentiality for the woman involved and subjects her to what may be perceived as discriminatory treatment. However, one of the most important aspects of dealing with any HIV antibody positive person is preservation of confidentiality because of the cruel stigmatisation of the infection. There is a real danger that if our policies threaten confidentiality women most at risk of HIV infection will stay away and deliver out of hospital because of their fear of exposure and their distress at the treatment they receive.[4] Finally, restricting our focus primarily to issues of infection control may distract us from the need to educate ourselves about the psychosocial and physical impact of this information in order to improve the quality of care we can offer to what is likely to be an increasing number of women.[5]

RISKS TO THE HEALTH WORKER

HIV is not highly infectious to health workers in the normal course of their duties as long as a high standard of hygiene is practised and this knowledge should form the basis for infection control policy.

A recent prospective study of 150 health care workers in the United Kingdom who had been accidentally exposed to HIV, either by needle stick injury or exposure to body fluids, showed no evidence of seroconversion.[6] However, in addition to health care workers enrolled in prospective studies, through world wide investigation, 8 persons who provided care to infected patients and denied other risk factors have been reported to have acquired HIV infection. Three of these health care workers had needle stick exposures to blood from infected patients and 2 were persons who provided nursing care to infected persons. Although neither of these sustained a needle stick injury, both had extensive contact with blood or other body fluids, and neither observed recommended barrier precautions.[7,8] The exact route of transmission of the remaining 3 persons is not known though all had direct contact of their skin with blood from infected patients; all had skin lesions that may have been contaminated by blood, and 1 also had a mucous membrane exposure.

It appears therefore that the risk of transmission of the virus to childbirth attendants is extremely low though not zero. No childbirth attendant has been reported to have caught this virus through occupational exposure.

Because there will sometimes be unidentified carriers of HIV and because routes of infection are well identified and easily prevented, the heart of any infection control policy is to treat blood and other body fluids from *all* persons as potentially infected for HIV and other blood-borne pathogens, i.e. universal precautions should form the foundation for our clinical care.

CHANGES IN CARE

As well as considering changes in practice we must be prepared to examine our attitudes about this virus, to the women who may be infected by it and the ways in which they may have acquired it. If we are unable to approach people with tolerance and respect, we are unable to offer them care.

Antenatal care

History taking at the booking clinic is probably the most opportune time to raise issues about high risk activity and part of the routine interview should elicit factors such as past intravenous drug abuse by the client and/or her partner.

All women need information which will help them identify "risk activity" so they can protect themselves and others from infection. Women look to midwives as a source of this information and we are often in a privileged position of learning about a woman's lifestyle and anxieties about her sexuality. We must be able to provide the information, counselling and advice.

If a woman identifies herself as someone who may have been exposed to the virus then the availability of testing should be brought to her attention. In every instance where the test is requested, precounselling is essential and must include discussion on the nature and limitations of test information, the consequences of a positive result including social, employment and insurance implications, and possible implications for the current and future pregnancies. Testing should only be offered as a way of providing options for women and not as a protective mechanism for staff.

Considerable psychological and emotional morbidity may occur in a person on learning that a HIV antibody test is positive. This is especially so when the test is conducted without consent or precounselling.[9] It is paramount that HIV antibody testing should only be offered within an institution where pretest counselling is available. We must ask ourselves however if obstetricians and midwives are adequately prepared and skilled to offer this service. The question of training of staff and the costs involved in the training for this still needs to be addressed.

The identification of large numbers of HIV antibody positive pregnant women will need the development of skills and facilities which are as yet unavailable. Seroprevalence studies will at least help to identify the scale of the problem. Therefore, before routine testing is even considered, we have a responsibility to prepare for its impact on the women and infants as well as on our services.[10]

Any woman who expresses a desire to be tested should be offered written as well as verbal explanation about the test and it is essential that she is given adequate time to make her decision.

Preservation of confidentiality is critical and this should apply to the woman's interest in being tested as well as the test itself. To maintain this, the client's identity and the possible diagnosis should not be revealed, so numbers or codes rather than names may have to be used. Thought should be given to the widespread practice of biohazard labelling of notes and specimens and whether this constitutes a breach of confidentiality. The application of universal precautions should preclude the need to use these. Care must always be taken to protect the woman's identity from inappropriate disclosure both inside and outside the hospital.[11]

When a person is found to be seropositive or diagnosed as having symptoms of HIV disease the period immediately afterwards is usually characterised by shock, acute anxiety, depression and often impulsive despair. It is therefore crucial to provide a lifeline after a positive result is given to the woman. Antenatal clinic staff must have a clear network of support workers who can be readily reached in case of need. It is questionable whether most antenatal clinics have this sort of facility.

Subsequent care

Whether or not the woman decides to continue her pregnancy, she will need the services of a skilled counsellor. This is a service which is becoming rapidly overstretched. We need to consider who will be undertaking the job of counselling pregnant women, who is going to train these counsellors, and who will pay for their training.

The woman who decides to continue with her pregnancy will have the additional anxieties about the health of her baby and about its future care should she become sick.[12] Intravenous drug abuse and the chaotic lifestyle often associated with it may present additional problems. It would be kindest to offer this woman continuity of care, preferably by one midwife and/or obstetrician with monitoring of the HIV infection by the clinical virologist and it would be desirable for this continuity of care to extend throughout the period in hospital. This system will give the woman the opportunity to develop a relationship with a small supportive team which can be responsive to her particular needs.

Antenatal care should include discussion with the woman of the concept of infection control and the potential risk to others through sexual contact and exposure to blood. Information about condom use should be an integral part of this discussion. If she or her partner have been intravenous drug users, education about the hazards of shared equipment should be given.

In preparation for labour, she should be made aware of appropriate measures to be taken in the event of spilled blood or amniotic fluid so that any spillage will be dealt with quickly. It is advisable to raise this issue with all women during their stay in hospital since all blood and amniotic fluid should be considered potentially infected.

Postnatal care

The emphasis during the postnatal period must be on self-care which is facilitated by midwifery staff.

It is not essential that the woman has a single room nor separate toilet facilities. It should be remembered that *all* blood from *any* women should be dealt with promptly in the recommended way[13] and if this policy is followed, the need for separate toilet facilities is overcome. The provision in toilets of alcohol wipes for women to disinfect toilet seats prior to use may be a way of ensuring good hygiene.

There is no need for staff to wear protective clothing unless there is likely to be exposure to blood. All soiled maternity pads must be disposed of either by incineration or by placing in a polythene bag for disposal and the midwife should have no need to perpetuate the past practice of removing a soiled pad for inspection. If she needs to touch the perineal area, gloves should be worn.

Transfer of this woman's care into the community should be discussed with her in advance because she will need to make decisions about informing others who will be involved in her care. Such discussion may give her the security of knowing that information about her HIV status will not be divulged indiscriminately. The notes that accompany her home and the discharge letter to health visitor, community midwife and general practitioner should not contain documentation of her HIV antibody status. It is worth mentioning at this point that where computerised records are used, it is particularly important that HIV antibody status is not part of the record.

It is important, once she returns home, that she has access to a support network. This may exist within her own family and friends or may need to be sought through one of the voluntary organisations. Presently, there is a shortage of groups catering for women. The services of a counsellor may be of particular value in helping her to tell those people close to her of the diagnosis.

The postnatal period for all women can be stressful, physically and psychologically. For the woman with HIV infection, this period is likely to be further complicated by isolation, grief, loss of self esteem, guilt and fear for her physical health as well as that of her child.[14] Our care should try to identify and ameliorate the impact of these on her.

Our ability to give the kind of holistic care outlined still needs to be developed. The authors have recent experience of a woman going through her third pregnancy. She had been discovered to be HIV antibody positive during her first pregnancy. In spite of the care received during that first pregnancy (she miscarried in between), she felt unable to attend for antenatal care this time because of feelings of guilt, fear of breach of confidentiality and poor self-esteem. Consequently, she delivered her baby at home, unattended by professional staff. When professional staff did arrive, she did not disclose her positive antibody status. For reasons which are undoubtedly very complex, this woman has been unable to come to terms with her infection and the implications of this for her life choices. Our previous care failed to identify and respond to this problem constructively. The incident also illustrates the need for universal blood and body fluid precautions because even when someone knows herself to be HIV antibody positive, she will not necessarily declare it.

STAFF SAFETY

Before discussing recommendations for staff protection, it should again be emphasised that there will always be unidentified carriers of HIV. Therefore, all health care workers must adopt safe procedures at all times to avoid exposure to infection. We must all adopt certain "ground rules" which apply when dealing with any client:

i. Sharps

The main risk of transmission of the virus to staff lies in needle stick and other puncture injuries and therefore efforts to reduce the likelihood of these occurring are essential. Needles must never be re-sheathed and these amongst other sharp instruments must be disposed of in the approved containers. To avoid the risk of a sharps injury in the foot, in case an attendant drops a used syringe and needle or sharp instrument, full shoes must always be worn in patient areas.

It is recommended by Centers For Disease Control (Atlanta, USA), that gloves be worn when performing venepuncture and for all other vascular access procedures.[15] Whether or not this recommendation should be accepted for use in maternity units in the United Kingdom is debatable. Firstly, it would be extremely costly and secondly, gloves do not necessarily improve technique or prevent spillage. Venepuncture technique is to be criticised if there is any blood spillage at all.

ii. Barrier precautions

Routine use of barrier precautions to prevent skin and mucous membrane exposure with blood, liquor and vaginal secretions should be part of any infection control protocol. For example, the practice of leaving the left hand ungloved when performing speculum and vaginal examinations is unacceptable. Gloves, however, must be changed after each use and before leaving the room. There is a tendency when staff are wearing gloves for them to forget that their hands are contaminated and thereby they become agents of cross infection.

Any cuts or lesions on the hands must be protected by a waterproof covering when in patient areas.

iii. Good housekeeping

Housekeeping practices should be of the highest possible standards including regular wiping down of all surfaces with detergent solutions and regular cleaning of all equipment. Any blood or body fluid spillage should be wiped up immediately and that area cleansed thoroughly with the recommended solutions.[16]

iv. Linen

All fouled linen (blood or body-fluid soiled) should be disposed of in the recommended alginate bags before sending for washing. Gloves should be worn when fouled linen is handled.

v. Accidental exposure

When accidental exposure to blood or body substances occurs, this should be removed immediately by thorough washing of the area with soap and water. Eye wash facilities should be available in all patient areas in case of splashes to the eyes. These practices do not constitute a change in procedure and should always have taken place.

CONCLUSION

A major change demanded of us in response to HIV infection is a tightening up of our "risky" clinical practices. One of the difficulties in motivating people to do this is that to date, we have little idea of the prevalence of HIV infection and most midwives and obstetricians have seen little evidence of it. However, whatever the prevalence, there is no excuse for a haphazard standard of infection control. Procedures must carry minimum risk to clients and staff alike.

A second change required of us is to shift our focus from the virus itself, to the needs of the person infected by it.

Whatever changes individual maternity units decide to make, we have a responsibility to ensure that:
— all staff are educated and able to meet the challenge of HIV infection constructively.
— the woman's confidentiality is protected at all times.
— measures of infection control are inoffensive to women.
— precautions are universally applied in order to reduce to a minimum the risk of exposure.
— staff do not allow judgemental attitudes to interfere with care of the woman or her infant.
— testing is employed in the interest of the woman and not for staff protection.

Midwives and doctors working in the maternity services could make a valuable contribution to the care of women and babies affected by HIV infection and in preventing its spread. To achieve these aims, we need to continue to challenge bad practices, ignorance and irrational fears. We also need to educate and support women who are at risk of or have acquired HIV infection. These women will carry on with their lives after being in our care and what they take away in terms of information, awareness and support will influence the difficult decisions which they will be required to make in the future.

REFERENCES

1. *AIDS and HTLV-III. The control of infection pack.* Paddington & North Kensington Health Authority & North West Thames Regional Health Authority 1986.
2. Krasinski K, Borkowsky W, Bebenroth D, Moore T. Failure of voluntary testing for human immunodeficiency virus to identify infected parturient women in a high-risk population. (Letter) *N Engl J Med* 1988; **318**: 185.
3. Bedarida G, Cambie G, D'Agostino F, Ronsivalle MG, Berto E, Grisi ME, Magni E. HIV IgM antibodies in risk groups who are seronegative on ELISA testing. *Lancet* 1986; **2**: 570-571.
4. Brierley J. Human immunodeficiency virus: the challenge of a lifetime. *Midwives' Chronicle & Nursing Notes* 1987; **11**: Supplement: x-xiii.
5. DHSS. *Quarterly figures on AIDS.* Press release. 1988 January.
6. McEvoy M, Porter K, Mortimer P, Simmons N, Shanson D. Prospective study of clinical, laboratory, and ancillary staff with accidental exposures to blood or body fluids from patients infected with HIV. *Br Med J* 1987; **294**: 1595-1597.
7. Grint P, McEvoy M. Two associated cases of the acquired immune deficiency syndrome (AIDS). *PHLS Commun Dis Rep* 1985; **42**: 4.
8. CDC. Apparent transmission of human T-lymphocytes virus type III/lymphadenopathy-associated virus from a child to a mother providing health care. *MMWR* 1986; **35**: 76-79.
9. Miller D. ABC of AIDS. Counselling. *Br Med J* 1987; **294**: 1671-1674.
10. Miller D, Jeffries DJ, Green J, Harris JRW, Pinching AJ. HTLV-III: Should testing ever be routine? *Br Med J* 1986; **292**: 941-943.
11. *Nursing guidelines on the management of patients in hospital and the community suffering from AIDS.* Second report of the RCN AIDS working party. London: Ruislip Press, 1986.
12. Pinching AJ. HIV, AIDS and pregnancy. *Matern Child Health* 1987; **5**: 146-150.
13. Levi A, Houghton D, Jenner E. Nursing infection control aspects of care. In: *The management of AIDS patients.* Eds. D Miller, J Weber, J Green. Basingstoke: Macmillan Press, 1986: pp.93-108.
14. Wofsy CB. Intravenous drug abuse and women's medical issues. In: *Report of the Surgeon General's workshop on children with HIV infection and their families.* Eds. BK Silverman, A Waddekk. Rockville: US Department of health and human services, 1987: pp.32-34.
15. CDC. Recommendations for prevention of HIV transmission in health-care settings. *MMWR* 1987; **36**: No.2S.
16. Advisory Committee on Dangerous Pathogens. *LAV/HTLV-III—the causative agent of AIDS and related conditions.* Revised guidelines. 1986.

Safety of invasive procedures in diagnostic antenatal and intrapartum care

Dr J.B. Scrimgeour

In patients known to be HIV positive and in those who are in a high risk group although not HIV positive, the actual indication for any invasive procedure must be re-evaluated. It may be that the added possible risk of HIV infection to the fetus or to the attendants outweighs any advantage to be gained by doing the procedure. It is essential that the person planning to carry out the invasive procedure is aware of the clinical situation and able to deal with the sensitivity of HIV positive patients. The more invasive procedures should be carried out by experienced staff and preferably those who also have been successfully trained in the counselling of such patients.

PERMISSION FOR THE PROCEDURE

The indications for the procedure must be fully discussed with the patient and, if necessary, her partner. Formal permission forms may be a local requirement for the patient's signature but it is mandatory that the notes contain written confirmation by the doctor concerned both that the procedure has been described to the patient as well as its objectives, its risks and the consequences should the test prove to be abnormal. The preliminary counselling may well take a much longer time than the procedure itself.

GUIDELINES FOR ALL OBSTETRIC INVASIVE TECHNIQUES

The Operator

1. Any open wounds of scratches, particularly of the hands of the operator, should be covered by a closed, unperforated, watertight plaster. Better still, a similarly experienced but unblemished operator should take over.

2. The operator must avoid as far as humanly possible the spillage of body fluids or tissue—blood, amniotic fluid, urine, cervical mucus or chorionic villi, on to anything other than disposable or sterilisable equipment.

3. The operator should wear gloves for venepunctures but for other invasive procedures should also wear an impermeable gown or apron. Where a possibility exists of splashing of body fluids, a double mask, goggles and cap should be worn.

4.   Surgical rubber single use gloves should be used as those have a standard specifying strength and are 97% free from perforations. Plastic disposable gloves are *not* recommended as they frequently give way at the joins.[1]

5.   Disposable linen should be used wherever possible.

Syringes and needles

Syringes and needles must be disposable. Stocks should be kept in a secure place, inaccessible to patients. After use, *needles should not be re-sheathed.* Used needles and syringes should be placed in a container strong enough to prevent it being pierced by the point of a needle; the container should not remain in the consulting room and should not be allowed to become full. When ready for incineration the container should be placed in a double strength plastic bag of a conspicuous colour known to all staff as "high risk" and labelled accordingly. The portering staff should then be notified and asked to remove it immediately.

Specimens

1.   Needles must be removed from syringes with the utmost care. The fluid must be gently discharged from the syringe and external contamination of the specimen container avoided. If this does occur it must be dealt with by disinfection.

2.   The container must be securely closed. If any leakage occurs it must be discarded. The specimens must be clearly labelled by whatever system is recognised locally to indicate a danger of infection.

3.   The accompanying request form must clearly indicate knowledge or suspicion of HIV infection and *must be kept separate from the specimen container* to avoid contamination.[2]

4.   In the interests of confidentiality, the patient's name on the specimen container or the laboratory form should not be visible to the casual oberver.

5.   Specimens should *not* be sent to the laboratories without an agreement between the clinician and senior laboratory staff. Specimens sent by post must have the inner wrapping, the actual container and the request form all labelled to identify the danger of infection. They must be packed in accordance with the recognised regulations for the postal transmission of any pathological specimen. For international postage, the revised conditions required by the Infectious Perishable Biological Substance Service must be observed. Details may be obtained from Postal Headquarters, 33 Grosvenor Place, London SW1X.

Accidental puncture wounds in staff

This matter is dealt with in greater detail elsewhere in this volume. These wounds must be dealt with immediately by removing the glove and washing liberally with soap and water while encouraging bleeding. Any puncture wound or contamination of broken skin or mucous membranes must be reported promptly to and recorded by the person with overall responsibility for the work.

DIAGNOSTIC ANTENATAL INVASIVE PROCEDURES

Venepuncture

In medical practice, this is the most common invasive procedure but the frequency with which it is carried out can also lead to poor or careless technique. If the technique is poor the operator will put himself/herself at risk when dealing with an HIV positive patient.

1. The patient must understand the reason for the procedure and give permission for it to be carried out.

2. Usually the cubital fossa is chosen as the site for venepuncture but this may need to be avoided if skin wounds, skin infection or rashes are present. An unblemished area of skin with a well filled vein should be selected.

3. Surgical gloves should be worn.

4. The skin must be wiped with a fresh pre-packed swab saturated with 70% v/v isopropyl alcohol. The area is allowed to dry.

5. A single-use pre-packed sterile syringe and needle is used.

6. Once the required volume of blood is obtained the tourniquet is released and the needle withdrawn. Pressure to the puncture site is applied by the patient using a sterile cotton wool swab. The puncture wound is covered by a waterproof dressing and the cotton wool discarded into a "high risk" disposal bag.

7. The needle is gently removed from the syringe and immediately inserted into the puncture-proof bin. The blood is slowly and carefully discharged into the appropriate container(s). The syringe is then also immediately put into the bin.

8. The container(s) are then appropriately identified with the patient's name and a "high risk" hazard label, then inserted into a plastic bag; the request form is completed and put into a separate bag similarly labelled; both bags are now put into a third bag also labelled "high risk" ready for delivery to the laboratory.

9. Gloves may now be removed.

10. The laboratory should now be forewarned of the specimen's arrival if this has not already been done.

Amniocentesis

In patients in whom this is indicated there is a higher risk to the attendants as another body fluid, amniotic fluid, may contaminate the area of the procedure. It must be assumed that if the patient is HIV positive the virus is likely to be present in the amniotic fluid.

A preliminary ultrasound examination by an experienced ultrasonographer is an essential preliminary to this procedure. From this the gestational age will be confirmed; the presence of a multiple pregnancy detected; confirmation of fetal life and, the actual location of the placenta obtained; and finally the site of an accessible pool of amniotic fluid demonstrated. Contact between the transducer and the maternal skin is improved by the use of a contact gel; this should be applied by the ultrasonographer from a plastic bottle or tube rather than by a brush from a large container. The latter has been used in some units for olive oil but the use of a communal brush is no longer considered appropriate and in the case of HIV positive patients must not be used.

During the procedure it may be necessary to watch the progress and position of the tip of the needle on the ultrasound monitor. It is therefore possible that some amniotic fluid may spill on to the patient's skin, the aqueous gel and thus on to the transducer. If this occurs the transducer should be wiped clear of any obvious gel, fluid or blood using a dry swab and then cleaned with a swab soaked in 70% isopropryl alcohol. The transducer should then be allowed to dry for 10 minutes before being used for the next patient.

Before proceeding it must again be confirmed that the patient understands the nature of the test, its risks and its limitations. A formal permission slip is signed by the patient and witnessed by the operator if that is the local requirement.

Hands and forearms are scrubbed as for any surgical procedure and gown and gloves donned. The area of the proposed puncture site is cleaned with hibitane in spirit and disposable drapes arranged accordingly. Areas of skin puncture, infection and rash are avoided. A 22g lumbar puncture needle with a stilette is used at the predetermined angle and depth. The stilette is removed and the amniotic fluid gently aspirated. If amniotic fluid is not obtained simultaneous ultrasound examination as described above is helpful but the change of contaminating the transducer is present. The sample is dealt with in the same manner as for blood, the syringe and needle are disposed of and the drapes also incinerated.

Chorionic villus sampling

This may be performed via abdomen or *per vaginam*. If the operator is equally skilled in both techniques and access is equally easy for either route in the HIV positive patient it would be preferable to choose the transabdominal route because HIV has been isolated from cervical secretions.[1]

The technique for the transabdominal route will be the same as for amniocentesis except that it will always be necessary to have simultaneous ultrasound tracking of the needle. Once the tip of the needle is placed in the correct spot of the chorion suction is applied, usually via a 10 ml syringe. It is essential that the syringe is firmly attached to the cannula; otherwise the two may suddenly come apart and blood spray around the assembled operators. For this reason it is preferable for cap, goggles and double mask to be worn.

If a transcervical route is the only possible option then care must be taken to make the cervix and the canal as aseptic as possible. Hibitane in spirit can be dabbed on the area and allowed to act before the cannula is inserted. This technique should only be used in such high risk patients when no other option— including waiting until 16 weeks gestation and performing an amniocentesis—is acceptable.

Fetoscopy, fetal blood sampling, placentacentesis and cordocentesis

These invasive procedures are carried out usually on patients with a very high risk of having a child with an identifiable genetic abnormality. Should the patient also be HIV positive even greater problems for the fetus are present. Should such techniques be necessary they should be carried out in a large centre whose staff are thoroughly experienced in the procedures and equally able to interpret the results obtained. The most vital part of the procedure is that the consultant to whom the patient is referred is informed that the patient is HIV positive and he can then act accordingly.

DIAGNOSTIC INTRAPARTUM INVASIVE PROCEDURES

Cardiotocography

Using the external transducer an adequate signal should be obtained unless the patient is obese. The transducer will require aqueous gel to obtain good contact. When the membranes are ruptured it is possible that amniotic fluid reaches the transducer and particularly the elastic waistband. It will be necessary to ensure that the transducer is thoroughly cleaned following delivery and sterilised in the manner described for the transducer after amniocentesis.

A scalp electrode should not be used unless absolutely essential as this involves an open wound of the fetus in a contaminated area.

Amnioscopy

This is now seldom used in the UK, and in the HIV positive patient should be avoided.

Artificial rupture of membranes

When this is indicated particular care should be taken in its performance as amniotic fluid may stream out with some force if puncture of the membranes coincides with a contraction. The operator should be in full theatre clothing including Wellington boots. Cap, double mask and goggles must be worn. If the instrument to be used to puncture the membranes is sharp then two pairs of gloves would minimise the chance of an accidental puncture of the glove. Following the procedure all the soiled, disposable linen and gowns should be sent in appropriately identified "high risk" bags for incineration. Surgical instruments are sent for sterilisation.

Intra-uterine catheters and fetal blood sampling

Those techniques should be avoided in such high risk patients unless absolutely essential.

CONCLUSION

The management of the HIV positive patient in pregnancy is particularly difficult when invasive procedures are indicated. Care must be taken with any body fluids both to protect the fetus and the attending staff.

REFERENCES
1. *Report of the RCOG Sub-committee on problems associated with AIDS in relation to obstetrics and gynaecology.* Royal College of Obstetricians and Gynaecologists, 1987: Para. 4.2.
2. Advisory Committee on Dangerous Pathogens. *LAV/HTLV III—the causative agent of AIDS and related conditions.* Revised guidelines. 1986: Para. 31.

Special precautions in delivery suites and operating theatres for normal labour and delivery and operative delivery including episiotomy

Mr C.N. Hudson

Just as bereavement induces a recognised sequence of emotional and psychological reactions—shock, denial, anger, depression and so forth—so the response of health care workers in obstetrics to the problem of HIV infection follows a broadly similar, but nevertheless quite distinct pattern. The emotions that we have had to contend with in attempting to draw up guidelines for obstetric and midwifery practice may be summarised as "denial, resentment, irrational fear and complacency". In their own way each has proved counter-productive and difficult to overcome. We have heard something of the problems in relation to antenatal and postnatal care, where the picture has been similar.

The general principle has emerged that if, in the average clinical situation, the level of clinical hygiene is raised and scrupulously maintained, there is little cause for paranoia. The exception, small print to this timely and necessary general advice, is exposure to blood. Of all clinical disciplines, midwifery (and we use the word in the old fashioned context to include obstetrics) probably carries the highest risk of exposure to uncontrolled blood spillage. The pattern of the emotional responses is easy to follow: *denial* is immediate—"AIDS is a male disease and is irrelevant to the health care of women alone"; *irrational fear* is the first response once the validity of denial is broken; *resentment* is the reaction of a professional group to the fact that events outside its control should have a direct impact upon its clinical activities; *complacency* is perhaps the most insidious of all, in that the attitude runs something like this, "There may be a problem: there are things which need to be done when the problem is around, but the problem is not around with us; it may be in the United States, Africa, Scotland, London, wherever, but not here, so we need not bother."

The Royal College's Sub-Committee (see Appendix) had to steer a median course between these various reactions. In all the debates it has been very difficult to quantitate the risk to health care workers. By all reckoning this must be very low; nevertheless, the penalty for materialisation of this risk is extremely serious and may, for our professions, include the need to cease from this particular professional practice. We, therefore, took the view that *no reasonably avoidable risk is acceptable.* Our aim has been to advocate measures in routine practice to eliminate as far as is possible, personal contact with blood.

A.   *Primary contact* is by splashing, aspiration or by personal contact with blood on tissues, such as placenta, or maternal or neonatal skin. It is easy to overlook the fact that the recently delivered infant is heavily contaminated with maternal blood until such time as it has been adequately cleaned. This is of particular importance to paediatricians and others involved in neonatal care.

B.   *Secondary contact* involves contamination by blood of clothing, linen, (including drapes and swabs), furniture (including beds) and technical equipment (such as monitors and their straps). The risks are obviously less but involve others remote from primary clinical care such as domestic staff and laundry workers.

Neither of these objectives is proving easy to achieve. For years the practice of midwifery has paid lip service more to antisepsis than asepsis. Over the years Dettol has given way to Hibitane as the main armament. The use of gowns and masks has been traditional because of the historical spectre of puerperal fever of streptococcal origin, but with recession of the virulence of streptococcal infection the necessity for much of this has been questioned. Much of the impetus for this change has come for ideological reasons as part of the process of "demedicalisation" of midwifery. Masks and hats disappeared from delivery suites more than a decade ago; more recently there has been a move to dispense with the use of surgical gowns except for operative deliveries.

The Royal College's Sub-Committee, in its report, which was endorsed without comment in this respect by Councils of both the Royal College of Obstetricians and Gynaecologists and the Royal College of Midwives, recommends a reversal of this trend. The latest recommendation in the United States is that full protective clothing, including visor and mask should be worn for all obstetric procedures and deliveries. In this country we have adopted a typical but illogical British compromise that protective clothing should be adopted for high risk HIV situations as it is for Hepatitis B, but that for ordinary purposes facial covering should be omitted. Judging from some adverse reactions to a simple return to the use of protective gown and overshoes the compromise was apposite in the present United Kingdom context. We are nevertheless aware that the trend foreshadowed by the American recommendations may become pertinent one day, but the time is not yet.

Another feature of clinical practice ripe for revision is mouth-operated aspiration. This has been used for the pipetting of fetal scalp blood samples as well as traditionally the oropharyngeal aspiration of the neonate both during and after delivery. As far as fetal scalp sampling is concerned modern capillary tubes can acquire an adequate sample for pH studies by capillary attraction alone. For oropharyngeal neonatal aspiration, mechanical suction in hospital practice is easily provided; but for the community and domiciliary midwifery the best substitute for mouth-operated suction is still to be determined, the choices lying between a foot-operated suction pump or a simple bulb syringe.

As far as secondary contamination is concerned, although there is general approval of the principle that blood spills should be contained and decontaminated early, the advice concerning overshoes and protective footwear has likewise come in for adverse comment. This reaction has likewise stemmed from a current trend in operating theatre suite management, which places much less emphasis than formerly on the infectivity of the floor. Elaborate rituals for stepping over lines, tacky mats and changing trollies are gradually being eliminated; by the same token, surgeons and others with blood stained boots, have been remarkably cavalier, and, at times, frankly unhygienic in their social behaviour in the immediate post surgical phase. Boots and overshoes in the delivery suite are seen as trappings of uniform and therefore, perhaps, threatening and "dehumanising" in this environment; the phrase "chilling" was used in this respect, and I quote directly from a somewhat irresponsible article in the *Sunday Times*.

Other features of delivery suite protocol which have been subject to recommendations have also had a mixed reception. We are concerned that the practice of bleeding the cord to obtain a cord blood sample directly into a tube commonly leads to soiling of the outside of the tube. This is an unacceptable lack of hygiene for laboratory staff. Our initial suggestion that a needle and syringe is preferable overlooked the fact that the needling of a slippery cord with an elusive vessel was a clear recipe for a needle stick injury, obviously the most important complication to be avoided. A proposal for bleeding into a tube using a plastic funnel to avoid soiling was a compromise which was suggested. Unfortunately this method is inappropriate for certain haematological investigations, namely those associated with haemoglobinopathy, for which needle aspiration is required. A no-touch technique has therefore been devised using two clamps or sponge holders.

Finally we come to the handling of products of conception, namely the placenta and membranes. The placenta is often preserved for histological examination; it certainly should be in any case of abnormal delivery, especially preterm labour. At other times there is a widespread practice of preservation of the placenta for commercial purposes. In all cases it should be inserted into an appropriate container so that the outside is not contaminated. The Department of Health is currently examining the conditions under which the commercial process is handled to be certain that there is no risk of inadvertent transmission of viral infections. Occasionally amnion is used as temporary skin cover and indeed, in gynaecological practice for lining the cavity after vaginal extirpation. It has now been determined that the same rules should apply to amnion donation for grafting as for any other tissue donation. Mere exclusion of known high risk groups is insufficient in this context.

OPERATIVE OBSTETRICS

In general, differing only in degree from those of normal midwifery, operator soiling is much more likely with complex deliveries in the lithotomy position. Most obstetricians are trained to conduct such deliveries in a sitting position, as this provides some safeguard against a slippery neonate falling from the attendant's grasp. Under these circumstances full protective footwear is really essential if soiling of the operator's shoes and stockings is to be avoided.

There is a risk of forearm contamination in several obstetric manoeuvres, namely manual removal of the placenta, bimanual uterine compression, internal podalic version and breech extraction and reposition of an inverted uterus. Insertion of the whole hand into the genital tract will inevitably produce major soiling of the forearm of the operator. In the past these situations were managed by the provision of elbow length gloves. A possible answer may be the provision of surgical gowns with impervious arms and bibs. There is a case that all obstetric units should change to these for obstetric operations as a matter of some priority.

TECHNIQUE OF DELIVERY

As far as the technique of delivery is concerned we reviewed the evidence available to date, which is discussed elsewhere, and have concluded that there is no indication at present to advocate elective Caesarean section in the interests of the fetus merely because the mother is known to be HIV positive. We appreciate that these data are scanty and it is most important that further data are collected. It is sensible, however, to avoid traumatising fetal skin during the course of delivery and it may be prudent therefore to avoid fetal scalp sampling and internal electrodes for cardiac monitoring. It is arguable that obstetric forceps might be safer than the vacuum extractor as the likelihood of skin trauma is less.

PERINEAL INJURY

Repair of an episiotomy and lacerations provides some difficulties, the redundancy and flaccidity of the recently parturient vagina means that site exposure for episiotomy repair is difficult and the operator often has to rely on tactile direction of the needle. Although personal injury is rare, in most surgical needle sticks occurring between two participants, glove puncture is common. The greater availability of wider retractors in the delivery suite may be a measure required to diminish this risk.

CONCLUSION

.In summary therefore, there has been a range of recommendations to improve the level of hygiene to spilled blood across the spectrum of midwifery together with a recognition of further special precautions whenever the HIV risk is appreciated to be great. Most of these have involved a measure of controversy and their universal acceptance will not be easily achieved. Experience overseas suggests that the present measures should only be regarded as interim and more intensive protective measure may yet be advised in this country for routine obstetric practice.

The most important message to get across to all health care workers in this situation is that we need to achieve a psychological attitude to spilled blood as equivalent to that of faeces, and if we can achieve this we will not readily allow personal contact nor will we leave it uncleaned on soiled footwear, walked around changing rooms, coffee rooms and corridors. The battle for hearts and minds always is the most difficult to win and this one must commence now.

Discussion

Chairman: Dr F.D. Johnstone

JOHNSTONE: There is one point on which the speakers differed, and that is the question of whether we are operating a one-tier or a two-tier system. Miss Brierley felt that it should be a one-tier system, whereas Dr Scrimgeour was talking about people who are already identified as being positive and are being treated differently.

LUCAS: I would like to bring up the concept of risk. What one normally means in statistical or epidemiological terms when one uses the word "risk" is the mathematical relationship between the number of adverse effects with the number of subjects in the population itself. If the number of adverse effects is zero, then it is impossible to talk about risk. There are large numbers of AIDS patients now and there must be as many health professionals who have looked after them. There have been a huge number of health professionals who have been bathed from head to foot with blood without any observable adverse effect. Are we talking about that zero risk at present, or have there been other reports of transmission? If there have not, how long do we need to go on studying the population before we can relax with the present procedures?

HUDSON: I think that there are two points which have to be made. Firstly, the risk is extremely low. On the other hand, whatever it is, it is almost impossible to determine because of the time lag before such an occult event would become apparent. It is perhaps easier to relate to the needle stick injuries. If someone has had a needle stick injury from an infected person, then he goes for testing. But it will take a very long time before epidemiological evidence will give us proof or otherwise of a very small risk.

JEFFRIES: We can quantitate that risk itself in terms of the risk of inoculation injury with HIV positive material, at a confidence limit of 95%. 0.76% of inoculation injury is known HIV positive material. I should like to make two other points related to this. One is that a number of us have seen the appearance of AIDS as an opportunity to review all our practices. On occasions in the recent past I have found myself talking to hospital engineers and plumbers. The plumbers have got to go in and unblock the sink on an infectious disease ward where there may be a salmonella case etc. I think that the advice that is coming through now is sensible not only in terms of HIV, but also of Hepatitis B where the hit rate we know is between 20 and 30%.

The other point is about the one-tier or two-tier approach. It goes against the grain for me as a microbiologist to accept the two-tier approach. I run a laboratory, and for years I worked in a part of London where we had Lassa fever, smallpox and the highest Hepatitis B rate in the country coming through our hospital. I have seen a biohazard system working over the years. I now see it starting to fail. I now see that the biohazard impact has been diluted out by hepatitis and now by HIV. I think the time will come very soon where we will abandon the two-tier approach across the board. We will have to assume that all blood and body fluids are potentially infectious. The Centers for Disease Control are recommending a single-tier approach for the United States, so I think that it will come here. The important thing is that any guidelines are interim guidelines. Hopefully we will be updating them as time goes by.

SHARP: I am sure that we all agree with Dr Scrimgeour when he says that we want a "higher order of clinician" to deal with the patient. Yet later he made a reference that gave the impression that undergraduates in Edinburgh were doing venepunctures on HIV positive patients. In Sheffield that is not the case.

SCRIMGEOUR: I had better correct that because it is not the case in Edinburgh either. When we consider HIV positive patients, what we are looking for is the kind of staff who are that much more experienced than the students, than the resident and sometimes even the junior registrar. Similarly in the auxiliary professions we would like to see those patients dealt with by the sisters or senior staff nurses. Could I just come back to the two-tier system? Are we now going to change our tune and say that we should not separate out the HIV positive patients for special care?

JEFFRIES: Can I throw the question back to you Dr Scrimgeour, and ask if you think that you could sell that to your staff? I do not think that I could sell that to our laboratory staff at present. What I am saying is that we are moving in that direction; I do not think that we are there yet.

JOHNSTONE: The gloves are going to cost £8.00 a pair. It could be an enormous economic burden.

BRIERLEY: We are happy to adopt a one-tier infection control system, but I would hate to see the midwives dressed as suggested. I think that if we are going to adopt a one-tier infection control system it must be reasonable.

JEFFRIES: That is the point. What we have got to decide is what our staff will accept as the level of that single-tier, and whether we can educate them and convince them that we really are dealing with skin/mucous membrane exposure. The point made by Mr Hudson about the need for protection of the forearms does not just apply to obstetrics, and we may well have to spend money on gowns that do not allow penetration by body fluids. There may well be a need for all surgeons, all obstetricians, everyone engaged in basic procedures to have at least that sort of protective clothing in addition to gloves.

HARVEY: We referred to stickers on notes. In my hospital Hepatitis B is identified by a magenta sticker and HIV is identified by a black sticker. I would like to enquire from others what they feel about identifying labels and what we should do about them.

HUDSON: We have a common sticker which does not specify the nature of the disease so it does not raise any particular comment when used in an HIV situation.

SCRIMGEOUR: We use a sticker which just reads "risk of infection", red on a yellow background. At one point in Edinburgh we were going to put the equivalent of your black sticker on the front of the notes. We have got to have somewhere inside the notes an indication that this is a very important part of the care of that patient.

HARVEY: That is exactly my worry because it is on the front, and I would quite like to change it. The problem is that if it is not on the front of the notes, then it does not always get seen.

BRIERLEY: If we did have a one-tier system then there might not be a need to put that sticker anywhere.

SOUTTER: If HIV and Hepatitis B are spread in similar ways, and Hepatitis B is a more infectious agent than HIV, can we extrapolate from the known rates of infection of Hepatitis B in medical or midwifery staff, to arrive at what we might expect in HIV?

JEFFRIES: The figures are available for acute Hepatitis B. Perhaps Dr Glynn might like to comment because the figures are kept under the auspices of the public health authority. Do remember that we are talking about acute Hepatitis B, not Hepatitis B at the carrier stage. That is more certainly underreported. There are recognised high risk areas in medical health care practice in general in this country. Pathologists and post mortem technicians are the highest in terms of risk. As far as I understand there is no obvious excess of Hepatitis B in obstetric or midwifery staff.

GLYNN: I cannot give you the figures for Hepatitis B carriers. Concerning the two-tier system, I do not think it is going to be particularly risky because the figures on HIV spread to health care staff indicate that the risk at the moment is low even in areas of high prevalence, so low as to be virtually negligible. But even a small risk is not really acceptable. I do not think that you are going to get much quantitative help from the figures for Hepatitis B. I think that we are moving toward, and in some places we already have, a one-tier system. The trouble is that if no real threat appears, one tends to get complacent. People resent being forced to take complicated precautionary measures that they do not perceive to be necessary.

HARE: I was quite impressed by the "compromise" midwives' gear. I am quite surprised that the working party did not recommend that the labour ward should be treated as the operating theatre is; that is, an area where one changed one's clothes on entering and changed again when going out. Also, is infection spread by bath water?

HUDSON: There was a certain division of opinion in the working party in that respect.

HEDGE: Dentists in my hospital who work in a clinic for HIV positive patients wear full protective clothing, and have found that it is quite acceptable to the patients if they are told what it looks like beforehand and the reasons why it is necessary.

SPIRO: I have a comment about the procedures that we have been required to follow in handling the baby in the community, during health visits. We must wear surgical gloves whenever examining the baby in case the baby passes urine, faeces or vomit. I would hope that we would feel that sort of thing is unnecessary. But a large number of health authorities are adopting this measure. There is also the confusion over which antiseptics are appropriate. There does not seem to be any consistency in the advice we are given.

Maternal resuscitation, haemorrhage and shock—the obstetrician's viewpoint

Professor W. Thompson

INTRODUCTION

Although the great majority of pregnant patients will have an uneventful pregnancy and delivery, significant complications involving haemorrhage can occur at any time resulting in maternal shock necessitating urgent resuscitation. In such circumstances health care workers will be expected to respond rapidly undertaking clinical procedures and operating under extreme pressure. As inadvertent skin puncture with a needle or scalpel used in an infected patient is the principal mode by which HIV can be transmitted to a surgeon or nurse it is essential that all staff are familiar with hospital procedures designed to protect them from exposure to body fluids. In the absence of routine antenatal testing for HIV it is preferable that all obstetric units adopt routine policies for practitioners and familiarity with these will improve efficiency in use when an emergency arises.

OBSTETRIC HAEMORRHAGE

Obstetric haemorrhage is still one of the gravest medical emergencies, accounting in relative terms for significant maternal morbidity and mortality.[1] The causes of significant obstetric haemorrhage are listed in Table 1. Bleeding from the

Table 1

Major causes of obstetric haemorrhage

SPONTANEOUS ABORTION
ECTOPIC PREGNANCY
ANTEPARTUM HAEMORRHAGE — Placenta Praevia
— Abruptio Placentae
POST-PARTUM HAEMORRHAGE

pregnant uterus, in particular, can rapidly become life-threatening and demand immediate control. In high risk cases, namely known HIV positive women and those with AIDS, it is accepted that barrier nursing must be used, but such precautions may result in a delay in initiating resuscitation. Emergency equipment which may have been removed from the delivery room must be readily available and fully operational with minimal delay. Once significant haemorrhage occurs, regardless of the cause, two large-bore intravenous drips (14-16 gauge) should be inserted. A central venous pressure (CVP) of Swan-Ganz catheter is an essential aid in the assessment of the patient, especially in the presence of shock; the nominal pressure range is 5-15 cm of water. Immediate replacement of body fluids with dextran/saline should be commenced concurrent with a rapid bu. careful physical examination and relevant laboratory evaluation. Once the cause of the bleeding has been established specific therapy is instituted as outlined below.

Abortion

Spontaneous abortion (at present defined in British Law as termination of pregnancy before 28 weeks gestation) is by far the commonest cause of bleeding in pregnancy; it is usually a complication of the first trimester and at least 20% of pregnancies will terminate in this way. There is no evidence to date that HIV positivity *per se* will increase the incidence of abortion, but associated risk factors such as drug abuse can result in lethal abnormalities. In cases of threatened abortion in which fetal viability is confirmed by ultrasound and the bleeding is not excessive, the patient should be advised to rest at home. If she is HIV positive she should be carefully consulted regarding the advisability of continuing with the pregnancy, in view of the known risks.[2] When the abortion is inevitable there is usually significant blood loss requiring hospitalisation and blood transfusion. An ultrasonic scan should be performed and if this shows retained products of conception it will be necessary to evacuate the uterus under general anaesthesia.

Ectopic pregnancy

The incidence of ectopic pregnancy is probably increased in HIV positive women; a proportion of this population will be prostitutes with pelvic inflammatory disease. Tubal rupture will result in significant intraperitoneal haemorrhage and thus necessitate urgent resuscitation and laparotomy.

Antepartum haemorrhage

In later pregnancy the most important causes of severe haemorrhage are placenta praevia and abruptio placentae. All patients with a major degree of placenta praevia should be admitted to hospital; conservative management to ensure fetal maturity before delivery may involve a prolonged period of nursing in the antenatal ward. Delivery by Caesarean section can usually be planned and this procedure must be undertaken by senior and experienced staff.

Abruptio placentae, or the separation of a normally situated placenta, may require resuscitation and delivery as soon as possible. Effective resuscitation requires rapid replacement of blood volume and fresh whole blood will reduce the risk of disseminated intravascular coagulation as a complication.

Postpartum haemorrhage

The most dangerous time for the mother is the third stage of labour; the uterus must contract, expel the placenta and constrict the blood vessels to arrest bleeding from the placental site.

If the placenta is retained, in association with excessive bleeding, manual removal under general anaesthesia will be necessary and full protection using a waterproof gown or long arm gloves must be worn as the procedure will involve intrauterine exploration.

Special problems can arise when dealing with deep vaginal lacerations or tears of the cervix. The sutures are frequently inserted blindly using the index finger to guide the needle through the tissue and thus ensure accurate placement at the apex of the wound. This will inevitably increase the risk of needle stick injury. It is therefore advised that good lighting and adequate assistance is available to provide wide exposures of the wound edges and sutures can then be inserted under direct vision.

NON-HAEMORRHAGIC OBSTETRIC SHOCK

The common causes of 'shock' not directly related to haemorrhage are listed in Table 2. Urgent resuscitation involving invasive procedures will be necessary to deal with such complications and it is imperative that staff are not only trained to deal with the problems but receive instruction in the use of protective gear to avoid contact with body fluids. The prognosis for survival in patients with established AIDS, already debilitated and anaemic, will be much worse when pregnancy is complicated by such disorders.

Table 2

Causes of non-haemorrhagic obstetric shock

— Amniotic fluid embolism
— Mendelson's Syndrome (inhaled vomit)
— Thromboembolic Disease
— Uterine Inversion
— Eclampsia
— Bacteraemic Shock

Amniotic fluid embolism

This rare but lethal condition usually occurs in labour associated with strong uterine contractions in the presence of intact membranes. Cardiorespiratory collapse is likely and urgent resuscitation will be necessary to reduce maternal mortality. Invasive procedures such as tracheal intubation and insertion of central venous pressure monitors will expose staff to the risk of contact with saliva and blood. Thus protective clothing should be worn. In the acute situation these measures may be inadvertently overlooked and in haste needle stick injuries are more likely to occur.

Mendelson's syndrome

The inhalation of stomach contents during general anaesthesia or in severely debilitated patients in pregnancy can lead to profuse bronchospasm, pulmonary oedema and eventually cardiac failure. The risk of this life-threatening complication can be greatly reduced by the routine administration of a simple alkaline mixture such as magnesium trisilicate during labour. H_2 blockers such as ranitidine may also be used in women at high risk of needing Caesarean section. If the complication does occur urgent treatment is necessary to avoid the risk of sudden deterioration. This will include full oxygenation, intermittent positive pressure ventilation, aspiration of any foreign material from the lungs and drugs to reduce bronchospasm.

Thromboembolic disease

This serious complication of pulmonary embolism is commoner during the puerperium and results in chest pain, sudden collapse or death. The condition is more likely to occur in debilitated patients such as those with AIDS who may be confined to bed. Invasive procedures such as venography are frequently used to confirm the diagnosis and it may be necessary to perform pulmonary embolectomy. Full protective measures as previously discussed will be necessary to protect staff from exposure to blood.

Uterine inversion

Acute inversion of the uterus may occur spontaneously or be produced by methods employed to expel the placenta. This rare complication can generally lead to profound shock. Rapid replacement of the uterus is essential and as this will involve intravaginal and intrauterine manipulation, protective clothing, including a waterproof gown, should be worn.

Eclampsia

This acute emergency is most likely to occur in a patient previously affected by pregnancy-induced hypertension; however it can occur without warning at any time during pregnancy and up to 48 hours after delivery. Maintenance of an airway during the convulsion is an essential part of treatment and may therefore involve risk to staff from exposure to saliva or trauma from bites. Although HIV can be recovered from saliva of persons with symptomatic and asymptomatic HIV infection the risk is low of transmission from this source.[3] Follow-up investigations of health care workers who were bitten by patients with AIDS revealed no evidence of HIV seroconversion.[4] Two nurses who performed cardio-pulmonary resuscitation on a patient with AIDS-related complex[5] and 63 health care workers performing or assisting in procedures on HIV-infected patients that involved direct exposure to saliva resulted in none developing antibody to HIV.[6] Eclamptic patients during or following the convulsion are frequently incontinent of urine and this will present an additional risk factor to staff who may come into contact with the body fluid during resuscitation measures. HIV has rarely been isolated from urine of infected patients,[7] and there are no known cases to date in which contact with urine in the occupational setting has resulted in transmission of HIV. In spite of this it is advisable that health care staff avoid extensive exposure to the urine of HIV-infected persons.

Bacteraemic shock

This condition in obstetric practice occurs most often in association with septic abortion. The infection may also originate from the urinary tract, especially if there is an in-dwelling urinary catheter, or from an intravenous plastic cannula. Such infections would be more common in patients with AIDS and the situation would again be more serious in pregnancy as it is known to result in immunosuppression *per se*.[8] Thus aggressive therapy will be necessary to prevent and treat infections in pregnancy such as *E Coli* known to cause bacteraemic shock. The condition can be further complicated by disseminated intravascular coagulation leading to a clotting defect.

The treatment of bacteraemic shock will require infusion of large volumes of fluid, given under central venous pressure monitoring, to improve tissue perfusion. Massive doses of intravenous hydrocortisone have also been recommended but the use of this in patients with impairment of cell-mediated immunity may lead to further complications and has not been fully evaluated.[9]

CONCLUSIONS

In dealing with an obstetric emergency involving massive blood loss and/or shock, carefully planned measures designed to protect staff from exposure to blood, body fluids and needle stick injury may be forgotten in the haste to cope with a life-threatening situation. Protective measures should not be so cumbersome as to delay response when urgent resuscitation is necessary and staff should be adequately trained and familiar with such hospital procedures.

REFERENCES
1. Department of Health and Social Security. *Report on Health and Social Subjects, 29. Report on confidential enquiries into maternal deaths in England and Wales 1979-81.* London: HMSO, 1986.
2. Pinching AJ, Jeffries DJ. AIDS and HTLV-III/LAV infection: consequences for obstetricians and perinatal medicine. *J Obstet Gynaecol* 1985; **92:** 1211-1217.
3. Ho DD, Byington RE, Schooley RT, Flynn T, Rota TR, Hirsch MS. Infrequency of isolation of HTLV-III virus from the saliva in AIDS. (Letter) *N Engl J Med* 1985; **313:** 1606.
4. Drummond JA. Seronegative 18 months after being bitten by a patient with AIDS. (Letter) *JAMA* 1986; **256:** 2342-2343.
5. Saviteer SM, White GC, Cohen MS. HTLV-III exposure during cardiopulmonary resuscitation. *N Engl J Med* 1985; **313:** 1606-1607.
6. Gerberding JL, Bryant-Le Blanc CE, Nelson K *et al.* Risk of transmitting the human immunodeficiency virus, cytomegalovirus and hepatitis B virus to health care workers exposed to patients with AIDS and AIDS-related conditions. *J Infect Dis* 1987; **156:** 1-8.
7. Levy JA, Kaminsky LS, Morrow WJ, Steiner K, Luciw P, Dina D, Hoxie CJ, Ohiro L. Infection by the retrovirus associated with acquired immundeficiency syndrome. Clinical, biological and molecular features. *Ann Intern Med* 1985; **103:** 694-699.
8. Larsen B. Host defence mechanisms in obstetrics and gynaecology. In: *Clinics in Obstetrics and Gynaecology, Vol. 10.* Ed. D Charles. London: Saunders, 1983; pp.37-64.
9. Weinberg ED. Pregnancy-associated depression of cell mediated immunity. *Rev Infect Dis* 1984; **6:** 814-831.

Maternal resuscitation, haemorrhage and shock—the anaesthetist's viewpoint

Dr D. A. Zidemann

Maternal resuscitation is a relatively rare event (8.9 deaths per 100,000 total births). It is impossible to assess accurately the total problem as reports only record those mothers who did not survive, and not those who did survive but required resuscitation. Despite its rarity, maternal resuscitation should never be delayed because of lack of training, experience or equipment. In the situation where a possible or proven HIV infective patient has been identified this should not provide any reason for delay. Resuscitation must begin immediately, with or without equipment, by whomsoever discovers the cardiac arrest victim. Any delay may lead to morbidity and mortality of either mother or fetus or both.

In a few cases the possibility of a cardiac arrest during pregnancy can be predicted. Pre-existing heart disease, either congenital or acquired, or a pre-existing arrhythmia are the most obvious causes. Myocardial infarction and cerebrovascular accidents are now seen more often in younger women. Pre pregnancy investigation and treatment of such patients may be the possible cause of their positive HIV status. Pregnancy-induced hypertension and toxaemia are well known, but should they be allowed to progress untreated can result in cardiopulmonary arrest.

Probably the most common cause of cardio pulmonary collapse during pregnancy is aorto-caval compression from the gravid uterus. The first manoeuvre in resuscitating the pregnant mother is therefore to displace the uterus sideways either by pulling it manually to one side or more simply turning the patient on her side. A simple wedge placed behind the mother's back may be enough but the rescuer must be sure that any aorto-caval compression has been released. If this manoeuvre is not successful then the patient's airway must be opened, breathing assessed and expired air respiration (mouth to mouth respiration) commenced. Although saliva is known to carry the HIV virus, we are assured by the virologists that there is no significant risk of acquiring a serious viral infection from mouth to mouth respiration. Nevertheless, there are a wide variety of mouth pieces/airways available to the rescuer. However, many such devices do not perform to expectation and nearly all require some formal training on a repeated basis for their use to be effective. Current opinions suggest that it is better to use a device that does not have an intra-oral portion, thus doing away with the need to place anything inside the mouth. The mouth to mask technique or the use of a simple viral filter are good examples. With ventilation established the pulse of the victim must be carefully assessed. Chest compressions must be commenced immediately if no pulse is present. The effectiveness of chest compressions with the patient in the lateral position has not been properly validated. Should compressions be required it would probably be more appropriate to roll the patient back onto a wedge or to place the patient on her back and to displace the uterus manually. Again it is vitally important to minimise aorta-caval compression. There are no implications for the HIV positive patient with regard to chest compression.

Reviewing advanced life support techniques in detail is beyond the scope of this paper. If the patient, following the basic life support described above, has not responded, then an intravenous cannula should be inserted into the major vein, the patient should be intubated and the neonate delivered by emergency Caesarean section. Resuscitation of the mother should be continued and the surgeon may wish to consider internal cardiac massage (by dividing the diaphragm and pericardium and squeezing the heart directly) from within the abdominal cavity. HIV positive precautions for these invasive procedures have been fully described elsewhere in this volume.

All resuscitation equipment must be properly cleaned and disinfected after use. The resuscitation bags, masks and laryngoscopes can be heat sterilised. All disposables should be carefully packaged in properly marked containers before disposal.

Finally, it cannot be emphasised enough that cardio pulmonary resuscitation of a suspected or proven HIV positive mother should not be delayed for the want of equipment nor the fear of infection. None of the basic life support procedures are risk factors. Only proper education and training will ensure that such patients are not provided with a second rate service.

REFERENCES

1. Evans T. *ABC of resuscitation*. London: British Medical Journal, 1986.
2. 1985 National Conference on cardio pulmonary resuscitation (CPR) and emergency cardiac care (ECC). Standards and guidelines for cardio pulmonary resuscitation and emergency cardiac care. *JAMA* 1986; **255:** 2905-2989.
3. Lee RV, Rogers BD, White RM, Harvey RC. Cardiopulmonary resuscitation in pregnant women. *Am J Med* 1986; **81:** 311-318.
4. Safar B, Bircher N. *Cardiopulmonary cerebral resuscitation*. Philadelphia: Saunders, 1988; pp 350-351.

Discussion

Chairman: Dr F.D. Johnstone

JOHNSTONE: Certainly these are very major obstetric and resuscitative problems, even if uncommon.

THOMPSON: I have not seen a great many drug abusers and their bad veins in Belfast. Is this a problem with resuscitation?

ZIDEMAN: It is not such a problem. Most of our staff are quite competent in putting the needle in the external jugular vein, which is not a vein which is often attacked by drug addicts.

JOHNSTONE: We have had 2 patients who have been given inhalational anaesthetics because they had already attacked the jugular vein.

THOMPSON: What about the acute emergency situation, after an accident, or haemorrhage in the labour ward? The recommendations are that minimum requirements should be mask and gloves.

SCOTT: One of the obstetric emergencies that we have seen in Miami was a mother who had acute respiratory distress because of severe pneumocystis pneumonitis who ended up in the medical intensive care unit. She was several months pregnant and elected to deliver the baby by induced labour. The mother died 2 or 3 days later. That baby was severely premature but was not affected. Another lady with a similar presentation did survive the pneumocystis and did ultimately deliver by normal vaginal delivery. But the major emergencies have occurred around the medical emergencies rather than being associated with acute haemorrhage or acute problems around the time of delivery.

ZIDEMAN: This is exactly the problem. The physician is reluctant to touch them because they have primary respiratory disease. The obstetrician thinks that it may be too early or may be too late in another sense. The anaesthetist has them on intensive care. The surgeon is not interested, and so it goes down the line. The patient ends up with an HIV positive label; nobody comes to see her, because nobody wants to see her. The biggest problem about this is that they are seen often by junior staff.

SCRIMGEOUR: If a patient collapses in the labour ward you as an anaesthetist would almost prefer not to know what their HIV status was, because it really is not going to make the slightest bit of difference to how you are going to manage the patient. Is that fair comment?

ZIDEMAN: Yes.

LUCAS: It seems in fact that if you want to be a health professional looking after sick people who could suddenly die on you, you mustn't worry about the possibility of personal risk.

ZIDEMAN: There is tremendous fear of this disease. People may withhold medical treatment because they are frightened, and probably unjustly so. You have to be aware of the risks that you are taking, and whether you in your own mind can justify it. It requires training to get over that.

JOHNSTONE: The keynote for this session has been that no reasonably avoidable risk is acceptable. The discussions have led us to a position where we are leaning towards a one-tier system where there is great awareness of risks, but that our practice is the same for all patients. At the moment the guidelines differentiate two standards of risk for various reasons such as acceptability to staff and expense. These are to be seen as interim guidelines which will be reviewed as more information becomes available in the future. At the moment we are working towards a higher standard of care for all patients in our practice generally, and examining a number of areas which we have not thought very much about to date.

SECTION V

HIV AND HEALTH CARE WORKERS

Risk of transmission to other patients and staff

Mr A. J. W. Sim

INTRODUCTION

A considerable fear of health care workers at all levels is that they will be infected with HIV from a patient. Less well documented are the concerns of non-infected patients about the possibility of being infected while in hospital. The results of infection with HIV are dire in terms of the health of the individual and because of the way society views those infected. It is therefore not surprising that debate about these forms of transmission exists.

TRANSMISSION FROM PATIENT TO PATIENT

The possibility of this mode of transmission is important when determining where HIV patients should be nursed during their hospital stay. There is no recorded incidence of transmission of HIV from patient to patient in a surgical ward. Casual contact with other people does not result in transmission of HIV and in a ward run by alert staff there should not be any possibility of cross-contact with body fluids of an infected patient. For practical purposes this mode of transmission should be ignored, and HIV-infected patients can be nursed, albeit with appropriate precautions, on an open surgical ward.

ACCIDENTAL INOCULATION IN HEALTH CARE WORKERS

Accidental inoculation of infected blood can cause seroconversion from HIV. It is uncommon and the likely risk of acquiring HIV infection from a single needle stick injury is less than 1%. Other exposures to infected material may also be responsible for seroconversion. The Cooperative Needlestick Surveillance Group[1] which collected data from 283 participating centres in the United States reported on 938 health care workers who had either parenteral or mucous membrane exposure to blood or other body fluids from patients known to have AIDS or AIDS-related illnesses. Fifty-six percent occurred in the patient's room or the ward, 22% in intensive care units, 11% in operating theatres, procedure rooms or mortuaries; 4% in 'emergency clinics' and 7% in laboratories. Seventy-six percent of the exposures were from needle sticks or cuts from sharp instruments. Two female nurses were seropositive; one injured with a colonic biopsy needle was positive on a blood sample taken 287 days after exposure, the other was seronegative within 30 days of a deep needle stick injury but was positive at 6 months.

A prospective study of 150 health care workers with occupational exposure to infected body fluids carried out by the PHLS Communicable Disease Surveillance Centre[2] in the UK failed to reveal any seroconversions to positive. These exposures occurred in nurses (61%), doctors (21%), laboratory workers (5%) and other health care workers (13%). Injuries from needles or other sharp instruments occurred in 76 individuals, 60 of whom were nurses or doctors.

Isolated reports of confirmed seroconversion in health care workers have identified transmission by needle stick injury on 4 occasions and via skin lesions on 3.[2] The needle stick injuries have been: an actual inoculation of blood,[3] a deep muscle injection with a wide bore needle,[4] an injury without apparent injection of blood[5] and a relatively superficial needle stick injury with a needle contaminated with pleural fluid occurring at the time of thoracocentesis.[6] Infection has occurred in a laboratory worker with the same virus with which he or she was working.[7]

There are a number of other incidents which have led to the identification of seropositive health care workers in whom the infection could have been acquired by occupational exposure. Proof is lacking and caution must be exercised in interpreting these events.

A surgeon, operating in Zaire (1972-1977) developed diarrhoea, weight loss, cutaneous anergy, pneumocystis carinii pneumonia and oral candidiasis and died in 1977 with respiratory insufficiency. She had worked under primitive conditions and reported seeing at least 1 case of Kaposi's sarcoma. She died from a disease which involved immune deficiency and could have been AIDS; the HIV infection could have been contracted from an infected patient.[8] Another young surgeon has died in 1988 from AIDS, believed to have been acquired occupationally in Zimbabwe.

One dentist out of 1309 dental workers without any known risk factors (94% of whom reported accidental skin puncture during dental treatment) has been found to be infected.[9]

Health care workers, apparently without any other risk factors, who are seropositive and in whom needle stick injury has occurred have been reported.[10,11] Lack of knowledge about their preinjury or immediate postinjury HIV status mean that infection cannot definitely be attributed to "occupational" injury.

Surgeons recognise that they are at risk of contracting infectious diseases from patients on whom they carry out operations. This is exemplified by transmission of the hepatitis viruses. Surgery has developed protocols of precautions to protect those involved in operations on known infected patients. Despite this, surgeons continue to be infected by their patients and the fact that a surgeon can contract HIV infection and subsequently die with AIDS gives rise to considerable concern.

IDENTIFICATION OF PATIENTS WITH WHOM PRECAUTIONS SHOULD BE TAKEN

At the present time it is both incorrect and unacceptable to carry out routine HIV antibody tests on all patients undergoing surgery (with or without their permission). The accuracy of the present HIV antibody test is such that a positive antibody test in an at-risk person is likely to be true, but a positive result in a non-risk person is likely to be false. It may take as long as 3 months for an individual who has been infected with HIV to become antibody positive and this "window" must be taken into account in interpreting a negative antibody test. The moral and social implications of identifying an individual as being infected with HIV are such that at the present time considerable thought must be given to the possible legal and ethical consequences of testing an individual without consent, however strong the medical imperative to do so may appear.

Fundamental to medical and surgical practice must be the identification of individual patients who are thought to be in one of the at-risk categories. At the present time the infection has remained within the high risk groups; whether it will in the future remains to be seen. It is encouraging that there have not been larger numbers of HIV positive patients reported from low risk heterosexual populations. Even though an individual may be in a high risk group, for him or her to become infected it is necessary to have taken part in a high risk activity. In taking a history appropriate questions to alert the medical practitioner to the possibility of an individual being in a high risk group should become part of routine practice. Once it is apparent that a patient may be from a high risk category more direct and specific questions relating to activities must be asked. These questions have to include ones relating to anal intercourse, promiscuity, sharing of needles, whether an HIV antibody test has been done and the result.

A practical policy for patients undergoing surgical procedures is as follows: if a patient is considered at risk of having HIV infection, but his status is unknown, the taking of blood for HIV antibody testing should be discussed with him. If he agrees to such a test then counselling about the significance of the result should be undertaken. If the patient does not agree, and the surgical procedure to be carried out is not of a major type, then the patient should be managed as if he was HIV positive. If a major surgical procedure is to be undertaken on a patient who is considered to be at risk of HIV infection and the patient refuses testing then the surgeon responsible for the management is in a dilemma. He should carefully consider whether he is willing to carry out the procedure (with or without appropriate precautions), or whether he is going to test the patient without his consent. As mentioned above, if the latter course is taken the surgeon must have considered the consequences (medical, social and perhaps medicolegal) of identifying a patient as being infected with HIV.

Although a contentious issue, testing for disease without prior consent is not new to surgical or medical practice; only rarely is permission sought before testing potential carriers of the Hepatitis B virus. However, the fact that uninformed testing has occurred in the past is not necessarily a reason for condoning it now or in the future. The rationale behind testing before major surgery is based on the perceived or real risk of occupational infection associated with a probably greater chance of accidental injury and greater exposure to infected body fluids during prolonged and sometimes difficult procedures.

An alternative form of management is to treat every patient as if they were infected. By doing this it would not be necessary to consider HIV antibody testing, nor would it be necessary to identify patients as potentially infected.

There are a number of reasons why this would not be an appropriate strategy at present: intellectually it is unsatisfactory as we know that even in the high risk areas the majority of patients are not carriers of HIV; practically it would have the effect of reducing the number of operations that could be carried out per operating session; economically it would almost certainly be more expensive. If the infection spreads through the community and identification of at risk populations is no longer possible it may be that the only pragmatic solution would be to move towards treating every patient with precautions and techniques which would ensure the maximum level of safety for the surgeon.

PRECAUTIONS FOR HEALTH CARE WORKERS IN THE PRESENCE OF KNOWN OR SUSPECTED HIV INFECTION[12]

Health care workers who at any time in their practice use sharp instruments in the presence of body fluids, particularly blood, would be unwise to ignore this viral infection. Not enough notice is taken of the hepatitis viruses, and health care workers do contract hepatitis as an occupational disease. In general terms the precautions used when managing patients with hepatitis infection should be employed for those known to have HIV infection.

As far as possible ward management should be no different from the management of a patient not considered to be infected. In those patients with open wounds or discharge of body fluids, nursing must be carried out in a fashion which ensures not only protection of the nurse from possible infection but also the correct disposal of contaminated materials.

Segregation of at-risk patients in separate infectious disease wards or side rooms of surgical wards should be reserved for those who request it and those in whom continuing discharge of body fluids before or after surgery make rational and sympathetic nursing impossible on an open ward. Attention must be paid to the feelings of other patients and attempts should be made to protect the infected patient from the irrational prejudices of others.

Any person involved in a procedure which involves sharp instruments and body fluids who has a skin lesion, whether it be a cut or a skin disease (i.e. eczema), should ensure that the lesion is reliably covered. If this cannot be guaranteed then they should not expose themselves to the possibility that infected material will come into contact with the break in the skin and should not be involved in the procedure.

During all invasive procedures individuals should consider wearing plastic aprons, disposable gowns, a visor or glasses and gloves. Disposable drapes should be used. Unprotected sharp instruments should be avoided. Meticulous attention to detail and a no-touch technique should be employed wherever possible. All needles whether used for blood sampling, drug administration or for inserting an intravenous cannula should, with any other disposable sharps, be discarded, without re-sheathing, into a safe container for incineration. These measures will reduce the possibility of skin contact with contaminated blood and other fluids and should decrease the incidence of injury with sharp instruments, but the major effect will come from the atmosphere of extra attention to detail created by adopting these precautions and techniques.

In the operating theatre, all unnecessary equipment should be removed and only personnel directly involved in the operation permitted in the operating theatre. The anaesthetist and his assistant must wear gloves, a gown and either glasses or a visor. Great care should be taken with the insertion of intravenous cannulae. The introducing needle along with any other disposable sharps should be discarded without re-sheathing, into a safe container for incineration.

The surgeon, his assistant(s) and scrub nurse should wear plastic aprons, disposable gowns, a visor or glasses and 2 pairs of gloves (normal size and one size larger). Plastic overshoes can be worn over existing theatre footwear, but if not, all boots or clogs should be left in the operating theatre at the end of the operation. Disposable drapes should be used.

At the end of the procedure the operators should discard all disposable garments into appropriate receptacles before leaving the theatre. The floor of the operating theatre should be mopped with appropriate hypochlorite solution and special care taken with any major spillages of blood.[13]

The patient should recover from her operation either in the operating theatre or a recovery area where the staff are fully versed in care of the HIV infected patient. Once back on the ward, nursing care should be the same as for any patient after surgery. If there are blood stained dressings these should be covered or replaced using the precautions listed above.

TECHNIQUES

The instruments used will be the same as for an operation carried out in a noninfected patient. Surgical technique should be essentially unaltered with the following exceptions:

(a) Unprotected sharp instruments should be avoided; for example more use should be made of scissors than knives.

(b) If appropriate, stapling devices should take the place of needle and suture, particularly in bowel anastomosis and skin closure.

(c) Haemostasis should be meticulous and a no-touch technique employed when possible.

These measures will reduce the possibility of skin contact with contaminated blood and other fluids and should decrease the incidence of injury to the operators by sharp instruments.

ACCIDENTAL INJURY

If accidental injury does occur during surgery the wound should be cleaned immediately with soap and water, it should be made to bleed and then dressed appropriately. The incident should be reported to the Control of Infection Officer. Blood should be taken from the injured individual and stored for future testing should the need arise. If the accident has occurred in an at-risk patient whose HIV status is not known then blood should be taken from the patient and stored; the patient should be informed of this once she has recovered from her operation. Such an injury is likely to cause considerable distress to the individual involved, and every effort must be made to allay unnecessary fear of HIV infection, bearing in mind that it may take up to 3 months for seroconversion to occur. Any acute viral type illness occurring after an injury is likely to cause anxiety and it is at this time that definite knowledge of the HIV status of the patient may be of value in managing the injured individual. The medicolegal situation regarding compensation following occupational infection with HIV is as yet undefined.

THE FUTURE

The potential for acquiring infection during care of patients infected with hepatitis and HIV and perhaps other retroviruses is something to which surgeons should give considerable thought. Accidental injury at the time of surgery should be relegated to the past; efforts should be directed towards protection of the surgeon and the development of techniques and instruments which minimise blood spillage and penetrating injury with needles, knives or other sharp instruments. Surgical gloves are punctured in as many as 30% of operations, and are therefore an inadequate protection for the surgeon. Penetrating injury with needle or knife occurs in as many as 15% of operations. Modern technology, expensive as it is, must be harnessed for the use of the surgeon. Ultrasonic dissectors/aspirators, lasers, tissue glues and staples should be used in routine surgical practice.[13] Then, and only then, will surgeons be able to exploit technological advances and play a part in the necessary development of safer and more sophisticated operating techniques.

Portions of this article are derived from articles written in *Surgery* and *Intravenous Therapy and Clinical Monitoring*.[13,14]

REFERENCES

1. McCray E. The Co-operative Needlestick Surveillance Group. Occupational risk of the acquired immune deficiency syndrome among health care workers. *N Engl J Med* 1986; **314:** 1127-1132.
2. McEvoy M, Porter K, Mortimer P, Simmons N, Shanson D. Prospective study of clinical, laboratory and ancillary staff with accidental exposures to blood or body fluids from patients infected with HIV. *Br Med J* 1987; **294:** 1595-1597.
3. Anonymous. Needlestick transmission of HTLV-III from a patient infected in Africa. *Lancet* 1984; **2:** 1376-1377.
4. Stricof RL, Morse DL. HTLV III/LAV seroconversion following deep intramuscular needlestick injury. *N Engl J Med* 1986; **314:** 1115.
5. Neisson-Vernant G, Arfi S, Mathez D, Leibowitch J, Monplaisir N. Needlestick HIV seroconversion in a nurse. *Lancet* 1986; **2:** 814.
6. Oksenhendler E, Harzic M, Le Roux IM. HIV infection with seroconversion after a superficial needlestick injury to the finger. *N Engl J Med* 1986; **315:** 582.
7. Palca J. Lab worker infected with AIDS virus. *Nature* 1987; **329:** 92.
8. Bygbjerg IC. AIDS in a Danish surgeon (Zaire, 1976). (Letter) *Lancet* 1983; **2:** 925.
9. Klein RS, Phelan JA, Freeman K, Schable C, Friedland GH, Trieger N, Steigbigel NH. Low occupational risk of human immunodeficiency virus infection among dental professionals. *N Engl J Med* 1988; **318:** 86-90.
10. Belani A, Dunning R, Dutta D, Jiji V, Rosen S, Levin ML, Berg R, Glassen D, Sigelman S, Baker S. AIDS in a hospital worker. *Lancet* 1984; **1:** 676.
11. Anonymous. CDC update: evaluation of HTLV-III-associated infection in health care personnel—United States. *MMWR* 1985; **34:** 575-578.
12. Jeffries D. Control of Infection Policies. *Br Med J* 1987; **295:** 33-35.
13. Sim AJW, Dudley HAF. Surgeons and HIV. *Br Med J* 1988; **296:** 80.
14. Sim AJW. IV therapy and HIV. *Intravenous Therapy and Clinical Monitoring* 1988; **9:** 140-145.
15. Sim AJW. AIDS and the surgeon. *Surgery* 1988; **59:** 1396-1401.

HIV-infected health care workers

Dr D. J. Jeffries

INTRODUCTION

Escalation of the epidemic of HIV infection has led to anxiety over the possibility that HIV-infected health care workers may present a risk to their patients. This issue entered the public arena in the United Kingdom in November 1987, in the case X v. Y, when a High Court judge made permanent an injunction against a national newspaper preventing the disclosure of the names of two doctors with AIDS undergoing treatment at a London hospital.[1] The extremely low risk of transmission of HIV by an infected doctor was considered to be far outweighed by the dangers of breaching confidentiality for those found to be infected or at risk. Only if absolute confidentiality could be guaranteed would doctors come forward for testing and seek medical attention and counselling if they were found to be infected. There are three major aspects to consider in attempting to evaluate the evidence supporting the assumption that the risks are minute: the danger of transmitting HIV itself, the possibility of transmission of opportunistic infections and the possible risks to the patient if a medical practitioner should develop dementia as a result of HIV encephalopathy. Although the public may perceive that these risks are particularly worrying in the context of an infected medical practitioner, they must also be considered for any health care worker who has patient contact.

POSSIBLE RISKS OF TRANSMISSION OF HIV

The major routes of transmission of HIV are well described and are: sexual transmission, transfusion of infected blood or blood products, use of contaminated syringes and needles by intravenous drug users, vertical transmission from mother to fetus and possibly by breastfeeding. There is also an extremely small, but proven, risk to health care workers who receive inoculation injuries or exposure of broken skin or mucous membranes to the blood of HIV positive patients. Although the virus has been isolated from a number of body fluids and tissues, only blood, plasma products, semen, vaginal fluids, donor organs and possibly breast milk have been implicated in transmission. Extensive studies of household contacts of AIDS patients and HIV positive individuals have shown that HIV is not spread by close, non-sexual contact even when kissing has been frequent.[2] There is no evidence for faecal-oral, airborne or salivary transmission of HIV. Thus, from the extensive epidemiological evidence now available, any

215

potential for transmission of an infectious dose of HIV from a health care worker to a patient must lie solely in the transfer of blood.

There has been no known case, anywhere in the world, of infection of a patient by a health care worker. This negative evidence must, however, be viewed with caution since if transmission were to have occurred it might not be detected because of the long time period between the episode of infection and the onset of disease. Epidemiological surveillance has allowed the identification of a risk to patients from health care workers infected with another blood-borne virus, Hepatitis B, which also produces disease after a prolonged period. Hepatitis B virus is much more infectious than HIV[3] and many of the reported nosocomial infections have resulted from dentists and oral surgeons working without gloves.[4]

In the complete absence of any evidence of transmission of HIV from health care workers to patients it is necessary to attempt to base an assessment of risk on the reports of occupationally acquired infection. Infections of health care workers resulting from parenteral exposure to needles used on HIV-infected individuals have been reported[5,7] as have 3 substantial exposures of either mucous membranes or inflamed, uncovered skin.[8] The total number of health care workers infected occupationally is remarkably small considering the enormous numbers of staff exposed during the present decade. The anecdotal reports in the literature cannot, however, be used to assess a rate of risk as the denominator is unknown. The best assessment of risk level comes from serological follow-up of staff exposed to blood of positive patients. Combining all the studies of documented percutaneous or mucous membrane exposure in which pre-exposure or contemporaneous serum samples were available, the upper 95% confidence limit for the risk is 0.76%.[9] This contrasts strikingly with the incidence of seroconversion of 12-17% following parenteral exposure to the blood of Hepatitis B carriers even after administration of hyperimmune globulin.[10,11]

Any risk of transmission from a health care worker could only arise from exposure to blood or serum if there is possibility of contact with the patient's blood or tissues. This situation could arise if the worker had unprotected cuts or sores on the hands or where injury occurs during an operative procedure. Simple hygiene and good clinical practice should ensure that no health care worker considers working unless hand lesions have been properly covered; the onus is on the supervisor to ensure that staff are properly trained and monitored in these matters. The danger of inoculation injury occurring during a clinical procedure will obviously depend on the occupational role of the person concerned. Surgical procedures involving cutting and stitching carry the highest risk of personal injury and the theoretical risk of bleeding into the wound. With the increasing awareness of a risk to the operator from the unidentified HIV carrier, health care workers carrying out invasive techniques will become increasingly careful to ensure that they do not inoculate themselves. This should lead to an increased awareness of the state of integrity of the gloves and thus make it much more unlikely than at present that the surgeon or dentist will bleed unknowingly into the wound. It is to be hoped that the present unsatisfactory standards of surgical gloves[12] will be improved and that there may also be developments in surgical techniques which will lead to less risk of inoculation.[13,14] If the worst situation should occur and an

HIV-infected surgeon bleeds into a patient's wound, the information cited above from published surveys indicates that the risk to the patient is very small.

Precautions to prevent transmission

In the United Kingdom the General Medical Council, the General Dental Council and the Central Council for Professions Allied to Medicine have all issued ethical guidelines for health professionals who know or believe themselves to be infected with HIV. These guidelines emphasise the need for health care supervision and counselling and should now apply to all health care workers who have patient contact.[15] Part of this counselling process will be detailed instructions concerning the nature of HIV and how transmission must be prevented or reduced to a minimum in the practice of the individual concerned. This counselling process may require the confidential advice of a senior colleague in an identical or parallel section of the profession to the infected health care worker. On the basis of this advice it may be necessary to recommend changes in techniques or possibly, in some circumstances, a move to a related field.

All health care workers (whether HIV-infected or not) should cover any cuts or abrasions with waterproof dressings before direct patient contact. If lesions are more extensive (e.g. weeping eczema, chapping or widespread lesions) gloves should be worn or consideration should be given to avoiding direct patient contact until healing has occurred. Gloves must be worn for any procedure involving likely contact with blood or tissues of patients and the operator should be constantly aware of the possibility that undetected penetration of the glove and underlying skin may have occurred. These measures form the basis of reasonable clinical practice for all health care workers and are no more than commonsense in the knowledge that any patient (or health care worker) may carry a range of blood-borne viruses apart from HIV (e.g. Hepatitis B virus, non-A non-B Hepatitis, HTLV-1, HTLV-2).

Testing and confidentiality

Routine testing of patients for HIV is not currently being recommended and medical practitioners have been strongly advised to seek fully informed consent from the patient before proceeding with a test.[16] A major concern, if routine testing were to be instituted, is the danger of breach of confidentiality and the likelihood that infected individuals would not come forward for medical care and counselling. Similar concerns must apply to health care workers and it is essential that they must be assured of total confidentiality if they come forward for testing and counselling. This offers the greatest safeguard for the public, for unless confidentiality can be guaranteed health care workers may not come forward to receive instructions on safe working practices fearing prejudice to their careers and livelihood.

POSSIBLE RISKS FROM OTHER AGENTS

Concern has been expressed that patients being cared for by health care workers who have AIDS or ARC could be at risk from opportunistic infections carried by them. Most such organisms are not transmissible from person to person, even in the contact found in health care provision. The term opportunistic implies the need for a state of compromise that is not present in the majority of patients. Indeed, the most severe infections experienced by AIDS patients are either endogenous in origin (e.g. cytomegalovirus, herpes simplex virus, varicella zoster) or are about in the environment and available to all (e.g. pneumocystis carinii, fungi). The infectious agents occasionally found in AIDS and ARC patients that do present a risk of infection to others, e.g. mycobacterium tuberculosis and varicella zoster virus, can be contained by the same provisions currently applied to all health care workers. Intestinal pathogens such as salmonella and cryptosporidia are only transmitted by the faecal-oral route and reasonable standards of hygiene, which should be practised all the time by all health care workers, should ensure that the patient is not infected. Here again, these measures can be reinforced as a result of careful counselling of staff known to be positive.

Cytomegalovirus has been suggested as an opportunistic infection that could present a hazard to patients, particularly women in pregnancy. Despite extensive serological studies, and detailed investigations using restriction endonuclease techniques when transmission has been suspected, there has been no evidence of occupational spread to or from health care workers. Indeed, the amount of virus excreted from patients with AIDS and ARC is small compared with that found in congenitally-infected babies. The lack of evidence of transmission of cytomegalovirus from neonates, transplant recipients and AIDS patients to the staff attending them means that there is no reason to exclude women in pregnancy from attending or nursing these patients. On this basis there is no logical reason to be concerned about possible transmission of cytomegalovirus from a health care worker with AIDS or ARC to his/her patients.

POSSIBLE RISKS FROM HIV-RELATED DEMENTIA

HIV is known to have the ability to invade the nervous system and cause progressive encephalopathy. There is naturally concern, therefore, that the mental capabilities of health care staff may diminish and lead to errors of judgement. Such concern may also be expressed for individuals in other professions, particularly if their work involves the safety of the public. An HIV-infected individual's frank dementia rarely occurs until the later stages of AIDS when the person is already too ill to work. Milder effects of mental disability such as forgetfulness, lack of concentration, etc. may develop in any individual for a variety of medical and psychological reasons. Existing procedures for dealing with matters relating to competence at work should safeguard the public against possible effects of mental deterioration in health care workers. Regular medical supervision of staff known to be infected with HIV coupled, if necessary, with psychometric testing, should allow the early detection of mental as well as physical decline.

PROTECTION OF HIV-INFECTED STAFF

An important reason for encouraging staff to come forward for testing if they believe they may have been at risk of acquiring HIV is to ensure that they are counselled with regard to exposure to other infectious agents. While the asymptomatic HIV carrier appears to be at no significantly increased risk from active immunisation, those with AIDS and ARC may be well advised to avoid receiving live vaccines. Those who have never contracted measles and varicella may decide to avoid contact with patients in the early stages of these exanthema and if exposure has occurred it may be wise to consider the prophylactic use of specific immunoglobulins.

CONCLUSIONS

The low infectivity of HIV from casual contact and in a health care setting means that the public has little to fear if their health care attendants are HIV positive. The level of safety will be even higher if *all* health care workers are adequately trained and supervised to ensure that the best standards of hygiene are observed at all times. All health care professionals who know or believe themselves to be positive must seek HIV testing and counselling and this advice should be given to all health care workers.

REFERENCES

1. Dyer C. Doctors with AIDS and the "News of the World". *Br Med J* 1987; **295:** 1339-1340.
2. Gill ON. The hazard of infection from the shared communion cup. *J Infect* 1988; **16:** 3-23.
3. CDC. Recommendations for preventing transmission of infection with human t-lymphotropic virus type III/lymphadenopathy-associated virus in the workplace. *MMWR* 1985; **34:** 681-695.
4. CDC. Outbreak of hepatitis B associated with an oral surgeon-New Hampshire. *MMWR* 1987; **36:** 132-133.
5. Anon. Needlestick transmission of HTLV-III from a patient infected in Africa. *Lancet* 1984; **2:** 1376-1377.
6. Stricof RL, Morse DL. HTLV-III/LAV seroconversion following a deep intra-muscular needlestick injury. (Letter) *N Engl J Med* 1986; **314:** 1115.
7. Oksenhendler E, Harzil M, LeRoux J-M, Rabian C, Clauvel JP. HIV infection with seroconversion after a superficial needlestick injury to the finger. *N Engl J Med* 1986; **315:** 582.
8. CDC. Human immunodeficiency virus infections in health care workers exposed to blood of infected patients. *MMWR* 1987; **36:** 285-289.
9. Henderson DK, Saah AJ, Zak BJ, Kaslow RA, Lane HC, Folks T, Blackwelder WC, Schmitt J, LaCamera DJ, Masur H, Fauci AS. Risk of nosocomial infection with human T-cell lymphotropic virus type III/lymphadenopathy-associated virus in a large cohort of intensively exposed health care workers. *Ann Intern Med* 1986; **104:** 644-647.
10. Werner BG, Grady GF. Accidental hepatitis-B-surface-antigen-positive inoculations. Use of e antigen to estimate infectivity. *Ann Intern Med* 1982; **97:** 367-369.
11. Seeff LB, Wright EC, Zimmerman HJ, Alter HJ, Dietz AA, Felsher BF, Finkelstein JD, Garcia-Pont P, Gerin JL, Greenlee HB, Hamilton J, Holland PV, Kaplan PM, Kiernan T, Koff, RS, Leevy CM, McAuliffe VJ, Nath N, Purcell RH, Schiff ER, Schwartz CC, Tamburro CH, Vlahievic Z, Zemel R, Zimmon DS. Type B hepatitis after needlestick exposure: prevention with hepatitis B immune globulin: final report of the Veterans Administration Cooperative Study. *Ann Intern Med* 1978; **88:** 285-293.
12. Paulssen J, Eidem T, Kristiansen R. Perforations in surgeons gloves. *J Hosp Infect* 1988; **11:** 82-85.

13. Sim AJW, Dudley HAF. Surgeons and HIV. *Br Med J* 1988; **296:** 80.
14. Sim AJW. AIDS and the surgeon. *Surgery* 1988; **59:** 1396-1401.
15. Department of Health and Social Security. *AIDS: HIV infected health care workers. Report of the recommendations of the expert advisory group on AIDS.* March, 1988. HMSO.
16. B.M.A. Human immunodeficiency virus (HIV) antibody testing. Guidance from an opinion provided for the British Medical Association by Mr. Michael Sherrard Q.C. and Mr. Ian Gatt. *Br Med J* 1987; **295:** 911-912.

Discussion

Chairman: Miss J. Greenwood

WHITWAM: There has to be a dose relationship for infectivity. I know that if you get a little bit of virus you can probably deal with it. It would be very like bacteria. What about the dose infection relationship?

JEFFRIES: We have no solid information on infectious doses of HIV. In the case of Hepatitis B virus, infectivity has been quantitated in human volunteer experiments conducted by McCallum *et al* in Oxford, and Krugman *et al* at the Willowbrook School in New York State. It is known, with Hepatitis B that subcutaneous doses of as little as .00004 ml of icterogenic serum have produced infections. Following a documented case of occupational infection of a nurse in whom an estimated 0.5 ml blood was injected, some have assumed that a substantial volume of blood must be injected to produce infection. However, in some of the occupational infections described by Mr Sim, seroconversion followed minimal skin penetration.

TYLER: I have a comment with respect to semen. In patients who received semen from infected donors in Westmead, Australia there was no relationship between the amount of semen they received and those who became infected. There is also an anecdotal case where a 60 year old gentleman who had intercourse once a year (and at his age he would not produce too much in volume of semen), actually infected his partner following his own seroconversion after a blood transfusion.

WHITWAM: If you get a bit of blood in your eye, that could cause a problem.

JEFFRIES: I think it is reasonable to assume that the vascular membrane, the conjunctiva, which we know is a receptive site for respiratory viruses from volunteer studies in the past, and which we know from primate models is infectable with Hepatitis B, until proven otherwise, is an area where one could get infected with HIV. My advice would be to use eye protection.

WHITWAM: Should laryngoscopes used in anaesthesia be sterilised routinely?

JEFFRIES: The obvious answer is "yes". The Association of Anaesthetists is drawing up guidelines.

SCRIMGEOUR: May I pose a hypothetical question? Let us say that we are looking at surgeons working within a very high risk group of patients. At what point do you think that we should ask those involved in that sort of surgery to be screened themselves, just in case they get a needle injury or an accidental injection, and then seroconvert?

JEFFRIES: At San Francisco General they decided to do just that, and they tested all their staff. They found that the HIV positivity was confined to those who had known risk factors. I think that you would be very hard put to get your colleagues to come in for testing with all the implications at the present time.

SIM: My comments relate to the fact that I have not yet been tested, and have not to my knowledge put myself in a position whereby I could have been infected. I say that with a little more confidence than a lot of people do. I think you would do quite well to identify those people who have a risk of the virus. Those people who do not know are at greater risk than I am. Given the situation that I do injure myself, then I think I would have a sample taken and merely have it stored. I do not feel that the atmosphere in this country is appropriate for widespread testing at the present time. All you have to do is to look at an insurance form to see that it does not actually ask if you are HIV positive, it asks whether you have been tested. Until that atmosphere changes you are not going to get much voluntary testing.

SCOTT: This is an issue which has been debated and one of the points raised is that of transmission from health carers to patients. That is a large consideration because there is the question of why else one would want to test health care workers. Perhaps if there have been some problems identified, then that might be a reason to identify patients early and follow them up periodically with some form of neurological or psychiatric testing to ascertain that they are not deteriorating. The other experience that we have had in Florida is that of a surgeon who was identified as dying from AIDS and whose name was unfortunately revealed by the newspapers. A historical review of the patients he had dealt with was carried out; there were no patients who had seroconverted discovered in that group. That was an unfortunate incident both for the family and for the surgeon, but it did point out that the surgeon had not passed on the disease to any of his patients.

JEFFRIES: Thank you for pointing that out. He was operating for about 4 years.

MILLS: Has anyone looked to see if there was any correlation between HIV seroconversion after needle stick injuries and HIV antigen in the blood with which the person was injected?

JEFFRIES: I do not know of any data on that.

MILLS: I would have thought that it would be very relevant to when people seroconvert. If there is a high level of HIV antigen in the blood perhaps there is an increased risk of seroconversion.

JEFFRIES: It would be interesting to know that. I doubt though that the data are available. I think that if this problem continues then the opportunity will now be here because the antigen tests are now available. I would like to comment on Dr Whitwam's question of the infectious dosage. I do not know the ground rules of the infectious range of HIV. The pattern is normal in terms of the infectivity at different times following infection, and also the apparent susceptibility of individuals. It may well be that people vary in their susceptibility from day to day, and also that people have to be in a particularly receptive state to be infected by the virus. We know in fact that in the laboratory when you are growing the virus you have to activate the t cells. We know what that means in terms of individuals—that the t cells have to be in a particular state to establish an infection. There may be factors of that type.

MOK: Just to get back to Dr Scrimgeour's point, I wonder if people would like to comment on the practice at the City Hospital in Edinburgh where the doctors working with high risk patients regularly bleed themselves on about a 6-monthly basis and store the serum. In the event of a needle stick injury, or some such mishap, there is serum to fall back on to say whether they seroconverted before or after injury. They are not testing it, just storing the serum.

JEFFRIES: I think that is a reasonable approach. We recommend that people have storage of serum at least after an inoculation injury. In fact, we encourage serum storage, in general, for all who are working with HIV positive patients or material. There are some individuals who wish to be tested, and some who cannot rest unless they have a regular follow-up following inoculation injuries. You can cater for that. But confidentially, the names are not allowed to be known. I can understand the reassurance that this gives the staff and the value that might accrue in the future in assessing the risks.

McMANUS: We do that too for our staff. We bleed each other every 6 months and store it. I would like to comment on something that Dr Jeffries said about medical colleagues who are HIV positive. It does pose tremendous problems to those of us who look after them as patients. They think that they have the same degree of confidentiality that other patients do. They assume that I will not tell anybody that they are HIV positive. Obviously if I see their health deteriorating I will discuss the problem with them. We have to think of dementia. We know that some patients are diagnosed as having dementia and are put on AZT, and they become well again. So, when do I tell the Authority that I know a doctor who is not fit to practice? And if I am going to tell someone, whom do I tell?

JEFFRIES: If you are the confidential medical advisor of those doctors, then you surely know the machinery. If I saw that a colleague was going downhill, or who was dementing or whom I thought was drinking too much, there is machinery that I could turn to. Certainly, there is in this country. It is the "3 wise men". . .

McMANUS: Some of our patients could be dementing, but when they are put on AZT they function normally for several years.

JEFFRIES: I am not sure that psychometric tests are refined to a sufficient point that we can adequately assess ability. People tell me that the houseman who has been on duty for 48 hours performs similarly in psychometric testing to a dementing HIV positive patient.

GREEN: The issue of dementia is rather complicated. We have a very large study ongoing at the moment of HIV and AIDS involving psychometric study. Some of the tests we use are able to detect the fact that people were drinking the day before. So when you are next operating after a "hard evening" you may think that you are okay, but we could probably detect the following day that you are slightly impaired from what you should be. So there is not a difficulty in terms of sensitivity of the tests. One of the problems is the term "dementia" which gives the idea of senile dementia. It tends to have a long and slow progress. There is an excess of diagnosis in the United States for a variety of reasons—because of the samples and because of the techniques that have been used in certain studies. Rates of the appearance of HIV-related encephalopathy have been overestimated, I think. What tends to happen is that a great many patients whom we identify as having problems are having problems at a level which would not be greater than those you would have after having a drink before you went to see your patients. It is true that some patients progress to being quite severely impaired. Generally though by that stage there are other signs of quite serious ill health. For a doctor to have reached the level of dementia where one would be seriously concerned, one would probably be also seriously concerned about whether physically he is able to do his job. Dr McManus has also raised the very vexed issue of AZT. There is some question of the extent to which AZT reverses dementia, but it does seem that some people do get better again. So it is rather less of an obvious problem than it might be. You would certainly see other ways in which a doctor was not up to his job before he became encephalopathic to the extent where it affected his cognitive function.

SCOTT: One issue which was raised was the confidentiality of the results. Many times the personnel in our hospital centre who wanted to be tested have the dilemma of how they can be tested, and the results remain confidential. They really do not want their colleagues to find out the test results whether they be negative or positive. The other question that I have concerns a surgeon evaluating by history a patient who might be at risk. Although that is reasonable, one would have to decide what to consider "at risk" in terms of sexual behaviour or even drug use in the past. In terms of that surgery, have you thought about what kinds of histories one would consider as positive? Would it be anyone who has had anything other than heterosexual relationships? How would one deal with that historical information?

SIM: In terms of the largest population we feel that it is the picture of the male homosexuals. I think that if one goes along the line of questioning that I indicated, you would ask about marital status. In the end you may find that some one is male and that they have a male partner. If they are promiscuous, then you have a reason to ask them about anal intercourse. If someone has anal intercourse on a regular basis with large number of partners, then it is not unreasonable to consider that person at risk of HIV infection. So it does mean taking a history in a different way to what we have done in the past. If the infection remains in the "at risk" groups as it has at the present time, then the difficulties are not as great. This is not accurate nor is it precise, but I think that it is the best that we have at the present time. But there is still the problem of what to do with the homosexual who has been tested and found HIV negative. My attitude there is that I make a clinical decision. I talk to the patient and question him, and I decide whether he is at risk of being infected. I think we need to develop this concept of making a clinical decision about what our patients are.

Human immunodeficiency virus and blood transfusion

Professor J.G. Whitwam, Dr V. Chowdhury and Dr J.M. Hows

INTRODUCTION

It was recognised in 1982 that AIDS could be transmitted by the transfusion of blood and blood products.[1,2] Since then, more cases of HIV transmission through transfusions have come to light and counter measures have been undertaken to reduce this risk. This paper reviews the literature and describes some of these preventative measures with particular reference to the experience in the UK.

SELF-EXCLUSION OF UNSUITABLE DONORS

When the first cases of transfusion-associated AIDS were reported there were no screening tests to detect persons who had been exposed to the causative agent. A viral agent was suspected but not proven until 1983. Thus an immediate priority was to discourage donors belonging to high risk groups. In the USA in March 1983, the Food and Drug Administration (FDA) recommended that such people be asked not to donate blood or blood components.[3] Similarly in the UK in September 1983 the Department of Health and Social Security issued a pamphlet which was distributed to potential blood donors and a health education campaign was undertaken which stressed the dangers of the transmission of disease.

As information about AIDS continued to accumulate, in the UK a second leaflet was issued to blood donors in January 1985 describing persons at risk from AIDS.[4] Persons in these groups were requested not to donate blood and positive action was taken by ensuring that each potential donor received a copy of this second leaflet before donating blood. In 1985 there was evidence that certain donors were under the misconception that they might develop AIDS by giving blood. In order to counter this a statement that donors could not become infected by donating blood was included within the leaflet.

SCREENING TESTS

In March 1985 following the isolation and identificaion of HIV the first enzyme-linked immunosorbent assays (ELISA) to detect antibodies to HIV were licensed by the FDA for screening donated units of blood and plasma. It was reasonable to expect that once assays were available for the detection of anti-

HIV, problems for the blood transfusion services throughout the world would be greatly reduced, as potentially infectious donations could be eliminated. However, the screening tests raised further problems, both ethical and practical. These included:

1) the specificity, sensitivity and reproducibility of the test;
2) the possibility of false negative results;
3) the information given to blood donors with positive test results.

The first tests licensed by the FDA had impressive sensitivity and specificity with sensitivity being between 93.4 and 99.6%, and specificity from 99.2 to 99.8%.[5,6]

False-positive results occur from human error and presence of cross-reacting antibodies. False-negative results occur from human error, poor test sensitivity, test performance failure, and from samples drawn from infected but HIV seronegative persons. The sensitivity of the assay depends upon the threshold chosen as positive. Increasing the sensitivity decreases the specificity and increases the rate of false-positive results. At that time the prevalence of anti-HIV in the donor population was unknown, but theoretical estimates, based on a prevalence of 1 in 1000, indicated that 68-69% of all repeatedly positive donations were likely to be false-positive.[7]

This raised concern amongst the major blood centres in the USA on two counts: 1. How should such donors be counselled? 2. There could be a serious effect on donor recruitment as some potential donors might be reluctant to donate if they were aware of a significant false-positive rate, leading to concern about blood shortages.

It is current policy in the UK that positive or equivocal results on donor serum are repeated on at least 2 occasions and include a test on the plasma from the tubing attached to the blood pack. The donation is not used if repeatedly positive and equivocal results are obtained. Persistently positive or equivocal sera are sent to one of the designated reference laboratories established within the UK where confirmatory tests are carried out using different laboratory methods including Western blot. If the specimen is reactive in one assay system alone it is considered a false-positive.

Because of the significance of a positive anti-HIV result it is essential to inform the donor that the test is to be performed. This has been achieved in the UK by issuing a third leaflet in September 1985, in which donors were informed that their blood would be tested for antibody to AIDS and that they would be asked at sessions to agree to this test being performed; permission is subsequently obtained by asking the donor to sign a statement indicating his or her consent prior to donation. The leaflet also informs donors that in the unlikely event of a positive reaction they will be contacted by a doctor from the transfusion centre so that additional confirmatory tests can be carried out.[8] In at least one Regional Transfusion Centre, donors are asked to fill in a questionnaire, contents of which are treated confidentially, and which contains questions aimed at identifying high risk donors. Donations from such individuals are discarded irrespective of the results of screening.

In the UK anti-HIV antibody screening tests were evaluated by the Public Health Services Central Laboratory during March-October 1985. Three tests emerged as most suitable for screening blood in the UK. Two of these, Organon Teknika and Burroughs-Wellcome were subjected to an evaluation within the Blood Transfusion Service (BTS) and Manchester and Edgware Regional Tranfusion Centres (RTC) and both were found to be suitable.[4]

RESULTS OF ROUTINE BLOOD TESTING

Since laboratory testing for anti-HIV antibody began in the UK, by the end of January 1988 approximately 6.5 million blood donations had been screened. Amongst these, 94 have been confirmed anti-HIV antibody positive, an incidence of 1 in 65,000 donations or approximately 0.002% (personal communication Dr H.H. Gunson, NWRTC). None of these donations were transfused. Eighty-five percent of these positive donors were males and 15% were females. The majority belong to well recognised high risk groups in the same proportions as reported earlier.[3]

Since many donors give blood more than once, the frequency of anti-HIV positive blood donations is not an accurate estimate of the prevalence of HIV infection in blood donors. Thus, from February 1986, the number of tests on "new" donors i.e. those donating for the first time, has been recorded and until the end of January 1988 there had been 30 confirmed anti-HIV antibody positive results amongst approximately 750,000 donations. This gives an incidence of 0.004%. Analysis of the results in new donors in 3-monthly periods initially showed a reduction in frequency of confirmed positives,[8] but this trend was not significant ($p > 0.2$), and it appears from more recent data that lack of significance in the frequency of anti-HIV positives in "new" donors has continued (personal communication, Dr H.H. Gunson, NWRTC). The overall frequency of positive donations has been falling significantly as seropositive donors have been asked not to give further donations, and many seronegative donors continue to donate on repeated occasions.

The seropositive donors are not uniformly distributed throughout the UK. Of the first 72 seropositive donors, 29 were found in Greater London and 19 occurred in Scotland, where intravenous drug abuse was the commonest risk factor. The majority of the remaining 24 seropositives were found in centres with a large urban population. It is of concern that in the UK most of the anti-HIV positive donors belong to one of the high risk categories.[8] There have been similar findings abroad where some studies report that 81-89% of donors seropositive for HIV have a risk factor for HIV infection.[9] Considering the fact that these donors in the UK have been given written material describing the reasons not to donate blood (and those in the USA had signed a statement acknowledging that they had understood similar written information) it is important to determine why these persons had given blood. In the UK 58 of the 72 seropositive donors detected by screening until the end of February 1987 were asked why they had donated. The commonest reason given was that the donors did not believe that they were at risk (29 cases). Other reasons included: they had not read the leaflet (9 cases), they did not understand the leaflet (2 cases), peer pressure (7 cases), their specific risk factor (e.g. relating to Central Africa) was not contained in the leaflet given to them at the time of their donation (6 cases). Only 5 of the 58 admitted to donating blood merely in order to have the test result. Similar reasons were given by some of the seropositive donors in the USA.[3] It is important to identify the small number of persons at risk for HIV infection who continue to donate blood and to make additional efforts to educate them about the importance of deferring donation.

HIV INFECTION TRANSMITTED VIA TRANSFUSIONS

Until the end of December 1987, 64 HIV antibody positive persons, other than haemophiliacs, have been infected via blood or blood component transfusion in the UK.[9] These cases are virtually confined to donations collected before routine anti-HIV antibody testing was introduced or to transfusion received abroad. Furthermore, until the end of February 1988, 27 cases of AIDS resulting from blood/component transfusion have been notified in the UK.[10] Amongst these cases there have been 11 deaths out of 18 cases in which transfusion was received abroad and 8 deaths out of 9 cases in which transfusion was received in the UK. These figures are considerably smaller than those reported from the USA, where as of December 7th 1987, 1,171 transfusion-associated cases of AIDS had been reported to the Communicable Diseases Center, Atlanta.[10]

In 1984 it was reported that some patients with AIDS were viraemic but seronegative.[11] Since anti-HIV screening began, there has been a small number of cases in the UK, in which an anti-HIV positive donor was found to have been negative on a previous occasion, but in only one instance has a single donation led to seroconversion in 2 recipients who are currently asymptomatic. Recipients of products from the other non-positive donors have not shown evidence of seroconversion. These donors were probably anti-HIV negative at donation in view of a sufficiently long gap for seroconversion between the positive result and previous donations (personal communication Dr H.H. Gunson, NWRTC).

A recent American study reports on 13 persons seropositive for HIV who had received blood from 7 donors, who were negative for anti-HIV antibody at the time of donation, but subsequently seropositive.[5] Twelve of the recipients had no identifiable risk factors for HIV infection other than blood transfusions. On assessment 8 to 20 months post transfusion, HIV-related illness had developed in 3 of the recipients, and AIDS had developed in 1. Six of the 7 donors reported risk factors for HIV infection, and 5 had engaged in high risk activities or had had an illness suggestive of an acute retroviral syndrome within the 4 months preceding their HIV seronegative donation.

An accurate estimate of the frequency of HIV-infected donors who are negative is difficult, since information is scant about the time elapsing between infection with HIV and the appearance of anti-HIV detectable by an ELISA method. Two studies in homosexuals have shown this interval to be between 16 and 47 days,[12] and between 2 and 3 weeks.[13] For parenteral exposure 4-7 weeks has been estimated as the most likely period,[14] although antigen has been detected 9 months prior to seroconversion in a study of haemophiliacs.

THE RISK OF TRANSFUSION-ASSOCIATED AIDS AND HIV INFECTION

The incubation period has been reported to be between 15-60 months,[8,11] but some studies quote figures up to a mean of 15 years. Furthermore, the incubation period has been reported to be generally shorter in children than adults.[5,11,15]

Mathematical models have been devised to predict the risks of transfusion-associated AIDS and HIV infection.[16,17] Estimates predict that there were approximately 12,000 people still alive in 1987 who had received a unit of blood infected by HIV in the USA. These people are at risk for AIDS and AIDS-related conditions and may also transmit infection to others.

Thus, some secondary transmission might possibly be avoided by identifying and counselling infected transfusion recipients. Blood-banking organisations in the USA have begun "look-back" programmes to identify previous recipients of blood, from donors who tested for HIV antibody after screening began. In one region 70% of recipients identified through such a programme were HIV antibody positive.[17] However, "look-back" programmes will be never be able to identify all infected transfusion recipients.

HIV ANTIGEN TESTING

Tests for HIV antigen, to identify infected but antibody negative individuals have been developed.[18] Some studies have suggested the likelihood of detecting only HIV antigen in low risk populations such as blood donors, is exceedingly small.[19,20] Limitations of HIV antigen testing include a high false-positive rate, the short duration of detectable HIV antigen in serum and the absence of detectable antigen prior to HIV seroconversion in a proportion of patients. At present HIV antigen testing is being evaluated in assessing prognosis or monitoring the effect of treatment on patients with HIV infection, but is not routinely utilised prior to blood donation.

HIV TYPE 2 AND 3 (HIV-2, HIV-3)

Studies in Western Europe[21-23] indicate that the HIV-2 virus has spread from West Africa. It is probably only a matter of time before HIV-2 reaches Britain.[25] HIV-3 has also been described previously.[24] It would seem that no commercial kit assay reliably detected both anti-HIV-1 and anti-HIV-2. It suggests, therefore, that both combined and separate assays are needed, otherwise HIV-2 infections must continue to involve careful Western blot studies or isolation and characterisation of the infecting HIV strain from each patient. Both these latter two techniques are not suitable for use as widespread screening measures.

AUTOLOGOUS TRANSFUSIONS

Since 1980 the fear of AIDS among the general population has created a new demand for autologous transfusion and a resurgence of interest among doctors.[25] As yet few laboratories in Britain provide the service, although it has been advocated.[26] Theoretically it may be true that autologous donation provides a safer alternative to volunteer donor blood. However, it should be remembered that there are other risks of transfusion, in particular errors of blood identification and those resulting from incorrect storage or handling of donations.

'DIRECTED DONATIONS'

An alternative to autologous transfusion involves patient selection of blood donors and is termed 'directed donations'.

The American Association of Blood Banks and the Council of Community Blood Centers in the USA have condemned such programmes, and there is no evidence to support the idea that 'directed donations' from family members, friends and co-workers, are safer than those available through the community blood bank. In addition, such a system may create intense pressure on family and friends who may therefore be untruthful about their ability to meet donor requirements. It should be remembered that most donations collected by transfusion services are subdivided into components i.e. plasma, platelets and red cells, each destined for patients with specific transfusion requirements. In this way any given donation may benefit several patients, with corresponding financial savings as well as savings in the total number of donations required.

RISK OF HIV TRANSMISSION FROM HETEROSEXUAL ADULTS WITH TRANSFUSION-ASSOCIATED HIV INFECTION

There have been reports from the USA that persons with transfusion-associated HIV infection have transmitted the virus to their sexual partners and newborn children.[18]

A group in the USA recently studied the families of some of the patients with transfusion-associated HIV infection.[27] They found 2 (8%) of 25 husbands and 10 (18%) of 55 wives, who had had sexual contact with infected spouses, were seropositive for HIV, but the difference between the sexes was not significant. Only one of the seropositive persons had had sexual contact with anyone besides their spouse since 1978, and in this case the contacts were not at increased risk for HIV infection. Compared with seronegative wives, the seropositive wives were older (median ages 54 and 62 years; p = 0.08) and actually reported fewer sexual contacts with their infected husbands (means 156 and 82; p > 0.1). Both these findings however, were not statistically significant. There was no difference in the types of sexual contact or method of contraception of the seropositive and seronegative spouses. Although most husbands and wives remained uninfected despite repeated sexual contact without protection, some acquired infection after only a few contacts. This is consistent with an as yet unexplained biological variation in transmissibility and susceptibility. There was no evidence of HIV transmission to the other 63 family members. As yet, there have been no reports to the CDC of an infection acquired by casual non-sexual contact.[29] However, one sibling of an infected young child in Germany has been reported to have become seropositive, suggesting that transmission from a young child may rarely occur.[28]

The rate of seropositivity amongst wives in the above study is similar to that reported in studies of wives of haemophiliacs (10/148 or 7%, and 3 studies each finding 2/21 or 10%), and of female sex partners of bisexual men (8/43, 19%).[27] However, the rate of transmission appears to be lower than that reported among "non-drug-using" female sex partners of intravenous drug abusers (32/76, 42%), infected "servicemen" (5/7 or 71%) and wives of patients in Miami (14/28, 50%) or Zaire (11/18, 61%).[27]

OPTIMUM BLOOD UTILISATION

In spite of the low risk of transmission of HIV from the transfusion of blood or blood products, the problem outlined above indicates that this cannot be considered a "no risk" situation. In view of the increasing demands for blood products and the problem of potentially infected donors there is a need to minimise the use of blood for surgical procedures, and to ensure that blood is not wasted. The following points are worthy of consideration:-

1. Patients can be transfused periperatively either with solutions of albumin, which due to the production process is free of risk for AIDS, or crystalloid or synthetic colloidal solutions, dextrans, gelatins (e.g. Haemaccel), starch (e.g. Hespan). The haematocrit can be reduced from normal values in excess of 40% to around 30% without reduction of oxygen delivery to the tissues, with little haemodynamic disturbance and only a small effect on the clotting system which has little clinical significance.

2. Many obstetric units maintain a pool of universal donor blood for emergency use; patients are grouped but blood is not ordered routinely for each patient.

3. Autologous blood transfusion would be satisfactory provided the total blood requirement is available. For routine surgery where 1-4 units will suffice, the requirement could perhaps be met. However, although small pilot schemes are in existence, the resources are not available for the general application of this type of facility. Even if resources were available, since the maximum storage time of blood is only 35 days, such a scheme could only apply to situations where previous experience shows that the blood requirement is limited to a maximum of 4 units. Deep frozen blood is available in a few institutions throughout the world and widens the possibilities for autologous blood transfusion, since a much longer period can be allowed for an individual to provide a small personal "blood bank". However such facilities are at present largely restricted to the storage of blood for transfusion in subjects with rare antibodies and for potential military use.

4. For non-emergency surgery, hospitals should introduce maximum blood ordering schemes.[29]

CONCLUSION

Current tests for positivity for HIV antibody and self-exclusion of the high-risk donors have effectively eliminated the majority of positive donations and it is still possible to state that the safety of blood transfusion in the United Kingdom remains exceptionally high. Although continued vigilance over the safety of the blood supply is essential, the risks of HIV transmission by a transfusion should be kept in perspective.

As most donors found to be HIV antibody positive belong to recognised high risk groups this highlights the need to continue to educate these groups about the importance of voluntary self-exclusion and the risk of HIV transmission to potential recipients. Furthermore, the prevalence of HIV infection, particularly in people outside currently recognised high risk groups, must be carefully and continually monitored.

At present there is no evidence that limited autologous donations or directed donations will provide any increased level of protection. Neither is routine HIV antigen testing warranted and infection with HIV-2 as yet has not been reported in the UK.

ACKNOWLEDGEMENTS

HIV is a rapidly developing subject and we wish to thank Dr H.H. Gunson of the Manchester Blood Transfusion Centre for generously contributing current data, not yet published, to this review and which is indicated in the text as personal communication.

REFERENCES

1. Anonymous. Possible transfusion-associated acquired immune deficiency syndrome (AIDS). *California Morbid Mortality Weekly Rep* 1982; **31:** 652-654.
2. Ammann AJ, Cowan MJ, Wara DW, Weintrub P, Drita S, Goldman H, Perkins HA. Acquired immunodeficiency in an infant: possible transmission by means of blood products. *Lancet* 1983; **1:** 956-958.
3. Ward JW, Holmberg SD, Allen JR, Ravenholt O, Davis JR, Quinn MG, Jaffe HW, Cohn DL, Critchley SE, Kleinman SH, Lenes BA. Transmission of human immunodeficiency virus (HIV) by blood transfusions screened as negative for HIV antibody. *N Engl J Med* 1988; **318:** 473-478.
4. Gunson HH. The blood transfusion service in the UK. In: *Proceedings of the AIDS Conference 1986.* Ed. P Jones. Newcastle upon Tyne: Intercept, 1986; pp.91-100.
5. Hilgartner MW. AIDS in the transfused patient. *Am J Dis Child* 1987; **141:** 194-198.
6. Fisher MC. Transfusion-associated acquired immunodeficiency syndrome—what is the risk? *Paediatrics* 1987; **79:** 157-160.
7. Osterholm MT, Bowman RJ, Chopek MW, McCullough JJ, Korlath JA, Polesky HF. Screening donated blood and plasma for HTLV-3 antibody: Facing more than one crisis. *N Engl J Med* 1985; **312:** 1185-1188.
8. Gunson HH, Rawlinson VI. HIV antibody screening of blood donations in the United Kingdom. *Vox Sang* 1988; **54:** 34-38.
9. *World Health Organisation Epidemiological Bulletin Summary* 1988, January 11th-15th.
10. PHLS. *Reported AIDS UK by transmission category. Communicable Disease Surveillance Centre leaflet* (APR/AID.A). Cumulative cases and deaths up to end February 1988.
11. Salahuddin SZ, Groopman JE, Markham PD, Sarngadharan MG, Redfield RR, McLane HF, Essex M, Sliski A, Gallo RC. HTLV-III in symptom-free seronegative persons. *Lancet* 1984; **2:** 1418-1420.
12. Cooper DA, Gold J, Maclean P, Donovan B, Finlayson R, Barnes TG, Michelmore HH, Brook P, Penny R, for the Sidney AIDS Study Group. Acute AIDS retrovirus infection. Definition of a clinical illness associated with seroconversion. *Lancet* 1985; **1:** 537-540.
13. Marlink RG, Allan JS, McLane MF, Essex M, Anderson KC, Groopman JE. Low sensitivity of ELISA testing in early HIV infection. (Letter) *N Engl J Med* 1986; **315:** 1549.
14. Melbye M. The natural history of human T-lymphotropic virus III infection: the cause of AIDS. *Br Med J* 1986; **292:** 5-12.
15. Medley GF, Anderson RM, Cox DR, Billard L. Incubation period of AIDS in patients infected via blood transfusion. *Nature* 1987; **328:** 719-721.
16. Peterman TA, Lui KJ, Lawrence DN, Allen JR. Estimating the risks of transfusion-associated acquired immune deficiency syndrome and human immunodeficiency virus infection. *Transfusion* 1987; **27:** 371-374.
17. Anonymous. Human immunodeficiency virus infection in transfusion recipients and their family members. *JAMA* 1987; **257:** 1860-1861.

18. Allain JP, Laurian Y, Paul DA, Senn D and Members of the AIDS-Haemophilia French Study Group. Serological markers in early stages of human immunodeficiency virus infection in haemophiliacs. *Lancet* 1986; **2:** 1233-1236.
19. Lange JMA, Paul DA, Huisman HG, de Wolf F, van den Berg H, Coutinho RA, Danner SA, van der Noorda J, Goudsmit J. Persistent HIV antigenaemia and decline of HIV core antibodies associated with transition to AIDS. *Br Med J* 1986; **293:** 1459-1462.
20. Yaskanin D, Swanda S, Swenson S, Gilcher RO. HIV antigen status of high risk individuals. *Transfusion* 1987; **6:** 549.
21. Zuk TF. Greetings—a final look back with comments about a policy of zero-risk blood supply. *Transfusion* 1987; **6:** 447-448.
22. Werner A, Staszewski S, Helm E-B, Stille W, Weber K, Kurth R. HIV-2 (West Germany, 1984). (Letter) *Lancet* 1987; **1:** 868-869.
23. Ferroni P, Tagger A, Lazzarin, A, Moroni M. HIV-1 and HIV-2 infections in Italian AIDS/ARC patients. *Lancet* 1987; **1:** 869-870.
24. Brüker G, Brun-Vezinet I, Rosenheim M, Rey MA, Katlama C, Gentilini M. HIV-2 infection in two homosexual men in France. (Letter) *Lancet* 1987; **1:** 223.
25. Kay LA. The need for autologous blood transfusion. *Br Med J* 1987; **294:** 137-139.
26. James SE, Dodds R, Smith MA. Avoiding AIDS with autologous transfusion. (Letter) *Br Med J* 1985; **290:** 854.
27. Peterman TA, Stoneburner RL, Allen JR, Jaffe HW, Curran JW. Risk of human immunodeficiency virus transmission from heterosexual adults with transfusion-associated infections. *JAMA* 1988; **259:** 55-58.
28. Wahn V, Kramer HH, Voit T, Brüster HT, Scrampical B, Scheid A. Horizontal transmission of HIV infection between two siblings. *Lancet* 1986; **2:** 694.
29. Dodsworth H, Dudley HAF. Increased efficiency of transfusion practice in routine surgery using pre-operative antibody screening and selective ordering with an abbreviated crossmatch. *Br J Surg* 1985; **72:** 102-104.

Discussion

Chairman: Miss J. Greenwood

SCOTT: Even with serological testing of blood we have had 1 or 2 patients who have seroconverted even though the blood they received tested HIV negative. The donors were obviously in a "window" of time where they were probably negative for viral accretion but not yet antibody positive. Have you seen any instances like that?

WHITWAM: There are 6 in this country which could have been in that position, only 1 of which I have dealt with. Five are being followed up. The situation may, of course, change in the next few months or years. The point is that people discuss what might be the minimum use of blood required at the time. Do not use blood unless you have to. Surgery can be conducted at lower levels of haemoglobin than traditionally accepted. We operate on renal patients with a haemoglobin level of 5gm/dl.

ZIDEMAN: Even though we cannot say that most pregnancies are planned, can we say that we have usually got plenty of time for women to give their blood while they are pregnant? Is this the way of starting frozen blood for transfusion in this country with a known group of patients?

WHITWAM: I do not see why not. Are you suggesting that every woman who is pregnant should part with 1 unit of blood? It is going to have to be deep frozen if it is going to come out early in pregnancy. At what stage would you take it? If you want every woman in labour to have some available it would have to come off within the "window" of CPBA-1; it would have to come within 3 weeks of potential delivery. We could do that, but there is a logistic problem and it is bound to cost money.

SCRIMGEOUR: I would like to support the view of not having blood actually available for cold gynaecological surgery. Particularly looking back about 10 years ago to find out how many actual packets of blood were used in Edinburgh, we found out that the number was extremely small. Very seldom was a patient actually transfused with blood. In view of that finding we changed our regime, and when a patient now comes in to us for a straightforward hysterectomy or repair, serum is saved. If transfusion is required because something has gone wrong in the course of the operation, then at least we know what the group and antibody situation is, and you can get blood up to us very quickly.

WHITWAM: Yes, we have a complete list worked out now and we found out that in gynaecological operations the usage was about 30%. It has been very hard to educate people to this fact. Hopefully, all patients are tested for grouping including identifying abnormal groups, abnormal antibodies, etc. When you know the patient is coming in there is a pool of blood in storage which that patient could be compatible with. Within 15 minutes you can have the blood in the theatre. It makes sense. But of course in obstetrics blood transfusion is always an emergency.

JEFFRIES: Professor Whitwam, I have been wanting to hear that talk for a long time, because it is an important message to get over. I think that we must not be too parochial in terms of our views on blood supply; we are very privileged in this country to have blood that is very safe indeed. But surely the message needs to be given to the Third World where the background prevalence rate is so high in some areas. The question I want to ask you is a practical point, but it relates to the fact that I have responsibility for about 300 medical students, about half of whom go to Third World countries. They need to see AIDS and work with AIDS patients. But I recommend that anyone who is going to a high risk area take along a couple of packs of Haemaccell at the present time. Is it best kept refrigerated?

WHITWAM: It should not be so cold that it jells out. GPs up north have a little heater in the back of their car to keep it at about 3°C. Anything colder and it will jell out. It can stand heat, and in a hot climate it will last up to 8 days, and so climatic heat is no problem.

THOMPSON: To extend the discussion of blood transfusion for elective obstetric procedures, I would say that the vast majority of my colleagues transfuse very few elective Caesarean sections, because with modern ultrasound one can nowadays pick out the high risk cases such as the placenta praevia or the anterior placenta.

WHITWAM: I take the view that in obstetrics you never quite know until you open the uterus what is going to go wrong in there.

THOMPSON: But you have backup in any modern labour ward that is doing Caesarean sections. In the refrigerator you have at least 2 units or 4 units of O-negative blood and you are prepared to give that to any patient.

WHITWAM: I think that is very good policy.

THOMPSON: Would that get around your problem?

WHITWAM: Yes it would.

LUCAS: May I raise a concern that I have in paediatrics, that is the care of premature babies. It is not uncommon for these infants to receive more than 10 transfusions. That must make them a very high risk group. It is an unavoidable procedure in that group because they need the high oxygen transport in view of their critical lung disease. I wonder whether you have any suggestions. Theoretically should paediatricians be more at risk in looking after these patients who need to have several blood samples taken each day? Would it be feasible to organise things so that wherever possible such an infant should receive multiple stored transfusions from one donor?

WHITWAM: If it were possible to check the parents then it would be possible to take fresh blood from a parent at the time when it is needed. If it is serologically compatible then if the mother does not have HIV the baby is not going to get it.

LAMBERT: I am working in a situation where I am frequently faced by parents begging to give their own blood to their baby, but we cannot convince our local blood transfusion service to organise that for us. This would obviously be the best alternative in that situation. Someone also asked what happened in the Third World. It was one of the policies that we had in Uganda, that we would transfuse parents' blood to children in the absence of testing facilities. We also had auto-logous transfusion at the time of operation, that is extracting shed blood, filtering it and putting it back. The problem in the neonatal unit is a very real one, and it is one which we are going to have to educate our blood transfusion service about. We should be taking maternal blood, packaging it into small units of 10 or 20 mls, which is usually what we are transfusing, and storing it for the baby. There has got to be a rising awareness that blood is precious, and non-infected blood is very precious. It should only be used when necessary and treated with respect.

HARE: May I express my surprise again at your routine cross matching of blood for Caesarean sections. We crossmatch routinely for neither elective nor emergency sections. If senior people are present to make the decisions and perform the surgery, then both the need and the use of blood could be reduced.

WHITWAM: How many of you have been exposed in the course of your career so far to any major systematic lecture on blood substitutes, plasma, and the attempts to develop fluorocarbons and blood and haemoglobin packages?

SCRIMGEOUR: In how many places do they actually have blood crossmatched ready for all cold gynaecological surgery, for elective Caesarean sections, or for that matter for emergency Caesarean sections?

HUDSON: I think you would have to exclude cancer surgery because I think that most of us crossmatch blood routinely then.

WHITWAM: I must say that in obstetrics, when you look at neonatal and maternal mortality rates you cannot afford to cut any corners. If one mother died next year because blood was not available for whatever reason it would be a tragedy.

STEELE: In obstetrics local circumstances differ very greatly: seniority of staff, distance from a blood bank, problems of portering at night. I think that the principle is well stated, and I am sure that we would all go along with it. But I think that there have to be differences in units. Another point is that we are going to get resistance from patients to having blood transfusions, which may be an additional stimulus to the conservative.

SECTION VI

NEONATAL PROBLEMS

AIDS and neonatal resuscitation

Dr A. Whitelaw and Dr D.A. Zideman

INTRODUCTION

Neonatal resuscitation has been one of the great success stories of medicine in the past 20 years with many thousands of lives being saved. In the anxiety over AIDS, it is important that staff are not frightened into taking precautions which are so Draconian as to reduce the standard of resuscitation for neonates in general.

TECHNIQUES

Neonatal resuscitation involves the application of a number of relatively simple techniques based on a knowledge of pathophysiology. The first essential is clearing the airway by suctioning the pharynx and nostrils. This is not required in all newborn infants, but should be carried out if breathing is not immediately established. Amniotic fluid, lung liquid and mucus are normally present and may not cause much trouble. Maternal blood may be irritant and meconium can cause a severe aspiration syndrome if inhaled.

If breathing is not established after clearing the airway, ventilation can be started by face mask and bag. Most apnoeic infants can be ventilated this way if good technique is used and this is the approach advocated in the Swedish national programme for resuscitation of the newborn[1].

Infants who fail to respond to bag and mask ventilation require endotracheal intubation and ventilation. If the infant remains bradycardic after effective ventilation, external cardiac massage should be started and endotracheal adrenaline should be given.

In a small proportion of infants an emergency umbilical or peripheral intravenous line will be needed for the urgent infusion of blood volume expanders, glucose or sodium bicarbonate.

FREQUENCY OF NEONATAL RESUSCITATION

Approximately 5% of all births require some form of neonatal resuscitation. Even in a healthy population of mothers with good antenatal care in Lund, Sweden, 1.3% of infants had an Apgar score of 0-3 at 1 minute.[1] In most hospitals in the UK 2-3% of all neonates are intubated and ventilated at birth. In some hospitals there is a policy of electively intubating and ventilating all infants of less than 30 weeks gestation or less than 1000g birth weight.

IS THERE A RISK?

Although we know of no doctor or nurse becoming infected with HIV from neonatal resuscitation, there is a theoretical risk in all cases, as HIV positive mothers are not reliably identified antenatally. The infant is generally covered in maternal blood. Procedures such as endotracheal intubation involve close proximity between the resuscitator's face and the infant. Ventilation and suction involve potential splashing and spraying of body fluids into the eyes, nose and mouth of staff. Many staff have small breaks in the skin, some of which would not be thought of as "skin lesions".

CURRENT PRACTICE

A paediatrician is usually called to attend an "at risk" delivery. Although theatre clothes are worn in the operating theatre if delivery is by Caesarean Section, practice is different at a vaginal delivery. The paediatrician arrives in street clothes, rolls up his or her sleeves and washes hands. The paediatrician will have arrived from the special care baby unit, paediatric ward, out-patient clinic or emergency department. No mask, gown or gloves are used in the resuscitation. Inevitably maternal blood frequently covers the paediatrician's hands. Until very recently, the infant was usually sucked out by mouth suction through a mucus extractor with no barrier stopping fluid reaching the paediatrician's or midwife's lungs. The laryngoscope is cleaned in soap and water between cases and wiped with 70% isopropyl alcohol. Endotracheal tubes and intravenous equipment are all disposable. Careful inspection of a paediatrician's glasses after resuscitation has shown small spots of dried blood which had not been noticed during the procedure.

In the Swedish Agency for Research Cooperation with Developing Countries report on neonatal resuscitation, published in November 1985, no mention is made of HIV, or of special precautions, despite the fact that it was aimed at the countries now known to have a large reservoir of HIV. This highlights the fact that it is only very recently that paediatricians have started to think about the implications of HIV.

The Royal College of Obstetricians and Gynaecologists Sub-Committee report (see Appendix) contains recommendations for the resuscitation of infants born to mothers known to have HIV or to be at risk,[2] and for modification of routine practice. The doctor or midwife should abandon the use of mouth-operated suction. Gas Venturi and mechanically powered devices are generally available. Care must be taken to limit the negative pressure to -100mm Hg (-136 cm water) to prevent damage to the airway. For midwives doing home deliveries, hand or foot powered suction devices should be readily portable. In high risk situations it is also recommended that the doctor or midwife should wear surgical gloves, eye protection (either glasses or a visor) and be gowned over a plastic apron. A face mask and protective footwear are to be used. Care is to be taken that the bag and mask be sterilised at 95°C before and after use. Laryngoscopes are to be sterilised. The mattress and suction apparatus are to be disinfected with hypochlorite.

Particular care is to be taken when cutting the cord as spraying of blood can easily occur, as with cord blood sampling.

These recommendations have been widely accepted and seem to be carried out when mothers are identified antenatally as having HIV or being in a high risk group such as intravenous drug abusers. Mouth-operated suction has largely been abandoned at all deliveries whether high risk or not.

HIGH RISK OR ALL DELIVERIES?

As HIV positive mothers are not identified with certainty before delivery, should these elaborate precautions be taken to protect staff at all deliveries? Informal estimates of the frequency of HIV among London pregnant women are in the area of 0.3%. To apply all these measures to every delivery would be very time-consuming and expensive. Most worrying is the delay while apron, gown, gloves, mask, protective footwear and eye protection are put on. In the event of sudden unexpected asphyxia with no paediatrician present, we have the possible scenario of a paediatrician rushing from the other end of the hospital to a cyanosed, bradycardic infant in terminal apnoea and spending two minutes to dress before intubating the infant. As over 99% of such asphyxiated infants are born to HIV negative mothers, general application of the full precautions to all deliveries could well increase perinatal mortality and neurological damage from hypoxia.

There remains a need to protect resuscitating staff from HIV in the unsuspected case. We believe that full protection with gloves, gown, apron, mask, eye protection and protective footwear should be used by paediatricians called to all deliveries but *in emergencies, the minimum protection of gloves, mask and eye protection should be used.* This need not take long to put on. There must be regular checks to make sure that all the protective items are always immediately available beside the Resuscitaire wherever a delivery may occur.

We also think that in smaller hospitals there should be increasing emphasis on the experienced midwives in a delivery ward being competent at neonatal resuscitation. Such staff would be likely to be already protectively clothed and immediately available. If one such midwife were on each shift, resuscitation of the unexpectedly asphyxiated neonate would be quicker and safer.[3]

In summary, the risk of HIV necessitates some modification of neonatal resuscitation. The use of full protection for staff should not result in dangerous delays in intubation for infants at low risk of HIV if the minimum protection is used in emergencies. Nor should such precautions in any way reverse the tendency to sensitive and personalised care which has emerged in the last few years. Finally, taking care to prevent the spread of HIV will undoubtedly reduce the spread of other infections, to the neonates and staff. This will be true of the organisms we already know are potential threats such as Hepatitis B, but will also apply to organisms as yet unidentified.

244 Study Group: AIDS

1. Sterky G, Tafari N and Tunell R. *Breathing and warmth at birth.* Stockholm: Swedish
    Agency for Research Cooperation with Developing Countries, 1985.
2. *Report of the RCOG Sub-committee on problems associated with AIDS in relation to
    obstetrics and gynaecology.* London: Royal College of Obstetricians and Gynae-
    cologists, 1987.
3. Gamsu H. *Resuscitation of the newborn.* Working party of the British Paediatric Asso-
    ciation, Faculty of Anaesthetists, Royal College of Midwives and the Royal College of
    Obstetricians and Gynaecologists. London: FFARCS and RCOG, 1988.

Care of the normal newborn of the HIV positive mother

Professor C.B.S. Wood

INTRODUCTION

Faced with the emergence of AIDS the neonatologists will need to take stock of their practice and that of the neonatal team, and in consultation, the practice of obstetric and midwifery colleagues. While the disadvantageous social associations of AIDS may additionally load HIV positive mothers with further general obstetric risks, such as low birth weight and pre-term delivery, many babies infected with AIDS will not have overt medical problems, and they will require normal patterns of early neonatal care. In the general postnatal wards the normal objectives of neonatal care (Table 1) must be achieved for all babies, whether born to mothers who are HIV positive or negative. But where special measures are required for the baby of the HIV positive mother, these must be humane, economical, unobtrusive and supportive to the general morale of staff, and of course to patients. Although other patients will not know that HIV positive mothers are being cared for, they will gradually and increasingly come to realise that their presence will from time to time be inevitable. They must, therefore, have confidence in the manner in which wards are managed to secure the safety of themselves and their babies. The atmosphere in a modern postnatal ward is open, informal and supportive, features which may initially be at odds with the increased level of care required for the potentially HIV-infected baby. It may be easier to make the necessary policies for babies in need of special care or intensive care, where ward protocols are a regular part of daily routine, and special precautions or segregation are matters of routine management for other purposes.

Table 1

Objectives of newborn care

1. Physiological

Safe establishment of postnatal circulation and breathing
Detection of congenital abnmormalities
Monitoring of early progress — jaundice, etc.

2. General

Establishment of feeding
Establishment of bonding
Establishment of secure home care

245

ROUTINE WARD CARE

Appropriate ward routines are clearly described for the babies of HIV positive mothers in the RCOG Sub-Committee report on problems associated with AIDS in relation to obstetrics and gynaecology (see Appendix).[1] They are summarised as follows:

1. The baby should be cared for in the same room as the mother.
2. At birth, the use of the mouth-operated mucus extractor should be abandoned in favour of a bulb operated syringe with trap, or a mechanical or Venturi sucker using an 8 or 10 FG suction disposable catheter at a suction pressure not exceeding 100mm mercury. After delivery the baby should be washed free of blood, etc. with soap and water, the attendant wearing surgical gloves. If resuscitation is needed the doctor or midwife must wear reliable gloves, mask and eye protection.
3. Reliable gloves should also be worn while attending to the cord, performing heel pricks or vein punctures but not for routinely changing napkins, or cleaning away vomit, unless they are bloodstained. Alcohol swabs may be used to cleanse the cord stump. Needles should not be resheathed and they, along with syringes and stilettes should be placed in burn bins which are themselves enclosed in yellow bags.
4. Disposable napkins, which would then be placed in yellow plastic bags, should be used; female infants' napkins may be additionally contaminated by temporary bloodstained vaginal discharge. Breast pads should be treated similarly.
5. Blood samples for bilirubin should be placed in double bags and sent to the laboratory, appropriately labelled, rather than being estimated on the ward bilirubinometer or centrifuged. Guthrie test cards should also be labelled as 'BIOHAZARD' and placed in plastic bags.
6. Appliances used in the care of the baby need special attention:
    (a) Disposable paper tape measures should be kept for measuring the head circumference and then discarded after the baby has been discharged.
    (b) The baby's thermometer should be soaked in 0.5% chlorhexidine and 70% ethanol for 30 minutes and then allowed to dry.
    (c) Scales and stethoscopes should be cleaned with 0.1% sodium hypochlorite solution or 70% alcohol and then wiped with detergent.

However, there may be many advantages in a safe single-tier level of service for babies of all mothers irrespective of the mother's HIV status. Such an arrangement, using the following precautions obviates the risk of the baby of an HIV-infected mother receiving inadequate, patchy or hesitant care.

FEEDING

As bottlefeeding is safe in developed countries, and breast milk may have transmitted HIV, it is probably wise to advise that artificial bottlefeeding be used.[2] However, as vertical transmission[3] already may have occured, it is probably not be justifiable to insist if a mother is adamant that she wishes to breast-feed. In developing countries the risks of bottlefeeding may be so great that breastfeeding is always the preferred option. Breast milk banks have been phased out in many Districts because of the threat of AIDS.

MANAGEMENT ISSUES

Obstetric and neonatal staff must meet regularly to exchange information about HIV positive bookings or other high risk mothers who have been identified. All staff must receive regular briefings about the procedures outlined above, and they must be reassured that their duty of care can be discharged easily at no significant risk to themselves. Lack of information, lack of preparation and unmanaged anxiety are more likely to promote poor standards of practice, which in turn may lead to lower standards of care at delivery and perhaps unconscious discrimination against HIV positive cases.

CASE IDENTIFICATION POLICIES

More difficult strategic decisions surround the problem that recognition of high-risk mothers and their cooperation in HIV testing, with counselling, will not detect all HIV positive mothers coming to delivery. All ward procedures will need to be regularly reviewed and the procedures for neonatal care outlined above may gradually find themselves coming into routine practice for all infants.

FOLLOW-UP OF HIV INFANTS OF POSITIVE MOTHERS (Table 2)

While there is a need for close liaison with regional paediatric immunology and infectious diseases centres, it is likely that the most effective and humane care for mother and baby can be provided at District level, and where appropriate, shared with the general practitioners,[6] community child health medical staff and health visitors. Initially the status of many babies may be indeterminate. The infants cord blood should be tested for HIV antibody and virus antigen by the most reliable methods available and virus cultures set up. It may be valuable to test for p24 antigen[5] in cord blood—perhaps twice weekly during the first 4 weeks—to try to detect early viraemia, but this has not always been successful. Not all infected babies develop antibodies but this should be assessed at monthly intervals initially, with careful clinical review made initially at fortnightly intervals. Feeding, weight gain, and other symptomatology will be assessed regularly. Tests of lymphocyte function and enumeration of CD4 cells should also be performed initially and later on at quite wide intervals, or sooner if symptoms of AIDS begin to appear. The follow-up process will in itself engender an element of support and counselling, but inevitably some difficult moments will arise in discussing the early recognition that a baby is indeed infected and not merely the carrier of maternal IgG antibodies. The onset of symptoms may sometimes be long delayed and even if early viraemia is believed to have occurred, it may be many months before the status of the baby becomes clear.

Table 2
Special objectives of care for infants of HIV positive mothers

Determination of infection status of baby
Satisfactory counselling
Follow-up of growth
development
early detection of AIDS

REFERENCES

1. *Report of the RCOG Sub-committee on problems associated with AIDS in relation to obstetrics and gynaecology.* London: Royal College of Obstetricians and Gynaecologists, 1987.
2. Ziegler JB, Cooper DA, Johnson RO. Postnatal transmission of AIDS-associated retrovirus from mother to infant. *Lancet* 1985; **1:** 896-898.
3. Mok JQ, Giaquinto C, DeRossi A,Grosch-Wörner I, Ades AE, Peckham CS. Infants born to mothers seropositive for human immunodeficiency virus. *Lancet* 1987: **1:** 1164-1168.
4. Eglin RP, Wilkinson AR. HIV infection and pasteurisation of breast milk. *Lancet* 1987; **1:** 1093.
5. Von Sydow M, Gaines H, Sonnerborg A, Forsgren M, Pehrson PO, Strannegard O. Antigen detection in primary HIV infection. *Br Med J* 1988; **296:** 238-240.
6. Anderson P, Mayon-White R, General practitioners and management of infection with HIV. *Br Med J* 1988; **296:** 535-537.

Discussion

Chairman: Professor C. B. S. Wood

SHARP: I should like to direct a question to Dr Whitelaw. You mentioned the abandonment of mouth to mouth resuscitation. What are we going to offer Third World countries if not mouth suction?

WHITELAW: The problem of HIV is much worse in Africa than in this country, so I do not think that one can really advocate the general use of mouth suction in such countries. It would be very shortsighted to advise carrying on using these simple means because it would be likely to disseminate HIV further into the population. So I think you have to go to simple mechanical suction devices such as provided by a foot pedal. One does not necessarily need to use an electrical device to produce suction.

HARVEY: There was the suggestion that putting a syringe on the other end of mouth suction produced too much pressure, and might be damaging to the mucosa. I am not sure of the evidence for that, but that would otherwise be a simple way of dealing with the problem.

WILDAY: We have tried this in our unit, but it was absolutely useless.

GREENWOOD: I am not sure that we have settled that question, but the problem is that there are two pieces of equipment that have to be assembled. The Department of Health would like to find some easily operated one-hand instrument. Obviously the mouth-operated device was easier because it left you with two free hands. I feel that we should not just be discussing the situation in the Third World. It is very easy to say that in the labour ward or in the neonatal unit you have got suction at hand. What about the post natal wards, the GP units, and home confinements? I think it is too easy to say that mucus extraction is a Third World problem.

LUCAS: May I come back to something that Dr Zideman raised yesterday? On occasion you might do something that was to the detriment of the patient if you took time taking care to protect yourself. I think that it is something that we have not yet come to grips with properly. Who comes first—the doctor or the patient—in a situation where any delay at all would be detrimental to the patient? I feel very strongly about this. If one enters this profession one has to take professional risks.

WHITELAW: I think that the best example of this is — what would you do if an infant started bleeding profusely from the umbilical cord and there were no gloves to hand? If you have to stop a haemorrhage inevitably you get some of the infant's blood on you. Certainly, the North American experience is that the staff are protecting themselves and the patients have to come second.

WOOD: If you think back in the history of infection in surgical procedures and the problems of surgeons, surgical careers had a high mortality years ago, and hospitals are full of memorials to surgeons who died of what they caught in theatre. It ought to be possible gradually to improve our practice so that the dilemma which you mention emerges less and less. In other words, there should be more availability of protection on the wards. In the children's hospital where I spend most of my time, for even such low risk things as diarrhoea, the nurses are expecting to find themselves gloved at all times. Amazing though it may seem the Treasurer does not seem to mind paying for the gloves.

MOK: I think we all know that we have to protect ourselves and we also have to do our best for the infant and for the mother. But there will be cases we will fail to recognise. Could we come up with a bare minimum essential that will be acceptable to everybody?

WHITELAW: What we have been saying is that the same standard of care has to be the bare minimum. The protection which I was describing for the delivery room and the precautions which Professor Wood was describing in his post natal ward do represent the bare minimum. It is completely illogical and unsound to suggest that anything less than that is adequate now.

MOK: Would you apply that to every delivery?

WHITELAW: Yes.

ZIDEMAN: May I change the subject for the moment. There are adequate devices available and they should be in every hospital in this country as a backup to the electrical systems that are there already. There are adequate hand-operated suction units, one of which has been out for 4 years now. This is what I would recommend, and this is what the Council are recommending, for example, for a district nurse where a foot-sucker may be too large for her to carry. These units are available and I have seen some modern prototypes which are much smaller. These are quite powerful, but they can have their pressures limited so that they would be ideal for the neonatal unit. I totally endorse what Dr Whitelaw said in that it has to be 100% or nothing at all, but I still return to what Dr Lucas has said that there is going to be the odd one when you are going to be caught. And this may be the equivalent of the needle stick injury in normal practice in neonatal resuscitation. There is about to be published a document from the Faculty of Anaesthetists of the Royal College of Surgeons together with the BPA and a number of other authorities on training in neonatal resuscitation. Despite my pleas and a number of other people's pleas there is nothing on protection against this disease, and that worries me.[1]

SCOTT: I think that the combination of protecting oneself and taking care of the patient even in emergency situations is quite compatible. We have gone through this for several years now. I recall particularly one time when a child arrested on the ward and was given mouth to mouth resuscitation. In that situation we subsequently decided that all children who had HIV should have a blue mask and a bag at the bedside, and it changed our patterns. On the other hand it did not really change the care of that patient. I think it is a matter of understanding what relative risks are and recognising that if you do get blood on your hands on intact skin, washing it off is going to be protective, and is probably not going to put that patient at excessive risk. But you also have to institute in your hospital enough measures to protect the staff and the people taking care of patients.

HARE: About a third of calls for a paediatric resident to come to the labour ward for resuscitation are unpredicted, and due to the fact that they have delivered an unexpectedly flat infant. I think that you would all agree that to run from the paediatric wards and then spend considerable time changing out of street clothes into theatre clothes, putting on apron, gown, gloves, face mask, hood and so on could be interpreted as time lost in resuscitation of the baby. Even if that is to be so, should active resuscitation have to wait for the paediatrician? Could not people who are already on the labour ward and already changed do it? In other words, are you not really asking for primary resuscitation to become the prerogative of the obstetric resident or perhaps the midwifery staff who are there already?

WHITELAW: Yes, it is ·difficult already to guarantee a trained paediatric resuscitator 24 hours a day and 365 days a year in many of the smaller district general hospitals and isolated maternity hospitals. At the moment, with the developments in limiting junior hospital staff particularly at registrar level, I do not think that the situation is going to improve. It is therefore logical to think that the experienced midwives should have more of a role that they have had in the initial resuscitation of asphyxiated infants. In North-West Thames, for instance, this has been accepted and welcomed by the midwives and nurses on the Regional Perinatal Services Working Party although we still have to work out how one achieves an adequate level of training. But the principle is accepted that it will be the person who is already on the labour ward who would see this as a first aid procedure.

HARE: Including intubation?

WHITELAW: Well, that is debatable. The Swedish emphasis on resuscitation is not to train everybody to intubate. They, of course, have a geographically separated population, so they have in some places small hospitals where you cannot guarantee that there will be a neonatal paediatrician around all the time. They train people to do face mask ventilation as well as possible. They claim that only a very small number of babies need to be intubated. To try to intubate for 5 minutes and fail is much worse than to use the face mask.

LAMBERT: If you are training midwifery staff who are on site to do resuscitation you surely have to teach them intubation as well because a percentage of emergency calls to delivery suites are for presumed mucus aspiration. I think we have to rethink the whole question of neonatal resuscitation and one surely has to bring midwives and obstetricians into this field. My second point is that if one of the purposes of this Study Group is to come up with recommendations and proposals, then I think it is important that we are clear about who we are proposing should take the precautions that we are describing and which group of patients we use it on. If we follow the Green Book (RCOG Sub-Committee report, see Appendix) those proposals which you were quoting are stated only for the care of neonates of identified seropositive women. That is the point that we need to discuss further and on which we need to make firm proposals. My last question is what should we be doing about blood gas measurement?

WOOD: I think that we should be negotiating with the chemical pathology laboratory to provide us with a safe service, at least up to the level of our requirements.

LAMBERT: It is also a matter of reaching a biochemistry lab which may be a mile away from the unit. Obviously the problems in the breakdown of that kind of service are quite great.

HARVEY: I do not see that we can possibly provide proper intensive care without having the blood gas analysis on our units as we now have. On our main ward round of the week there is always a microbiologist and there is always a chemical pathologist. That is the moment when the other professions can influence us and we can influence them.

WHITELAW: Do we restrict these protective measures just to known HIV and high risk mothers? I think that the answer to that is "no". This is something that we are thinking of applying to the entire population and I do realise that this is extremely inconvenient and possibly detrimental to the infants of non-infected mothers. The noises that I am getting from nurses and junior hospital staff are that they want all mothers screened. They want to know who has the virus because the measures taken to deal with it are detrimental to the non-infected population. I do not say that this is my personal view; I am just saying that there are many nurses who are telling me this.

JOHNSTONE: I would be alarmed if I thought that there was a recommendation from a body such as this that there should be an inferior standard of care because of risks, which at the same time we are saying are extremely remote. We are talking about patient care, and I do not think that we should be compromising our standards in that at all. I was very interested in the mucus extraction paper, but I do not believe for a moment that babies are routinely having mucus aspirated. In fact, I wonder if you have a non-asphyxiated, non-meconium stained baby, whether this is a necessity.

WHITELAW: It is not a necessity at all, but it is a procedure which you need to have available.

ROTH: May I respond to the point made about the demand from staff for protection. I think that we have to go back to starting to educate people about the risks. I would be curious to know how many of those staff were protecting themselves against Hepatitis B infection which is far more likely to be a problem to them. I think that what we see reflected is bigotry towards the people who have suffered this infection. I do not think that we can allow ourselves to develop practices on the basis of that attitude. We have to put a very sharp focus on our own sloppy and quite revolting practices. I suspect that if we did it right and we did not have people leaving dangerous and infective material around that we could feel quite confident that we are not at any risk whatsoever.

WHITELAW: Yes, I quite agree with you, but I do not think that we can get away from the problem of the sudden, unexpected infant, covered in maternal blood, who is not breathing. Are you asking junior doctors who do not have time to put on gloves to get in there and intubate, and get more than just a few spots of maternal blood on them while resuscitating a baby in order to save a couple of minutes?

ROTH: I suspect that is what we are doing right now. And we are doing it not because there is any pressure to bear but just because they have not considered recent changes of practice.

WHITELAW: But the fact that we are doing it now does not mean to say that this is how it should be.

LUCAS: What I would hate to see is a lot of procedures which could be interpreted by people as meaning that they could always put themselves before the patient. I think that if we are going to suggest complex procedures for protection in every case, it is quite obvious that there will be innumerable occasions when a doctor cannot, in fact, protect himself. Are we going to specifiy that the patient comes first under those circumstances? Because if we do not, then I think that there really is a danger that legalistically-minded people might do things which were to the detriment of the patient, all in the name of a relatively minor risk.

LAMBERT: May we come back to your point about teaching people who are in on the situation — obstetricians and midwives — to do resuscitation and to do intubations. I think that does not mean that you are giving a second class service and we need a complete re-think about who does resuscitation and to whom we teach resuscitation. We expect a new SHO in paediatrics who has maybe intubated a few adults, or maybe not, to learn to be able to intubate babies efficiently and expertly. But we do not seem able to think that a midwife of 10 years' standing who has delivered babies every day could be taught to do the same thing.

ZIDEMAN: The document that I referred to before has dealt with this in considerable detail.[1] It does include the training in various strata of all doctors and nurses in the delivery room situation. That would include paediatricians at a very high level; it would include anaesthetists at that level because we are often involved; it would include the midwives, including intubation. It also includes obstetricians being trained to quite a high level as well to be able to perform procedures on babies. The document is due to be published in the next few weeks.[1]

SIMMONS: I would like to support what has been said about midwives. One has to recognise that 90% of all deliveries are done by midwives without any doctor being present. If there is a doctor present he is relatively inexperienced, either as a paediatrician or an obstetrician. They are all trained to be general practitioners, and so policies of safeguarding staff should be directed to midwives. In terms of training you have to remember that we are training very inexperienced doctors. What has been suggested in terms of gloves, etc. is precisely what midwives have been doing for years. What you are trying to do is bring a very young and untrained doctor up to the standard of a very highly trained and qualified midwife.

WHITELAW: I think that it would be more acceptable if we moved in the direction of consolidating the skills of people who spend their working time on the labour ward, and are correctly clothed and equipped for working all the time on the labour ward, and do not think in terms of relying on people rushing out of outpatients and onto the labour ward to provide first line resuscitation. I think that this would be a very advantageous policy for many reasons, not only for HIV, because it would mean that effective resuscitation would be available 24 hours a day. It is not at the moment. We should get away from the situation where somebody has to rush in and cover themselves with blood when they have not had time to be prepared. If somebody has done the initial resuscitation and they want to get a more experienced person then there should be time for that person to spend a minute or two preparing himself just as if you were doing surgery and you wanted a more senior person to assist you. You would not expect him to come in and not gown up and put gloves on.

REFERENCES
1. *Resuscitation of the newborn.* Report of the working party of the British Paediatric Association, Faculty of Anaesthetists (Royal College of Surgeons of England), Royal College of Midwives, Royal College of Obstetricians and Gynaecologists. London: FFARCS and RCOG, 1988.

Implications of human immunodeficiency virus for neonatal intensive care

Dr D. Harvey

As the epidemic of AIDS develops, it is expected that neonatal units will care for an increasing number of babies whose mothers have been infected with the human immunodeficiency virus (HIV).[1,2] However, it is likely that the maternity hospital staff will often not know that a particular baby is likely to have been infected;[3] thus, working practices must be developed to allow for this. HIV infection has major implications for those working in neonatal medicine and nursing,[4] since some of the babies will require special care for related neonatal conditions such as drug-withdrawal symptoms. Some will even need intensive care because of serious illness; for example, those born prematurely who may require mechanical ventilation.

It is of the greatest importance that the care of babies should come first and should not suffer because of the attempts of staff to protect themselves. Children's nurses and doctors have a good record of caring and this must not be damaged.

NEONATAL SPECIAL AND INTENSIVE CARE

Intensive care typically involves mechanical ventilation, often for many weeks, the monitoring of blood oxygen and bilirubin levels and the use of long catheters for intravenous feeding. There is therefore ample opportunity for the attendants to come in contact with body fluids from the baby. Since many risk patients may decline an offer of testing an antenatal sample of blood, the importance of using procedures in a neonatal unit which would allow staff to do their everyday work without worrying whether the baby might be HIV antibody-positive or not should be emphasised.

The advent of HIV infection has occurred at a time when the number of admissions to special care baby units (SCBUs) has been reduced.[6] When such units first became available in many hospitals in the 1970s, it was common to admit babies for observation after an abnormal birth. The number of such admissions has decreased in the last decade and should not exceed 10% of births. A concept has been developed of intermediate or transitional care in which a preterm baby is nursed at the mother's bedside instead of the SCBU.[7] The parents themselves are encouraged to do much of the work. This concept has particular relevance to babies who have HIV antibodies. Since many of the mothers of such infants are intravenous drug users (IVDUs), one must expect that many babies will show signs of withdrawal such as crying, irritability and convulsions.[8] Most of these babies need be treated only with simple sedation and swaddling, and this can be done in a special section of a postnatal ward. The relationship between the parents and baby needs to be particularly nurtured, and it is improved if one avoids separating the baby from the mother by admission to the SCBU.

Family-centred care for newborn babies in SCBUs has required a lot of work to achieve; it is important that this should not be lost in the next few years by over-enthusiastic adherence to strict protocols of isolation of the babies of HIV-infected women; such procedures must therefore be adequately evaluated.

The babies of mothers who are HIV positive are more likely to be of low birth weight and preterm, partly because of premature rupture of the membranes.[9] Babies of IVDUs are more likely to be small for dates and this may be one of the reasons why babies of HIV positive women are small. It is recognised that blood must be cleaned from a newborn baby immediately after birth, but hypothermia is a real risk and is particularly likely in the preterm.

About 1% of cases of AIDS are in children, but symptoms of HIV infection are unlikely to be present in the immediate neonatal period; they usually arise only after several months.[10] Clearly, any unusual infection must be carefully investigated; the pattern of infection at this age is different from that in older children or adults, and serious infection is common with the Group B streptococcus and *E coli*. Most neonatal units in developed countries have recently seen a marked increase in sepsis caused by coagulase-negative staphylococci, so it is not surprising that these organisms have been found in HIV-infected babies.[11]

CONSENT FOR TESTING A BABY'S BLOOD

The parent or guardian of a child under 16 years in England can give consent for a medical procedure, but it is recognised that a doctor may proceed in an emergency without consent, even if the parent has refused to give it.[12] The usual example given is that of a life-saving blood transfusion in the child of a Jehovah's Witness. It is clearly wise when there is time, to obtain consent, or when necessary to ask for the child to be made a ward of court.

It is not certain when an illness in a newborn baby would be a reason to consider testing for HIV. AIDS has not yet been recorded in the immediate newborn period, but many babies remain in an SCBU for a long time and unusual infections are common. When there is any suspicion that the baby might have HIV infection, the best plan would be to counsel the mother and with her permission, to test her blood first. Whether it is justifiable, in the best interests of a seriously ill baby with an unusual infection, to test for HIV antibody without permission requires a lot more thought and discussion.

CIRCUMCISION

Routine circumcision of newborn boys has a very long history in human society. It is practised universally by Jews, who are usually circumcised by special practitioners on the eighth day of life. Muslim boys are all circumcised before puberty and some ethnic groups from West Africa are also all circumcised. Where there is a religious indication for the operation, it is difficult to produce any good reason why it should not be done.

However, the arrival of HIV infection is a reason for avoiding any unnecessary operation which has the risk of bleeding, and this strengthens the arguments against routine circumcision. The operation is sometimes done in a rather cavalier fashion, even though it has been greatly simplified by the use of the plastic bell technique. Like any neonatal operation, a proper procedure should be followed even in a side room of the ward. Good analgesia must be used and an aseptic technique for which the operator wears a gown, gloves and a mask.

NEONATAL SURGERY

There is no reason to treat neonatal surgery any differently than other types of operation.[13] Proper precautions must be taken, and should be drawn up in each hospital. There has been a tendency to do more surgery in the SCBU itself rather than in the operating theatre. This only applies to very small babies receiving intensive care for whom a transfer to a distant operating theatre may cause hypothermia and disruption of mechanical ventilation. Several SCBUs in the UK now ask surgeons to close a patent ductus arteriosus in the unit itself rather than in the operating theatre. The operation usually takes less than half an hour and the neonatal team can continue monitoring any intensive care during and immediately after the operation. Some units have also allowed operations for necrotising enterocolitis to be performed in the incubator. This is more controversial since the laparotomy may reveal severe intestinal necrosis which requires a major resection. However, an enterostomy is often possible in the neonatal unit and can be done without disturbing a very ill baby unnecessarily with a journey. During these procedures the neonatal unit should have a proper drill similar to those used in an operating theatre; this should be written down so that it can be consulted when an operation is planned.

Small incisions for the insertion of long intravenous lines are often done under local anaesthesia in the SCBU, but most other surgical procedures would be done in the operating theatre.

TRANSFUSIONS

There are particular points to be made about blood transfusion in the newborn. Exchange transfusion is still often used for the treatment of severe neonatal jaundice and for anaemia in haemolytic disease; about twice the baby's blood volume is removed and replaced by bank blood. It is clearly important to deal carefully with any discarded blood.

It has become common to give small transfusions to tiny babies who require ventilation and oxygen therapy. This is to provide an adequate oxygen-carrying capacity in the blood and to give very preterm babies some adult haemoglobin instead of the fetal haemoglobin in their red cells at birth. Blood samples are frequently taken from such babies for blood gas analysis and for electrolyte estimations. Such samples represent a significant proportion of the baby's blood volume which is about 90 ml/kg and thus may only be about 50 ml in the smallest babies receiving intensive care. It is not surprising that anaemia results.

The indication for transfusion has changed gradually. At one time a haemoglobin estimation of 9 g/dl was regarded as an indication, whereas a value of 12 or even 14 g/dl is now commonly used. This rise has not really been properly evaluated, although it is logical. Further investigation is therefore needed to be certain that these transfusions are good practice, or whether their number might be reduced.

PROCEDURES FOR STAFF ON NEONATAL UNITS

Guidelines have been drawn up by individual hospitals to protect staff from being accidentally infected by HIV, even though it is recognised that the chances of this are slight. There does not seem to be any significant risk of hoizontal transmission in a neonatal nursery.

A greater awareness of the importance of hygiene will benefit newborn babies and prevent the accidental infection of staff; at present SCBUs are much more commonly presented with problems related to the more infectious Hepatitis B than to HIV. There are many units which believe in a one-level system of infectious precautions for dealing with patients in an SCBU. While the prevalence of HIV remains low in the obstetric population, constant encouragement will be necessary to keep up standards. Extra precautions for known infected patients could be used in addition, but may not be necessary.

It is frequently recommended that cracks on the hands should be covered with waterproof plasters. It is doubtful whether this is practical advice in SCBUs. Constant hand washing means that staff have many open lesions on their hands.

It is common to recommend that use of gloves to all staff who have come in contact with potentially infected body fluids, particularly blood, but in neonatal care the situation is not clear. For instance, after the heel prick done frequently for blood sampling in the newborn, it is very common to find that blood has become smeared on the collecting bottle or on the tester's hands. Conversely, because of the difficulty of setting up intravenous lines in tiny babies many junior paediatricians feel that they will have difficulty in inserting these essential infusions when they are wearing gloves.

A pilot study of the acceptability of gloves has been conducted in the SCBU at our hospital. The junior paediatric staff were assigned at random for 2 week periods to 1 of 3 options when setting up intravenous infusions or when taking blood. The initial options chosen were: no gloves, as in the past; the use of disposable polythene gloves; or the use of surgical latex gloves, which were worn for the whole shift and only changed if they became punctured. The surgical gloves were washed after touching each baby, in the same way as routine hand washing. The doctor's reactions to these options have been analysed by means of linear analogue scales and a semi-structured questionnaire.

None of the three options was popular. Wearing no gloves at all, when there was a risk of blood contamination, was no longer considered acceptable. The polythene gloves produced great difficulties as they interfered with setting up infusions and were difficult to put on. A typical comment was: "Blood went everywhere when I was taking a heel-prick sample". Such polythene gloves are liable to split along the seams and there is no British standard for holes in the material. They are, however, very cheap.

Latex surgical gloves were found to be suitable for even very delicate procedures, but those who used them complained that they were very uncomfortable to wear for the whole day, as sweat collected inside.

In order to provide a one-level system of infectious precautions, a strict minimum set of procedures should be instituted. Gloves should not be worn unnecessarily, so that ordinary body contact with an ill baby would not require their use. Gloves would be worn for any procedure involving blood letting; we suspect that disposable latex gloves will be best for this, but allowance will need to be made in the budget for each paediatric department. Gloves are already worn when sucking out endotracheal tubes, in order to prevent the introduction of bacteria.

Whenever there is a risk of being sprayed with blood, it seems best to wear some protection to prevent the blood reaching the mouth and eyes. A disposable mask should suffice for the mouth and it would be best for all paediatricians to wear glasses with refractive or non-refractive lenses as appropriate.

It is not certain whether there is a real risk of spraying during blood letting. It is possible that this might happen during radial artery punctures and more information is needed about this.

Many procedures in SCBUs are very invasive. These include the insertion of umbilical and radial artery catheters, setting up long intravenous lines, exchange transfusions, cerebral ventricular taps, and performing peritoneal dialysis. There are good reasons for thinking that such procedures need a full aseptic technique, and this would be considered good practices in most units. Therefore the operator should wear a gown, gloves, and mask; the addition of spectacles would now be considered necessary.

LABORATORY PROCEDURES

The RCOG report[14] recognised that the bilirubinometer, in which plasma bilirubin estimations can be done in the SCBU, was a potential source of infection. Very often the blood sample for estimation on the ward is taken into a glass capillary tube which is centrifuged and cut before the plasma is put in a cuvette. The problem is that the glass often splinters and the working surface in the ward laboratory is easily contaminated. Gloves should be worn for these estimations and careful consultations are necessary between the clinical and laboratory staff to be certain that correct procedures are being followed.

Blood gas analysis is also commonly required for ill newborn babies and is usually done in automatic machines in a side-room on the SCBU. It is very easy for serious blood contamination of the surrounding area to occur if proper procedures are not followed. It is very unlikely that it will be possible in most SCBUs for all samples of blood to be sent to the hospital laboratory for blood gas analysis, even in those ill babies who are known to be HIV positive.

CONCLUSIONS

HIV infection is bound to influence the work of those caring for ill newborn babies. More investigation is needed to develop satisfactory procedures and to evaluate them. The care of our patients must not suffer while this is being done.

REFERENCES

1. Peckham CS, Senturia YD, Ades AE. Obstetric and perinatal complications of human immunodeficiency virus (HIV) infection: a review. *Br J Obstet Gynaecol* 1987; **94:** 403-407.
2. Daniels VG. *AIDS: the acquired immune deficiency syndrome.* 2nd ed. Lancaster: MTP, 1987.
3. Landesman S, Minkoff H, Holman S, McCalla S, Sijin D. Serosurvey of human immunodeficiency virus infection in parturients: implications for human immunodeficiency virus testing programs of pregnant women. *JAMA* 1987; **258:** 2701-2703.
4. Sherr L. The impact of AIDS in obstetrics on obstetric staff. *J Reprod Infant Psychol* 1987; **5:** 87-96.
5. Inglis AD, Lozano M. AIDS and the neonatal NICU. *Neonat Network* 1986; **5:** 39-43.
6. Pharaoh PO. Childhood epidemiology: perspective and patterns. *Br Med Bull* 1986; **42:** 119-126.
7. Harvey D. *Parent-infant relationships. Perinatal practice.* Vol. 4. Chichester: Wiley, 1987.
8. Klenka BM. Babies born in a District General Hospital to mothers taking heroin. *Br Med J* 1986; **293:** 745-746.
9. Minkoff H, Nanda D, Menez R, Fikrig S. Pregnancies resulting in infants with acquired immunodeficiency syndrome or AIDS-related complex. *Obstet Gynecol* 1987; **69:** 285-288.
10. Mok JQ, Giaquinto C, De Rossi A, Grosch-Wörner I, Ades AE, Peckham CS. Infants born to mothers seropositive for human immunodeficiency virus: preliminary findings from a multicentre European study. *Lancet* 1987; **1:** 1164-1168.
11. Mejia FM, Kandall SR. Coagulase-negative staphylococcal sepsis in drug-dependent newborns who may be HIV-positive. *NY State J Med* 1987; **87:** 301-302.
12. British Medical Association. *The handbook of medical ethics.* London: British Medical Association, 1981.
13. Sim AJW, Dudley HAF. Surgeons and HIV (Editorial). *Br Med J* 1988; **296:** 280.
14. *Report of the RCOG Sub-committee on problems associated with AIDS in relation to obstetrics and gynaecology.* London: Royal College of Obstetricians and Gynaecologists, 1987.

Discussion

Chairman: Professor C.B.S. Wood

LAMBERT: I think that we should not abandon the implications of seeming to propose dual standards in our advice to breastfeeders. We have got to evaluate very clearly the evidence for transmission of HIV in breast milk because of long term implications of saying that in the West HIV-infected mothers should not breastfeed, but in the Third World—the developing world—it is acceptable because of the other problems associated with artificial feeding. This leaves a dual standard. Developing countries frequently look to the West and say that our standard is one to which they should aspire. If they then see 2 standards being given, that has much more far reaching implications. I wonder if you could say more about the evidence of the transmission of HIV in breast milk.

LUCAS: I totally agree with your first point. I share your discomfort about the recommendations that we have made in the West in terms of their implications for the developing world. We are faced with the fact that bottle feeding is associated not only with an increase in morbidity, but with a substantial increase in mortality in the developing world, whereas one is very hard pressed to detect any increase even of morbidity in bottle-fed babies in the West. So the dual standard is based upon existing data, and we cannot get away from that. As far as the evidence for HIV transmission is concerned, I was pilloried by Miss Wilday for saying that the evidence for HIV transmission by breastfeeding was weak, circumstantial and scanty. Recently my attention has been drawn to a number of reports concerning HTLV-1 transmission and I think that we now have to take that into account.[1,2] The evidence of HIV being transmitted by breast milk is based on 3 circumstantial case reports and on the presence of virus in milk. The virus invades the cellular and the cell free fraction of milk in quite high titres. I think that the transmission of other retroviruses in breast milk does require that we examine the situation seriously. The evidence is based on several studies showing a higher incidence of HTLV-1 infection in breastfed babies in Japan and the prevention of HTLV-I transmission by bottlefeeding. Eleven out of 24 breastfed babies became HTLV-I positive compared with 1 out of 11 bottlefed babies.

MOK: Dr Jeffries, are there any physical qualities that differentiate HTLV-I and HIV? What makes HTLV-I so efficiently transmitted?

JEFFRIES: Not that I am aware of. The physico-chemical characteristics of the whole family of retroviruses have been known and studied since 1911, and were well characterised in terms of certain members of the family in the 1960s. We knew early on after the discovery of HIV that HTLV-I and HIV are spread by similar routes and by similar risk activities. In terms of virus structure and morphology they show no differences that I know of.

HOWIE: The very important issue of what advice should be given on breastfeeding policy because of the presence of HIV in breast milk is very difficult. There are 2 questions that should be answered. First, what is the evidence that HIV in breast milk does cause the disease in infants? As you quite rightly said, this is not established beyond any doubt. The other question which mothers will ask is, "if there is virus in breast milk, can you assure us that its use is absolutely safe?" The answer is equally uncertain. It is impossible to reassure mothers on the basis of the current evidence. So we have got to take the second question into account when formulating guidance policies. It is the answer to that second question which has influenced the Department in its guidelines, although I accept the reservations which you put.

WHITELAW: Following on from those two questions, should we not strive to avoid the need for breast milk banks by having every mother with a sick or small baby lactating herself? I do not feel that we go as far as we could to achieve this, and with information, persuasion and assistance more could be done than is being done at the moment.

LUCAS: This presents a fundamental difficulty. In our multi-centre trial we leave it to the mother's choice to provide milk for her own infant. But feeding a fortified diet is better in all the outcome responses we have had, apart from enteral feed induction using donor breast milk. We just do not know about mother's own milk. It is very important to emphasise that we are not talking about full term babies; we are talking about premature babies with very special requirements. If we were to promote the use of mother's own milk much more with the result that more mothers might provide all of their own infant's requirements, we might not necessarily be doing them the best service. We are now starting another randomised study on the supplementation of mother's milk. That might be a good alternative, but it is much more dificult than giving a formula because the base diet varies a lot, and it is going to be difficult to calculate the safe amount of supplement for each particular baby. If we can demonstrate that we can achieve the same advantages from supplemented breast milk that we can achieve with formulae, then your argument will come into its own. What I would be worried about at the moment is promoting something which would be very useful in the early days up to a couple of weeks after birth, but which might not turn out to give the baby the best overall end result.

WILDAY: Perhaps one of the other considerations might be whether the mother really wants to do this. This is frequently a time of very great stress for the mother of a very small baby. I believe that midwives and neonatal nurses are now discussing with parents the value, the wisdom and the mother's desire to express breast milk from the very early days.

WHITELAW: I am impressed that that is happening at your hospital, but I personally do not think that most midwives on postnatal wards actually have this information on the advantages of mother's milk for low birthweight, sick babies. Most of this information is very recent, and giving the mother a choice would at the moment be inappropriate because it would not be an informed choice. Issues such as psychological feelings on whether she should breastfeed or not which are quite appropriate for a mother with a full term baby would be quite inappropriate for the mother of a baby in an intensive care unit. The balance is very different, and it must be presented in a totally different way to such a mother.

LUCAS: You can only advocate a policy if you have the data to support it. We now have data, so we can make a recommendation. We have left mother's own milk alone; we have no reason for promoting it. But we also have no reason for stopping mothers who wish to provide milk for their own babies. What we have done is to encourage mothers in their choice.

WHITELAW: But you said that human milk is better for starting off very small babies.

LUCAS: Yes, I think that we can encourage mother's milk in the beginning. I think that the AIDS scare might actually be an incentive as well.

LAMBERT: If you accept that theoretically an infant could be infected by HIV by ingestion, which is what we are saying, surely a logical extrapolation is that people who are preparing food are in a potential position to infect others. And that goes against all the advice which we have been given about casual contact. But this is a logical extension of what we are claiming in the case of breast milk. Have we looked at the hydrolysed milk formulae, such as Progestamilk, instead of donor milk?

LUCAS: That is a good suggestion. If we reach a position where we have to get rid of milk banks, then it is imperative that we find formulae that are better than the ones currently in use. That would be a very exciting research programme to find out what it is about formulae that makes them so much more poorly tolerated than human milk.

JEFFRIES: There are two main issues here: one is the HIV positive mother and whether she should breastfeed. Although I answered Dr Mok's question as well as I could, that there is no obvious physico-chemical difference or nature in the character of these 2 viruses, that does not mean that they behave the same biologically. The early data from the European Collaborative Study suggest that we are not getting babies infected with AIDS from breastfeeding, but it is too early to extrapolate from that. However, I do take Dr Lambert's point because I think it would be tragic if we see what I think is happening already. I have had messages given to me that in certain developing countries people are already advising mothers not to breastfeed because of the HIV risk. It would be tragic if that went ahead on the basis of extrapolations from the Japanese literature on HTLV-I as we have seen all the implications of artificial feeding. In terms of milk banking, I do not think that donor screening is ever going to be the answer. There is always going to be a false negative rate on testing. We are just starting to plug in HIV-2, but there is no doubt that it is in the country, and it cannot be picked up reliably in the screening tests. We now know that there is a carrier for HIV-2 in London who has no African links and there will be other viruses and retroviruses coming along; we already have HTLV-I. So I do not think that even leaving aside all the implications of how the screening is going to be carried out, that that is an efficient way to do it. When it comes to pasteurisation, Dr Lucas made a comment about virologists disagreeing in terms of inactivation of viruses. I do not really see that there is a problem there, because the experimental work is relatively easily done. The controversy to which I think he is referring is over the papers written on pasteurisation, or heat inactivation of virus at 56°C. The experiments that Roger Eglin did in Oxford[3] showed that using either cell-free or cell-associated virus the infectivity in good assay systems was removed. Now all we need is confirmation of Roger Eglin's work, then we know that we can pasteurise against HIV. At the same time we can plug HTLV-I into that. The virology can easily be straightened out. The question I would like to ask is, in terms of establishment of enteral feeding is there any difference between 56°C and 62.5°C in terms of the quality of the milk after treatment?

LUCAS: I cannot answer that question because we pasteurise our milk at 62°C, but having pasteurised it at 62°C which ought to be the more aggressive treatment, we have not got the protective effect. The data which I showed were for milk that had been pasteurised. I was delighted to hear what you have just said because I have talked to a number of other virologists who have expressed concern about human milk even after pasteurisation because the virus may survive. They point out that as a result of pasteurisation there is a reduction in virus by several log orders which is not the same as destruction, so that even if you could not detect it there might be some infectivity left. I would be delighted if virologists could reassure us that we can choose a time/temperature relationship that we know does not damage the microbial factors in the milk too much. If they could devise that for us we would then remove the recommendation for screening.

JEFFRIES: You will never get virologists to agree on this. But this anxiety seems to be a purely British phenomenon. There would be enough virologists in this country prepared to do this work. I have offered to look at milk from HIV positive mothers to see if we can do it.

SPIRO: I share Dr Lucas' concern about the lack of knowledge which many midwives have about the establishment of breastfeeding, and you still hear of mothers coming out of hospital who have been told to use the breast pump once or twice a day. The supply and demand message is still not getting through. Also there is the question of the possible use of oxytocic sprays. They do seem to be effective for some mothers in helping the milk get down. The second point I should like to raise is the question of high risk mothers. I am extremely concerned that we are putting out this information, and it is up to the individual health care professional to interpret who is the high risk mother who must be advised not to breastfeed. That worries me in that even some high risk mothers may not be infected with the virus at the present. Are we not a bit premature about putting forth this recommendation?

WILDAY: I think that I actually said seropositive mothers, not high risk mothers.

MOK: Given the fact that there may be HIV in breast milk, do we know what the normal neonate's pH is? Can that not inactivate the virus even if it is ingested?

LUCAS: There are more variations in gastric pH in the neonatal period than in virtually any other period in life. They start out with a level of 7 which reflects amniotic fluid being swallowed, and then you get a sharp drop followed by a prolonged rise. Eventually you will find a period of time when the gastric pH is almost anything you like. So that is the problem.

HUDSON: Could I direct one question to Miss Greenwood on the legal position over breast milk donation as determined by the Department of Health's publication on tissue and organ donation. Is that in the form of a directive, and are we obliged to follow the terms of screening which are suggested for other organs at present, or is it entirely facultative?

GREENWOOD: I do not have the data with me about donations, so I cannot answer that question. I would like to raise the question with Dr Jeffries, because he has said that donor screening is not feasible for breast milk donation. I wondered how far he would make that statement about the donation of any other organ in such a situation. My impression was that over donation of breast milk we would be following the principles that had been suggested for other organ donations.

JEFFRIES: Nothing is safe. If one has got a reliable inactivation process then that is always better than trying donor screening in any of these situations. I made the statement that blood is not safe in any country in the world at the present time. We are constantly looking to see whether HIV itself or HIV-1 is mutating so that we are getting an increase in false negatives. We know that we have HIV-2 in the community; we are debating whether we ought to be screening donors for HTLV-1. My point is that if you have got something that can be shown with a little more experimentation to inactivate these viruses in breast milk it will always be better than screening. Dr Mok's comment about pH and gastric juice was a nice ploy, but it looks as though you are not going to get much of an answer. But that probably is the answer to Dr Lambert's question. The gastric acid if it is below a level of pH2 is going to inactivate HIV.

WOOD: I should like to turn first to the problems of standards of care. Several people here have taken the view that it is an absolute priority that the standard of care of neonates is not varied. Whatever is our norm for an HIV positive mother, or merely a high risk mother or for an ordinary person, it should be the same. The overall priority should be that in all circumstances the care of the child should be correct and not qualified by consideration of risk to the attendant.

HARVEY: You said newborn. Can we say families?

WOOD: I am sure that we would agree with that. In order to achieve that I would have thought that a process of consultation between all the various professional groups which are involved in neonatal care should be established. That means that the procedures that we use will have to be looked at in quite precise detail. Suddenly we are going to find something about our particular unit, or the procedures or a particular protocol which has not been "dusted down" for 3 months, 6 months or 4 years, and which needs careful examination. There will be surprises. That is what goes on within a unit between professional groups, but there is also a need to consult with the supporting laboratory services because they have their own particular interests and views. They have their own very precise safety regulations. There is the control of infection nursing officer. How does she come into this? There is also the committee structure, the medical advisory structure in any district. There is the district management board and its general manager. Do we agree that detailed and careful consultation should take place? Should we not frequently review the guidelines? Most neonatal units have regular ward meetings, but might this not be more formal?

WHITELAW: I agree with you, but there are many things which neonatal staff are feeling under pressure about at the moment: the tremendous shortage of nursing staff, the fear of litigation, the retinopathy of prematurity, in some places the lack of equipment. Neonatal nurses are leaving the profession, and there is a very limited intake to the qualifying training course. I get the feeling that some neonatal staff see infants of intravenous drug abusers as just one more problem, and one that they could do without. There is a tremendous need for people like us to listen to these concerns and to defuse some of the slightly less realistic fears that staff have. Policies will not work unless time is spent having meetings like this.

WOOD: My feeling is that if consultation takes place properly then the levels of anxiety will fall and the levels of efficiency will rise. When a unit is run in such a way that opinions are sought out and advice acted upon things seem to work much better.

McELWEE: It is quite true that staff already do feel under pressure. I do not work in a neonatal unit or a special care baby unit, but I am very aware of their need for protection. Even as professionals, we are people too, and we have just as many attitudes, prejudices and bigotries as the general public. I think that in consultation we should be aware that sometimes our attitudes might get in the way of maintaining good standards of practice and making sure that everyone has the level of care to which they are entitled no matter what their background or social problem. If we recognise that we as professionals are actually people first and are no better than anyone else in terms of attitudes then we might be able to disguise them a bit better.

WOOD: Another point which we covered is the attempt to arrive at a simple standard of procedures, particularly with regard to resuscitation, so that we have a simple minimum. I do not think that we are going to be able to decide here and now what that is. This should be part of the consultation process in any particular district to decide who does what and how it is to be done, depending on the resources available and the level and quality of trained staff. Can we agree that it is desirable as far as possible to move away from always selecting the high risk case to generalise the minimum protective standard?

ROTH: Would it be possible to put a rider to that as well? It should be that the minimum standard is based on a minimum degree of extra care and a greater concentration on simple procedures such as bathing babies early on in their life and other measures to remove the basis for risk rather than putting up a protective barrier.

WHITELAW: Can I add one point with regard to the unexpected resuscitation of a baby where someone must spend 2 or 3 minutes trying to find an apron, gown, etc. while the baby is lying there. I wonder what people feel about a bare minimum not including an apron and gown, but firstly gloves as the most important item and then to include glasses and a mask. Could this be the bare minimum that we insist on for resuscitation—gloves, mask and glasses—not including changing clothing?

HARVEY: Why the mask?

WHITELAW: Because at resuscitation one is more likely to have a spraying of body fluids. You are suctioning, you are using positive pressure, so you need a face mask.

HARVEY: I am happy to accept that, but we had virological evidence that glasses were desirable. Are virologists happy that masks are also desirable?

JEFFRIES: One of the 3 contact cases as opposed to the inoculation cases of infection that have occured appears to have followed the splashing of blood into the mouth of the resuscitator. The mask is not, as you know, to prevent air flow, but to protect the lips in case of splashing. I agree with that comment. Gloves are by far the most important in terms of protection. At a second level in terms of splashing, eye protection and a mask are desirable. I would go along with you in terms of the basic protective clothing. Clothing protection comes further down on the list of priorities, to be used if there is time. Gloves should be first with eye protection and mask at a second level, and then clothing.

WOOD: Could I now ask you to think about the ward procedures which are best for the normal newborn? Can I take it that the general principles which have been presented earlier are seen to be practicable?

SHARP: You can refer to the working party report, because I think it is likely that we will include the report as an appendix to the proceedings so that it is available for people who have not seen it.

WOOD: As I recall there was no violent argument as to the procedures which were presented.

GREENWOOD: Except, Mr Chairman, that these were for the high risk cases. One of the principles that the revised document has to look at is, "do we still have two groups of recommendations for routine and high risk cases?" At the moment I cannot agree with what you are saying, and I am not sure what you are suggesting, whether it is to apply to the care of all babies or just high risk ones.

WOOD: We had thought that we would move towards a uniform pattern of care. Does it mean that the relevant paragraphs in the working party report should be generalised, or are they too difficult to generalise? It does not seem to me to be a particularly stringent or difficult style of practice.

WILDAY: I am not sure about the first sentence stating that the infant should be cared for in the same room as the mother.

WOOD: It means that in the apparently normal neonate this practice should be encouraged. The HIV-infected baby may be very often entirely normal.

MOK: This is when you identify it as being high risk.

WOOD: The question is whether these paragraphs should be generalised to describe a uniform standard of care, because it seems to me that they are not particularly demanding.

HUDSON: It is a logical extension if you take the view that single-tier care is preferable, although that is at variance with what we have recommended. It would be logical now to include this in general terms as suitable for single-tier care.

ROTH: There is a question with regard to this general policy. It is the question of the Guthrie tests. It is quite true that they do represent a biohazard and are handled in a fairly casual way. I also wonder whether the issue of banding them in plastic should be something that is universally applied. Also, given a greater awareness of the risks associated with blood and blood products, whether that again should not be a universal standard and not something that we need necessarily to label as such.

WOOD: In a way this relates to the principle of consultation which we have discussed. It involves trying to get people more aware of the usefulness of a standard procedure.

HARVEY: I am quite happy about surgical gloves for attending to the cord and doing heel pricks, but I really wonder whether it is practical or necessary for nappy changing and cleaning vomit. That sounds a bit excessive.

JEFFRIES: All these procedures are constantly under review. One starts out from a basis of logic. Everyone knows that blood is the highest risk fluid, but any body fluid can on occasion have blood or lymphocytes in it. So the first inclination is to say that contact with any blood fluid ought to be walled. Now we are coming back by implication to the position where there are body fluids which are recognised as being clearly of very low risk indeed. Bearing in mind all aspects of the equation we probably should not be recommending wearing gloves for contact with these other body fluids, but somebody has got to say so. The Hospital Infection Society has a working party which has been reconvened to discuss this among other issues. In terms of the other body fluids, I cannot speak for vomit because I do not think that anyone has looked at vomit in this situation. The virus has only been isolated once from urine. It has never been isolated from faeces. That does not mean a great deal, but I think you are right. We have got to be selective in the use of gloves.

STEELE: We may be in danger of contradicting ourselves because we have already said that we must inform the laboratory if high risk specimens were going over. Now we are suggesting doing away with the labelling of biohazards. Are the laboratories going to be happy with that?

WOOD: I did not think that we were going to do away with biohazards; I thought we were going to make procedures for consultation at a higher standard.

JEFFRIES: This is going to be changed in time; I am sure about that. I introduced the concept that we are going to be moving more and more towards a single-tier system. San Francisco has abandoned the biohazard labelling system altogether. I also said that I do not think that we are ready for that in obstetric practice or in the laboratory system in this country. In terms of consultation, informing the laboratory that an HIV positive sample may be on the way, is certainly not necessary in my hospital. There is an understanding at the moment that we will be sending a constant stream of HIV positive samples to the laboratory. It really depends on circumstances. In low prevalence areas it would be polite and sensible to do that. But at the moment, rightly or wrongly, our laboratory staff are relying on the biohazard for handling samples differently when they come into the lab.

WOOD: We had quite a good discussion on breastfeeding. We said that we saw a place for properly run human milk banks, that we might need to discover what the law says about human tissues and that we need to know more about the virology and infectivity, and the vulnerablilty of the stomach to ingested infected material.

We were cautious of the view that milk banks might survive if well run. As to advice about whether HIV positive mothers should breastfeed, that would vary depending on whether she was in the Third World or the developed world. I sense that there was a certain amount of tentative disagreement about that. Are you prepared to go along with a simple consensus that breastfeeding in the Third World should not be discouraged, but until the picture emerges more clearly in developed countries then it might be best to discourage breasfeeding among HIV positive mothers?

REFERENCES
1. Kinoshita A, Amagasaki K, Hino S, Doi H, Yamanouchi K, Ban N, Momita S, Ikeda S, Kamihira S, Ichimaru M. Milk-borne transmission of HTLV-1 from carrier mothers to their children. *Jpn J Cancer Res* 1987; **78:** 674-680.
2. Ando Y, Nakano S, Saito K, Shimamoto I, Ichijo M, Toyama T, Hinuma Y. Transmission of adult T-cell leukaemia retrovirus (HTLV-1) from mother to child: comparison of bottle- with breast-fed babies. *Jpn J Cancer Res* 1987; **78:** 322-324.
3. Eglin RP, Wilkinson AR. HIV infection and pasteurisation of breast-milk. *Lancet* 1987; **1:** 1093.

AIDS and human milk banking

Dr A. Lucas

INTRODUCTION

During the past 15 years there has been a re-emergence of human milk banking, to provide breast milk for preterm infants undergoing intensive or special care. In the past 2 years, however, a number of milk banks have been closed. There has been increasing concern amongst paediatricians that human milk may not meet the special nutritional needs of premature babies, and more recent anxiety that AIDS could be transmitted via breast milk. Indeed, public awareness about AIDS has reached a point where even parents occasionally object to their premature baby receiving banked donor milk.[1]

Clearly, current practice in this field needs to be reappraised. Two important questions emerge. First, are there good clinical grounds for maintaining a supply of donor breast milk for feeding premature babies? And second, how can milk banking be conducted so that both parents and the medical profession are reassured that the infants' risk of acquiring HIV has been essentially eliminated?[2,3]

FEEDING THE PRETERM INFANT: AN OVERVIEW[2]

When a preterm infant is born there is sudden loss of its continuous intravenous infusion of nutrients via the placenta, and cessation of maternal control over fetal metabolism, up to 4 months "too soon" in biological terms. The tiny preterm infant cannot suck effectively, it has an immature gut, and is born with low body stores of many nutrients which would normally accumulate during the third trimester, such as subcutaneous fat, bone minerals, trace metals and several vitamins. The birth of a premature baby disrupts a pattern of growth and nutrient accretion which is substantially different to that of the full term infant.[4]

The choice of diet for premature babies is not an obvious one. These infants are not fetuses, since, once born, they rapidly acquire metabolic and nutrient handling skills which would not have been seen at an equivalent stage *in utero;* yet, neither can they be regarded as full term with respect to their nutritional needs.

The use of raw maternal breast milk, has been favoured on the grounds of its specific composition, with high concentrations of semi-essential amino acids (cystine and taurine);[4,5] its low renal solute load and osmolality; the absorbability

271

of its fats;[6] its possible role in protecting against necrotising enterocolitis[7,8] and infection;[9-10] and finally, on the grounds that it contains non-nutrient factors, including a large range of hormones[11] and certain enzymes (e.g. lipase)[12] which might have biological importance.

It must be conceded however that these are largely theoretical arguments; many of the nutrient properties cited above may be achieved in a formula; the evidence that human milk protects (Western) preterm infants against infection, or necrotising enterocolitis is scanty; and finally there is no evidence to support the view that such non-nutrient factors as breast milk hormones would be biologically useful if consumed up to 4 months "too soon".

An opposing argument has been that if premature babies are to grow and accrete nutrients at the *in utero* rate, they need, compared with full term infants, more protein, energy, sodium, phosphorus, calcium, zinc, copper, iron and certain vitamins.[2] These theoretical, increased requirements, based on extensive physiological studies on newborn infants, have been met by a generation of special preterm infant formulae.[2]

Some neonatologists, committed to the use of human milk, have attempted to modify breast milk to meet the preterm infant's theoretical nutritional needs, either by separating and reconstituting breast milk to produce a human milk formula,[13] or by adding extra nutrients to breast milk, a procedure with potential problems in view of the great variability of the base diet. However, the principal problem faced by those wishing to use breast milk is the limited availability of mothers' own milk.[14] In 5 centres, we observed that about a third of mothers elected not to express milk for their infants and those who did supply milk, provided a median of under 50% of their infants' feed volume requirement. Thus, two thirds of the milk volume used by these neonatal units was a 'back-up' diet.[14] If this back-up diet is to be human milk, it needs to be collected from donors and banked.

HUMAN MILK BANKING

Human milk banking is a major undertaking. It involves collaboration between paediatricians, clinical bacteriologists and biochemists, hospital nursing staff, community midwives and health visitors and voluntary workers or organisations, such as the National Childbirth Trust. The canvassing and care of donors and the collection of milk from the community needs considerable planning and effort. In the hospital, a milk bank requires allocated space, special equipment, staffing and funding.[15]

Paediatricians involved in human milk banking have found themselves grappling with the types of technical problem solved by the dairy industry 40 years ago; and on the public health and clinical safety side, the field of milk banking has lagged well behind that of blood banking. It has been only in very recent years that milk banking has emerged as a relatively sophisticated discipline.

It is now known that human milk undergoes significant changes during the process of collection, processing and storage. Donor milk varies considerably in nutritional quality. If donor mothers express their excess milk, the fat and energy content will depend on whether donors provide 'foremilk' or 'hindmilk'.[16]

In this country, donors have been encouraged to collect so-called 'drip breast milk', which drips from the contralateral breast in significant quantities in about 20% of lactating mothers.[17] Drip breast-milk (which can be collected into a shell worn over the breast), like foremilk, has a very low fat and energy content (often under 50 kcals/100 ml, compared with 65-70 kcals/100 ml in expressed milk). While the milk is being collected it becomes contaminated with micro-organisms. In the neonatal unit, for convenience of microbiological monitoring, milk from multiple donors is usually pooled, resulting in cross contamination. Most units use pasteurised milk. Even accurate pasteurisation at 62°C for 30 minutes damages antimicrobial factors in milk such as IgA and lactoferrin[18] and inaccurate pasteurisation may result in almost complete loss of these components. Yet, the presence of these factors in breast milk has been a major argument for using it in clinical practise. Some units have used raw donor milk for this reason, but the safety and advisability of this approach has been debated.[19]

Whether used raw or heat-treated, donor milk is usually stored frozen, and the freezing and thawing of breast milk may damage nutrient and non-nutrient properties further. When human milk is instilled into feeding apparatus, fat may adhere to the sides of vessels and tubing resulting in significant caloric loss.[20] Finally, as milk is collected, processed and fed to babies, its exposure to light results in significant destruction of vitamin A and riboflavin.[21]

These practical and scientific problems, together with the organisational difficulties of running a milk bank, have put an onus on those undertaking milk banking to provide sound clinical evidence in its support.

CLINICAL TRIALS OF PRETERM INFANT FEEDING

Uncertainty over how preterm infants should be fed has resulted in a multiplicity of feeding regimes. The principal reason for this uncertainty has been that management policies have been based on information obtained from short-term physiological studies rather than from clinical outcome trials. In 1982, a large multicentre randomised outcome trial of early diets[22,23] was established to address the questions: do diets used in the neonatal period differ in their clinical safety and does the diet chosen influence long term development, growth or morbidity?

During the course of these trials nearly 1000 preterm infants, weighing under 1850g at birth, have been randomly assigned to their early diet, intensively monitored, and are being followed up indefinitely. The cohort has now passed its 18-months post-term follow-up period.

The initial dietary assignments were, in 3 of the centres, to banked donor breast milk or a special preterm formula as sole diets (trial 1); or, in babies whose mothers chose to express their breast milk (EBM), to banked milk and preterm formula, assigned randomly, as supplements to EBM (trial 2). In 2 further centres a standard term formula was compared with a preterm formula as sole diets (trial 3) or as supplements to EBM (trial 4).

Compared with infants fed donor milk, those fed a preterm formula gained weight, length and head circumference faster.[22] At discharge from hospital (at about 2000g body weight), preterm formula-fed infants had, as a group, maintained the centile for body weight that they were on at birth. In contrast, by discharge, donor milk fed infants had a mean weight below the 3rd centile for gestational age and could be classified therefore as 'failing to thrive'. Perhaps the most impressive difference in growth performance relates to the growth of the head. Using an equation for deriving brain weight from head circumference,[24] we have shown that in the first month, the increment in brain weight in babies fed a preterm formula was twice that seen in donor human milk (Figure I).

Figure I

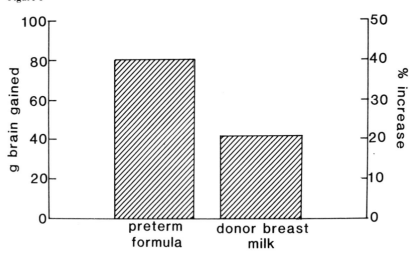

Brain growth in the first month in preterm infants (mean birthweight 1370g, range 600-1849g), fed preterm formula or donor breast milk as sole diets. Data represent g of brain tissue gained since birth (left y-axis) and % increment above brainweight at birth (right y-axis). These data are means, derived using an established relationship between head circumference and brainweight,[24] and based on our previously published data showing a significant difference in head circumference gained between preterm formula-fed and donor milk-fed infants.[2]

The preterm formula-fed babies have further advantages[23,25] compared with those fed donor milk in that they have a significantly lower incidence of severe bone disease due to insufficiency of dietary phosphorus and calcium and of jaundice which has been associated in other studies with handicap and deafness; they have half the incidence of severe hyponatraemia; they seldom develop the profound hypophosphataemia that is often seen with human milk, and they have been found to have a reduced incidence of a number of vitamin deficiencies.

Infants fed on a preterm formula are discharged home significantly sooner; babies born under 1200g and fed donor milk may take 50% longer to attain 2000g. Quite apart from the medical and social implications of this finding, it has obvious significance in terms of Health Service economics.

Of most importance, however, is the preliminary evidence emerging from our studies, that later in infancy those who were fed on preterm formulae have higher developmental scores than those fed donor milk. The significance of these findings in relation to later IQ and performance will be investigated at future follow-up periods.

HAVE THE THEORETICAL BENEFITS OF DONOR MILK BEEN ESTABLISHED?

On preliminary analysis (unpublished) of 30,000 patient-days for the 926 babies in our study, we have been unable to demonstrate that feeding pasteurised donor breast or indeed fresh maternal milk results in a reduction in the incidence of minor or severe infections. These data contrast with those from developing countries,[10] and indicate that such studies cannot be generalised to apply in infants undergoing intensive care in Western hospitals.

It has been proposed, largely on the basis of animal studies,[7,8] that fresh breast milk (with live cells) might protect preterm infants against necrotising enterocolitis, a disease associated with substantial morbidity. Our preliminary data suggest that raw maternal milk may result in a significant reduction in this condition. However, like others,[26] we were unable to demonstrate a significant benefit from pasteurised donor milk.

Preterm infants fed on milk formula have been shown by us to develop latent anaphylatic sensitisation to cows milk.[27] Preterm infants could be expected to be at risk for such sensitisation since their gut is relatively permeable to whole proteins[28] and they have reduced protein digestion, thus increasing their antigenic exposure. Our data, and those of many others, might suggest, on theoretical grounds, that preterm infants fed on formula would be more prone to future atopic disease than those fed breast milk. Yet at 18 months post-term our preliminary (unpublished) findings provide strong evidence, from a randomised prospective feeding study, that early use of human milk has no prophylactic effect on the later incidence of reactions to cows milk or other foods, wheezing or eczema.

CLINICAL APPLICATIONS OF DONOR MILK

When viewed in isolation, the above data would appear to have eliminated any requirement for human milk banking, and hence any need for concern about the transmission of HIV to preterm infants via donor milk. However, new data from our multicentre study have indicated that there are important applications for donor milk in neonatal intensive care.

A major difficulty in the care of very small, sick preterm infants, who are increasingly surviving with modern care, is the establishment of enteral feeding. The gut is functionally immature in the premature baby, especially before 28 weeks gestation, and enteral feed tolerance is limited. The need for early intra-venous nutrition may result in atrophic changes in the intestine[29] which compound this problem.

Whilst preterm formulae appear to have emerged as a major advance for the routine nutritional management of low birthweight babies, their use in small sick babies in the early days post-partum may be problematic. We have noted previously that babies fed such formulae, compared with those fed human milk, have an increased rate of vomiting, gastric stasis and constipation.[1] The latter

Figure II

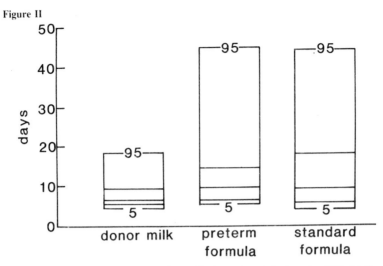

Days to attain full enteral feeds according to diet in preterm infants under 1850g birthweight. Data are represented in centiles; the horizontal lines in the data bar for each diet represent, from bottom to top; the 5th, 25th, 50th, 75th and 95th centile for the number of postnatal days to reach an enteral intake of 150 mls/kg per day. Randomised comparison of donor milk group (n=76) and preterm formula group (n=70) by Mann Whitney rank sum test; P < 0.001. No significant difference between preterm and standard formula.

may progress, on rare occasions, to frank obstruction requiring surgical removal of inspissated formula which has failed to progress along the gut, though with careful management and slow introduction of formula feeds this complication is probably avoidable.

The foregoing problems with formula feeds are reflected in a dramatic increase in the time taken to establish an infant on a formula (either preterm or standard formula), compared with that taken by a baby fed human milk (either donor or mother's own). This is illustrated in Figure II which indicates that the 95th centile for the number of days taken to establish an infant on full enteral feeds of banked milk (150 mls/kg per day or more) is 18 days; compared with a corresponding figure of 44 days for infants fed on preterm or standard formula. As a corollary, in units which do not have a milk bank, a formula-fed baby can be expected to spend considerably longer on partial parenteral nutrition, a procedure which is invasive, expensive, time-consuming and, above all, associated with a range of well-described metabolic, mechanical and microbiological hazards.[30]

RECOMMENDATIONS FOR THE USE OF DONOR BREAST MILK

Establishment of enteral feeding (up to 150 ml/kg per day) using donor milk (or mother's own milk, or a combination), is recommended prior to commencing with a preterm formula in the following circumstances:

a)   in all infants born under 28 weeks gestation

b) in preterm infants who have undergone prolonged total parenteral nutrition (more than 7 days)
c) in preterm infants recovering from necrotising enterocolitis
d) in infants who fail to tolerate formula feeds.

AIDS AND THE USE OF DONOR MILK

The evidence that HIV may be acquired by the neonate through the ingestion of breast milk is scanty and circumstantial.[31,32] The virus has been found in high titres in cellular and cell-free fractions of breast milk from infected mothers.[33,34] Occasional case reports[31,32] have identified mothers who have acquired HIV postnatally from a blood transfusion for post-partum haemorrhage, and whose breast-fed baby subsequently became HIV positive. These findings are difficult to interpret, since close contact between mother and infant might have resulted in HIV transmission by routes other than the gut. Perhaps more convincing are the data from primates and man suggesting that other retroviruses, including HTLV-1, may be acquired by breastfeeding[35,36] and that formula feeding significantly reduces the risk of transmission of HTLV-1 from mother to baby.[37] Currently, there is no published report on the acquisition of HIV in a premature baby fed either raw or pasteurised donor breast milk.

Nevertheless, it has not been possible to ignore current data, however scanty, on the risks of HIV transmission via breast milk, and some official bodies in Western countries[38] have recommended that HIV positive mothers should be advised against breastfeeding, though the application of this advice in developing countries has been much debated.[39]

Recommendations for milk banking practice

While the spread of AIDS via the enteral route remains an under-researched field, recommendations on appropriate milk banking practices must be regarded as provisional. Stringent control is justified because if milk banking is to survive in this country, convincing reassurance that donor milk is a safe diet must be provided.

a. Pasteurisation of human milk

The thermolability of HIV infectivity[40] and reverse transcriptase activity[41] at 56°C have been documented. Most units that pasteurise human milk to render it bacteriologically safe use a standard regimen of exposure to a temperature of 62°C for 30 minutes, followed by rapid cooling. Recently, a temperature of 56°C has been shown to be effective and this is employed in some units.[42] In either case, these regimens should result in inactivation of HIV. Recently Eglin and Wilkinson[43] examined the effect on HIV of pasteurising breast milk at 54.5-55°C for 30 minutes ('Oxford' pasteuriser, Vickers Medical) or 56-57.5°C for 33 minutes ('Axicare' pasteuriser, Colgate Medical). 10 mls of milk were removed from a bottle and replaced with 10 mls of tissue culture fluid containing 10^5 HIV infectious units/ml and 10^5 HIV-infected CEM cells/ml. Neither infectivity nor reverse transcriptase activity were detectable in the post-pasteurised samples, even after 14 days culture.

Recommendations:
a) Donor human milk intended for routine use should be pasteurised at a minimum temperature of 56°C for 30 minutes (see below for guidelines on the use of raw donor milk).
b) Accurate, purpose built and validated pasteurisation equipment should be used.
c) Mother's own milk need not be pasteurised for use with her own premature baby. (If a Western mother is known to be HIV positive, provision of breast milk and subsequent breastfeeding is not generally advised, though if a specific risk of formula-feeding was identified in an individual infant, after discharge home, a balanced appraisal would be required).

b.   Screening of donors

Pasteurisation of donor milk has been claimed by some workers to eliminate HIV infectivity from breast milk and hence obviate the need for donor screening.[43] However, virologists continue to debate this issue and some express concern that pasteurisation may reduce infectivity to levels which are difficult to detect, but not necessarily eliminate it. While any doubt remains, the safest policy would be to screen milk donors in pregnancy or post-partum, as practised for blood donors. Against screening donors is the argument that the number of mothers agreeing to supply milk would be reduced, and result in closure of some milk banks. In this instance a small and unknown risk of the infant contracting AIDS would have been traded for a more defined risk,[30] namely that smaller babies, which could not be supplied with breast milk, may be subjected to the potential hazards of more prolonged parenteral nutrition. However, if donor milk is used only in special circumstances as recommended above, much smaller amounts are required than when it is used as a routine diet; hence fewer donors would be needed than in the past.

Recommendations:
a) Potential donors should be screened by questionnaire, to ensure that they are from a low risk group.
b) In view of the foregoing arguments, it would not be inappropriate for donors to milk banks to be screened by blood testing during pregnancy or post-partum. However it is hoped that further virological studies on the efficiency of human milk pasteurisation will be forthcoming and perhaps obviate the need to screen donors. At present there are insufficient data for a firm recommendation on the need for screening.

c.   The use of raw donor breast milk

Many units collect breast milk in a casual way from mothers on postnatal wards. Such milk is frequently used in the raw state. It is clear that the practice of using such *ad hoc* donations is unacceptable. In those units wishing to use raw donor milk, a more stringent approach is required to ensure that the risk of HIV transmission is removed.

Recommendation:
If raw donor milk is to be used, it should be frozen and not released unless the donor's screening test is negative after the milk has been collected.

OVERVIEW

While banked donor milk has not emerged as an ideal diet for the routine feeding of preterm infants, either when used as a sole source of nutrition or when used in conjunction with maternal milk, in special circumstances donor breast milk has an important role in neonatal intensive care. When maternal milk is not available, it is the milk of choice for establishing very small or sick preterm infants on enteral feeds. Compared with formula-fed preterm infants, those fed on banked milk in the early days post-partum have less vomiting and gastric or intestinal stasis and hence a significantly more rapid transition to full enteral feeding with a correspondingly shorter period on parenteral nutrition. For these reasons, human milk banking should still be encouraged in larger neonatal intensive care units. Nevertheless, the possibility that AIDS may be transmitted via human milk has meant that a greater degree of stringency is required in donor selection and milk banking practice.

REFERENCES
1. Lucas A. AIDS and milk bank closures. *Lancet* 1987; **1**: 1092-1093.
2. Lucas A. Feeding low birthweight infants. In: *Textbook of Neonatology*. Ed: NRC Roberton. Edinburgh: Churchill Livingstone. 1986; pp 204-210.
3 Raiha NCR. Biochemical basis for nutritional management of preterm infants. *Pediatrics* 1974; **53**: 147-152.
4. Gaull G, Sturman JA, Raiha NCR. Development of mammalian sulfur metabolism: Absence of cystathionase in human fetal tissues. *Pediatr Res* 1972; **6**: 538-543.
5. Sturman JA, Rassin D, Gaull GE. Taurine in development: Is it essential in the neonate? *Pediatr Res* 1976; **10**: 415.
6. Fomon ST (Ed). *Infant nutrition*. 2nd Ed. Philadelphia: WB Saunders Co. 1974; pp 161-164.
7. Barlow B, Santulli TV, Heird WC. An experimental study of acute necrotising enterocolitis: The importance of breast milk. *J Pediatr Surg* 1974; **9**: 587-592.
8. Pitt J, Barlow B, Heird WC. Protection against experimental necrotising enterocolitis by maternal milk. 1. Role of milk leukocytes. *Pediatr Res* 1977; **11**: 906-909.
9. Gerrard JW. Breast-feeding. Second thoughts. *Pediatrics* 1974; **54**: 757-769.
10. Narayanan I, Prakash K, Gujral VV. The value of human milk in the prevention of infection in the high risk low birthweight infant. *J Pediatr* 1982; **99**: 496-498..
11. Sack J. Hormones in milk. In: *Human milk, its biological and social value*. Eds. S Firer, Al Eidelman. Amsterdam: Excerpta Medica 1980; pp 56-61.
12. Williamson S, Finucaine E, Elliott J, Gamsu HR. Effect of heat treatment of human milk on absorption of nitrogen, fat, sodium, calcium and phosphorous by preterm infants. *Arch Dis Child* 1978; **53**: 555-563.
13. Lucas A, Lucas PJ, Chavin S, Lyster RLJ, Baum JD. A human milk formula. *Early Hum Dev* 1980; **4**: 15-21.
14. Lucas A. Availability of preterm milk. *Lancet* (S) 1983; **1**: 1045-1046.
15. DHSS. *Report on health and social subjects: The collection and storage of human milk*. London: HMSO, 1981.
16. Lucas A, Lucas PJ, Baum JD. The Nipple Shield Sampling System: A device for measuring the dietary intake of breast fed infants. *Early Hum Dev* 1980; **4/4**: 365-372.

17. Lucas A, Gibbs JD, Baum JD. Human milk banking with drip breast milk. In: *Intensive care of the newborn II.* Ed. L Stern. New York: Masson, 1978; pp 369-379.
18. Evans TJ, Ryley JC, Neale LM. effect of storage and heat on antimicrobial proteins in human milk. *Arch Dis Child* 1978; **53:** 239-241.
19. Baum JD. Raw breast milk for babies in neonatal units. *Lancet* 1979; **2:** 898.
20. Brooke OG, Barley J. Loss of energy during continuous infusions of breastmilk. *Arch Dis Child* 1978; **53:** 344-345.
21. Bates CJ, Liu D-S, Fuller NJ, Lucas A. Susceptibiity of riboflavin and vitamin A in breast milk to photodegradation and its implications for the use of banked breast milk in infant feeding. *Acta Paediat Scand* 1985; **74:** 40-44.
22. Lucas A, Gore SM, Cole TJ, Bamford MF, Dossetor JFB, Barr I, DiCarlo L, Cork S, Lucas PJ, A multicentre trial on the feeding of low birthweight infants: effects of diet on early growth. *Arch Dis Child* 1984; **59:** 722-730.
23. Lucas A. Does diet in preterm infants influence clinical outcome? *Biol Neonate* 1987; **52:** Suppl 1; 141-146.
24. Cooke RWI, Lucas A, Yudkin PLN, Pryse-Davies J. Head circumference as an index of brain weight in the fetus and newborn. *Early Hum Dev* 1977; **1/2:** 145-149.
25. Lucas A. Baker B. Breast milk jaundice in preterm infants. *Arch Dis Childhood* 1986; **61:** 1063-1067.
26. Kliegman RM, Pittard WB, Fanaroff AA. Necrotising enterocolitis in neonates fed human milk *J Pediatr* 1979; **95:** 450-453.
27. Lucas A, McLaughlan P, Coombs RRA. Latent anaphylactic sensation of infants of low birth weight to cow's milk proteins. *Br Med J* 1984; **289:** 1254-1256.
28. Roberton DM, Paganelli R, Dinwiddie R, Levinski RJ. Milk antigen absorption in the neonate. *Arch Dis Child* 1982; **57:** 369-372.
29. Heird WC. Effects of total parenteral alimentation on intestinal function. In: *Gastrointestinal function and neonatal nutrition.* Ed. P. Sunshine. Columbus: Ross Laboratories, 1977; p 16.
30. Kerner JA, Sunshine P. Parenteral alimentation. *Semin Perinatol* 1979; **3:** 417-434.
31. Ziegler JB, Cooper DA, Johnson RD, Gold J. Postnatal transmission of AIDS-associated retrovirus from mother to infant. *Lancet* 1985; **1:** 896-897.
32. Lepage P, Van De Perre P, Carael M, Nsengumuremyi F, Nkurunziza J, Butzler J-P, Sprecher S. Postnatal transmission of HIV from mother to child. *Lancet* 1987; **2:** 400.
33. Thiry L, Sprecher-Goldberger S, Jonckheer T, Levy J, Van de Perre P, Henricvaux P, Cogniaux-le-Clerc J, Clumeck N. Isolation of AIDS virus from cell-free breast milk of three healthy virus carriers. *Lancet* 1985; **2:** 891-892.
34. Vogt MW, Witt DJ, Craven DE, Byington R, Crawford DF, Schooley RT, Hirsch MS. Isolation of HTLV-III/LAV from cervical secretions of women at risk for AIDS. *Lancet* 1986; **1:** 525-527.
35. McClure HM, Keeling ME, Custer P, Marshak RR, Abt DA, Ferrer GF. Erythroleukemia in two infant chimpanzees fed milk from cows naturally infected with bovine C-type virus. *Cancer Res* 1974; **34:** 2745-2757.
36. Hino S, Yamaguchi K, Katamine S, Sugiyama H, Amagasaki T, Kinoshita K, Yoshitta Y, Doi H, Miyamoto T. Mother-to-child transmission of human T-cell leukemia virus type-I. *Jpn J Cancer Res* 1985: **76:** 474-480.
37. Ando Y, Nakano S, Saito K, Shimamoto I, Ichijo M, Toyamo T, Hinuma Y. Transmission of adult T-cell leukemia retrovirus (HTLV-I) from mother to child: comparison of bottle- with breast-fed babies. *Jpn J Cancer Res* 1987; **78:** 322-324.
38. Rogers MF. Breast feeding and HIV infection. *Lancet:* 1987; **2:** 1278.
39. Baumslag N. Breast-feeding and HIV infection. *Lancet* 1987; **2:** 401.
40. Spire G, Dormant D, Barré-Sinoussi F, Montagnier L, Chermann JC. Inactivation of lymphadenopathy-associated virus of heat, gamma rays and ultraviolet light. *Lancet* 1985; **1:** 188-189.

41. McDougal JS, Martin LS, Cort SP, Mozen M, Heldebrant CM, Evatt BL. Thermal inactivation of the acquired immunodeficiency syndrome virus, human T-lymphotropic virus-III/lymphadenopathy-associated virus with special reference to antihemophilic factor. *J Clin Invest* 1985; **76:** 875-877.
42. Wills ME, Han VEM, Harris DA, Baum JD. Short time low temperature pasteurisation of human milk. *Early Human Dev* 1982; **7:** 71-80.
43. Eglin RP, Wilkinson AR. HIV infection and pasteurisation of breast-milk. *Lancet* 1987: **1:** 1093.

Breastfeeding and human milk banks— a midwife's viewpoint

Miss R.J. Wilday

INTRODUCTION

The possibility that human immunodefiency virus (HIV) could be transmitted through breastfeeding or breast milk has been identified. At present the degree of risk has not been determined, but the probability of intrauterine transmission is greater than that of transmission through breast milk. In situations where artificial feeding can be considered safe, known HIV seropositive mothers and those falling into high risk groups are probably best advised to use artificial formulae. However, midwives emphasise the importance of consideration of the circumstances, needs and wishes of mothers as individuals.

BREASTFEEDING—A MIDWIFE'S PERSPECTIVE

In the third report 'Present Day Practice in Infant Feeding', published by the DHSS,[1] the view that breastfeeding provides the most satisfactory form of feeding is reaffirmed, there is disappointment about the extent to which babies in England, Wales and Scotland are being breastfed.

The involvement of partners in the agreement of midwifery care plans is now widely recognised as essential. Much more time, therefore, needs to be spent in ensuring that informed choices are made, although it is recognised that some parents opt out of participation in decision making, being content to accept the advice and care on offer from the professionals available at the time.

The determination of midwifery policies in relation to HIV and AIDS is made extremely difficult by the lack of research. Infant feeding policies are apparently being determined in the absence of the findings of randomised controlled trials.

A questionnaire was distributed to Heads of Midwifery Services in England, Scotland and Wales in January 1988. Sixty-six completed questionnaires out of 80 distributed were returned. Twenty-five percent of the respondents stated that parents were known to have expressed concern about the safety of donor breast milk. This was particularly related to babies in special care baby units. Twenty-nine percent stated that their infant feeding policy had been changed due to an increased awareness of HIV and AIDS. Most of these changes related to the counselling of known HIV positive mothers about the 'risks of breastfeeding'. Advising these mothers to feed their babies with a milk formula in countries where safe, nutritionally adequate artificial milk formulae are available is irresponsible. It could also be argued that any changes in infant feeding policies would be premature, in view of the wide range of professional views expressed to date. In 1987, Alan Lucas wrote that "the evidence that AIDS can be contracted from breast milk is weak, circumstantial and scanty".[2] This view is supported by others who describe two cases of possible post-natal maternal - child transmission of HIV. They admit, however, that although both children had been breast-fed for over twelve months and human milk seemed the most likely source of infection, no attempt was able to be made to isolate HIV from the breast milk of either mother. Indeed, they suggest that "These cases should not discourage mothers from breastfeeding."

The description of a study which reviewed data on the first 83 infants enrolled in the European collaborative study of infants born to HIV positive mothers states that although numbers are too small to make any definitive statement they do add to the impression that the relative contribution of breastfeeding to HIV transmission is probaby small compared with that of intrauterine transmission.[2] A differing view by Hino et al in 1987 is that "refraining from breast feeding by carrier mothers with high titres of human T-cell lymphocyte virus (HTLV-1) antibody is a practical and the only available measure to break the endemic cycle of HTLV-1."[3]

Faced with these apparently conflicting viewpoints, is it any wonder that midwives, together with their medical colleagues, find difficulty in agreeing an infant feeding policy in which they can be confident of a sound scientific basis? Midwives wholeheartedly support the conclusion of the World Health Organisation's (WHO) Consultation on Breastfeeding/Breast milk and HIV Infection,[4] which begins "Breastfeeding should continue to be promoted, supported and protected in both developing and developed countries. The overall immunologic, nutritional, psychosocial and child-spacing benefits of breastfeeding to infants and their mothers continue to be important factors in determining the overall health of mother and child."[4]

From my discussions with midwifery colleagues in England, Scotland and Wales it is evident that the most widely accepted principles are that:—
(a) midwives should participate in defining and agreeing infant feeding policies;
(b) such policies should be based on experience and scientific evidence and reviewed on a regular basis as new evidence becomes available;
(c) agreed policies must be discussed in detail with all prospective parents enabling them to make an informed decision regarding the method of feeding most suitable for their baby;
(d) parents should be fully supported in whatever choice they make.

These principles apply equally to all mothers, not only those known to be HIV positive, in a defined 'high risk group'[5] or those who are highly motivitated and apparently demanding. The report of a WHO consultation on AIDS and the Newborn[6] states, "Where artificial feeding is safe it is preferred for HIV sero-positive women, but any recommendations concerning breastfeeding need to be carefully weighed against other neonatal hazards that may be introduced by abandonment of breastfeeding in an environment where bottlefeeding may not be easily and safely achieved."

In Europe it has been clearly demonstrated that milk formula feeding can be described as widely available and of effective nutritional value, hence the recommendation of the *Present Day Practice in Infant Feeding: Third Report,*[1] ". . . women known to be HIV antibody positive or those at high risk who have not been serologically tested should be discouraged from breastfeeding in the UK".

Midwives, however, have identified the importance of the consideration of each mother's individual circumstances. For example, the newly delivered HIV seropositive mother who is a drug abuser may not be considered able to sterilise feeding equipment or mix artificial formulae safely. She therefore may be more appropriately advised to breastfeed if she wishes to do so. "Only she can know the psychological and practical costs of either breast or artificial feeding in her situation, and there is little point encouraging her to adopt a course that she cannot sustain . . . Research in Africa might well show that some women transfer the antibody without active HIV, or that HIV in milk lymphocytes can immunise but not replicate, and thus breast milk might be therapeutic as well as protective."[7]

Midwives recognise the urgent need for further research into the risks of HIV transmission through breast milk and into the advantages and problems of breastfeeding babies of HIV seropositive mothers.

HUMAN MILK BANKS—A MIDWIFE'S PERSPECTIVE

During 1986, The National Childbirth Trust sent a questionnaire to all their breastfeeding counsellors asking them to report on the operation of milk banks in their areas.[8] The main aims of this informal survey were to assess the extent of milk bank closures in the light of anxiety of HIV contamination and to determine whether hospitals were attempting to ensure the safety of expressed milk by pasteurisation and/or screening of donors.

The findings of this survey, which appears to have covered approximately 60 hospitals, indicate the closure of 10 milk banks due to concern about HIV contamination. The findings also identify 3 needs:

(a) a central register of milk banks.

(b) new DHSS guidelines on the procedure for ensuring the safety of donated breast milk while preserving as far as possible the nutrients and immunological properties.

(c) clarification of where responsibility lies for screening donors.

I would suggest that midwives support the need for a central register of milk banks, but that the term 'milk bank' requires clarification. Some would define the term as the provision of the facility to collect, pasteurise, pool, freeze and store human milk for donation to babies in their own and other hospitals. Others consider that if mothers express milk for storage for their own babies, this also constitutes milk banking. Midwives would appreciate updated guidance from the DHSS relating to the safety of breast milk donation.

In 1987, questionnaires concerning the collection and storage of human milk were sent by the British Paediatric Association (BPA) to the Health Regions in the UK. I find that I am in possession of information from the same Health Regions covered by the BPA survey, but I have no means of determining whether the hospitals responding to both surveys were the same. None of the hospitals included in my survey routinely screened mothers for HIV during pregnancy or prior to milk donation. The lack of knowledge concerning the timing of seroconversion was identified as the reason for not screening mothers.

Seven (11%) of the respondents sought to identify high risk mothers by detailed questioning prior to milk donation. The screening of the expressed milk (EBM) itself for HIV is carried out in only 2 of the hospitals included in the survey.

Sixty-one (92%) of midwife respondents indicate that untreated (raw) EBM is fed to mothers' own babies, but any baby may be fed with raw donor milk in 4 hospitals (6%). Raw milk is used only for specific babies, for example babies with necrotising enterocolitis or following gut surgery in 5 hospitals (8%). In some instances consent is first obtained from parents.

In 16 (24%) of the hospitals EBM is pooled. Expressed breast milk appears to be pasteurised routinely in only 14 (21%) of the hospitals included in the survey. In 2 of the hospitals EBM is boiled.

The practice relating to the collection, treatment and storage of human milk has changed in 28 (42%) of the hospitals included in the survey as a result of increased awareness of HIV. In 19 units (29%) the collection and pooling of human milk has ceased (10 since late 1986). Five units (8%) changed their pasteurisation techniques in 1987 as a result of the Oxford research.[9] Two units have introduced more detailed selection of donors and another 2 are proposing specific screening for HIV prior to donation. Practice and policy in relation to the collection, treatment and storage of human milk is under review in a further 6 units.

In summary, the surveys have highlighted:

(a) regional variation in the use of donated human milk in England, Scotland and Wales;

(b) declining use of donated milk, partly due to a fear of HIV/AIDS and partly due to the development of formulae for babies of low birthweight;

(c) change in pasteurisation techniques;

(d) closure of some milk banks;

(e) need for clarification of the term "milk banks";

(f) need for a central register of milk banks;

(g) urgent need for updated information and guidance in relation to the safe collection, storage and use of human milk.

CONCLUSION

There is need to maintain an awareness of the developments in knowledge in relation to HIV/AIDS in midwifery practice, to implement good breastfeeding techniques and to communicate with and counsel parents about the choices of infant feeding whatever their serological status. It is essential to ensure that donors of EBM have been serologically screened for HIV prior to the donation. The availability of appropriately effective pasteurising machines in human milk banks must be ensured, and written procedures agreed relating to the use of breast pumps and pasteurisers incuding cleaning techniques and methods of quality control. It is important that donor mothers be informed if their personal details are to be stored on a computer.

ACKNOWLEDGEMENTS

I wish to thank my midwifery colleagues, Professor Forfar, President of the British Paediatric Association and the Royal College of Midwives librarian.

REFERENCES

1. DHSS. *Present Day Practice in Infant Feeding: Third Report.* Report on Health and Social Subjects 32. London: HMSO, 1988.
2. Senturia YD, Ades AE, Peckham CS. Breast feeding and HIV infection. *Lancet* 1987; **2:** 400-401.
3. Hino S, Sugiyama H, Doi H, Ishimaru T, Yamabe T, Tsuji Y, Miyamoto T. Breaking the cycle of HTLV-I. Transmission via carrier mothers' milk. *Lancet* 1987; **2:** 158-159.
4. *WHO Special Programme on AIDS statements. Breastfeeding/Breastmilk and Human Immunodeficiency Virus (HIV)* 1987, August; p 2.
5. *Report of the RCOG Sub-committee on problems associated with AIDS in relation to obstetrics and gynaecology.* London: Royal College of Obstetricians and Gynaecologists, 1987.
6. WHO Health for All 2000. *AIDS and The Newborn.* Report on a WHO Consultation. Copenhagen, 1987; April, 6.
7. Minchen M. *AIDS and infant feeding. What are the choices?* 1987.
8. National Childbirth Trust. *Milk banks survey reveals few closures.* Breastfeeding Promotion Group News, New Generation, 1987; p 30.
9. Eglin RP, Wilkinson AR. HIV Infection and pasteurisation of breast milk. *Lancet* 1987; **2:** 1093.

Discussion

Chairman: Mr C. Hudson

HUDSON: Miss Greenwood, are you able to talk to us about the latest information from the Department of Health on the quality of gloves and what is going to be available?

GREENWOOD: I can say that the Technical Division of the Department is looking at the standards of gloves. As Dr Harvey said, the opinion is that cheap disposable gloves, are actually not satisfactory as they split quite often. There is also discussion about goggles versus glasses, and whether we could find some cheap glasses which would probably be the price that Dr Harvey has just mentioned, but there is no immediate information.

MILLS: Could I amend that, because the DHSS has been liaising with me. They have sent out a consultative document and have said that I could talk about it. Essentially it looks at latex examination gloves. The acceptable quality was looked at in various ways. From the point of view of perforations (which I think is what most of us are interested in) the acceptable level is 1.5% which are allowed to have a hole in them. There is a balance between the cost of the gloves and acceptable quality levels. I have looked at costings on the latex disposable gloves of acceptable quality as against the plastic disposable ones, and they are approximately 3 times more expensive. Could I put in a plea that people who have any cuts on their hands should cover them with waterproof plasters. It is a very simple measure and you will find that even in an emergency situation you have some protection on your hands.

MOK: I want to ask Dr Harvey if there were any repercussions from his staff when it was found out that they had been doing exchange transfusions on a baby who was HIV-infected? My contention is that identifying a child as being at risk of HIV infection sometimes leads to detriment of the care of that infant. If they had known this situation before would they have raised the criteria for exchange transfusion?

HARVEY: In reply to your first question, there was a great deal of anxiety on the unit when it occurred. What I did, and what we have seen the senior nursing staff do, is to meet all the staff and discuss the occurrence. I said that the most important thing was the care of the mother, the baby and the family. The panic subsided when we shared the worries that were there, and all the staff wanted to be tested. With regard to the second question about raising the criteria for transfusion—I very much hope not.

MOK: May I just quote from my experience? There was one infant who was identified as high risk only because the father was seropositive. The guidelines in Edinburgh state that a paediatrician should, if at all possible, be called to the delivery. In this case the SHO arrived to find an asphyxiated baby who was flat. The SHO was not allowed to touch the baby because it was not thought that he was a "paediatrician". So they waited for the registrar to arrive while the baby lay there flat because they knew that the baby was high risk.

The other instance was one of twins. The second twin was polycythaemic and actually had a fit in the first 12 hours of life, but did nor receive a plasma transfusion. So I put it to you that sometimes identifying a high risk patient can be detrimental.

HARVEY: I accept that and it makes me very sad, but I think that clearly this is one of the things that the more senior people in a unit have got to recognise and deal with.

MOK: Getting back to the point that has already been raised, can we just have minimum protection that everyone will use for all babies and stop talking about the identification of high risk babies?

HARVEY: I totally agree with that.

STEELE: Following on, may I just ask that some recognition of the financial implications be given. If we put forward recommendations which would be extremely expensive they will rebound and create a great deal of antagonism, particularly among colleagues who are not particularly sensitive to the need for protection in gynaecology. If we are recommending minimal precautions they should be a reasonable minimum and certainly not over the top. Otherwise they will be very difficult to defend. If every expenditure that we ask for is at the expense of something else we all know what that means in the Health Service at the moment.

SPIRO: I should just like to put the mother's point of view. We have been talking about protection of staff, but in one of Dr Harvey's slides we saw a sibling touching the baby. It would be a great pity if we got away from the relaxed special care baby units that we now know, where siblings and relatives can come in and touch the baby. If they are seeing staff gowned up and gloved, they are going to feel uncomfortable and worried.

HARVEY: You will know that I totally agree. As I have said, I do not think that gowns are necessary; I think that we can develop a minimum very simply. I accept the cost factor, but I expect that it is gloves for blood letting procedures to protect against contamination with blood, and glasses where there is likely to be spraying, as well as proper surgical precautions when doing something like a circumcision or putting in an arterial catheter.

SECTION VII

GYNAECOLOGY AND HANDLING OF SPECIMENS

Gynaecological surgery

Miss E. M. Campbell

INTRODUCTION
This paper addresses issues relating to the nursing care of patients with HIV or AIDS in the operating theatre, with particular reference to gynaecological procedures, although the principles can be applied to all surgery.

STATISTICS
The gathering of statistics has been extremely difficult. Of the 3 largest hospitals in Lothian, I can find only 1 which routinely keeps a note of all patients treated as "high risk" in the operating theatre.

There is no regulation requiring collection of this information, so data recorded depend upon local policies. In the 1 hospital where data were available there were 8 cases over a 6-month period, but 4 were gynaecological cases—3 for termination of pregnancy and 1 for sterilisation. The reason that this information is available at all is the result of chance, as the system was set up about 15 years ago to monitor what was then only a very occasional "high risk" case. Perhaps the time has come for all theatres to be more vigilant about the recording of such data and to store the information centrally to allow for adequate planning.

"RISK"
Theatre staff rely almost entirely upon the medical staff to inform them that a patient is in a "high risk" category. In some places, theatre nurses may be able to collect such information personally, or the nursing staff on the ward may warn the theatre staff. Occasionally only the movement of the "high risk" box down the corridor may alert the theatre staff to a potential case. Generally, however, it will be by luck rather than good planning, which seems less than satisfactory.

SCREENING
There seems to be no official view of which patients should be screened before surgery, but rather it is decided on the basis of the patient's history. If the patient refuses a blood test, but the medical staff regard her as a potential risk, she will be treated as such in theatre anyway. This is reasonable of course, as a negative result cannot be regarded as conclusive in these circumstances. So many "high-risk" procedures will be implemented without proven necessity.

In some theatres patients will not always be informed that they are being

293

treated as "high risk" unless they are to be awake during the procedure and may be aware that precautions are being taken. This situation also seems worthy of further study.

Possible evidence to show that minor and non urgent surgery might accelerate the disease process[1] might lend argument to the view that patients should know that they are being tested, in case they wish to decide against surgery.

The "high risk" grouping includes Q fever, Hepatitis B and of course HIV infection and AIDS.

PROCEDURES

It would seem that theatres less involved with such cases have a tendency to dramatise the situation, whereas those more often involved treat precautions as a matter of routine. The danger is that without vigilance complacency may be allowed to develop. The Royal College of Nursing has published the general principles for the management of patients with HIV infection[2] and the National Association of Theatre Nurses is preparing guidelines for theatre staff. The principles of managing such cases involve the reduction in the use of resources to a minimum and the possibility of cross-infection to the lowest realistic level. There are 10 main principles:—

Resources management.

i)	*people*	Staff in theatre should be reduced to a minimum with those inside theatre remaining in and those outside remaining out.
ii)	*skill*	Experienced people should form the team.
iii)	*time*	The team should be familiar with procedures.
iv)	*equipment*	The minimum of furniture and supplies should be retained in the theatre.

Cross-infection

v)	*scheduling*	The case should be placed at the end of the list.
vi)	*protection of theatre staff*	Appropriate disposable clothing should be available and worn correctly. This includes suits and gowns which should be water-repellent, hats, gloves and visor-type masks or goggles in addition to suitable footwear.
vii)	*protection of other staff*	Wound dressings should be impervious to exudate and drainage should be 'closed'.
viii)	*cleaning*	There are well-defined guidelines on cleaning of equipment, walls/floors and spillage with a named chemical disinfectant.[3]
ix)	*disposal*	Methods of dealing with waste material including specimens, sharps and instruments must be clearly defined and all necessary equipment available.
x)	*environment*	The theatre should be left undisturbed after cleaning to allow for the appropriate number of air changes to take place. An hour is thought to be the minimum but the theatre is often left free overnight. The rules will differ for areas which do not have a suitable ventilation system.

The greatest areas of dissent are those relating to chemical disinfection and the period of time for which it is necessary to leave the theatre undisturbed following cleaning. The most recent DHSS recommendations suggest sodium hypochlorite rather than glutaraldhyde. There is also a difference of opinion about the need to leave the theatre free following cleaning, but this issue seems to be more related to dissipation of the smell and irritation of the chemical disinfectant rather than to principles of cross-infection.

Information about the action of the virus continues to change, but there is not an ensuing flexibility of action in relation to "high risk" procedures. Staff generally prefer instructions to be unequivocal and it is often a lengthy process to alter recommendations in the light of new information.

TESTING OF PATIENTS
Surgeons meeting in Atlanta, Georgia have expressed a great concern about the risks of contracting AIDS from patients in theatre.[1] Although there was considerable argument against compulsory testing it seemed that the proposal received a large measure of support. But if testing ever became compulsory for patients in order to protect the staff, at which point would it become compulsory to test staff in order to protect the patient? If, for example, the theatre nurse is stabbed with a scalpel by a surgeon, she will possibly bleed into the patient. If she has HIV/AIDS, the patient will be at risk and not the theatre nurse. If mandatory testing were to be introduced and some theatre staff were found to be infected, what restrictions would be put upon them?

GOOD TECHNIQUE
Greater attention must be paid to good theatre technique as this is the single most effective way of reducing risk. Some aspects of technique, or indeed basic theatre facilities, which have received greater attention recently, include the following:

i)   All staff in theatre who are likely to be handling blood should wear gloves.

ii)   All theatres should have adequate ventilation systems. In older theatres this may be difficult especially if the only way to ventilate the theatre adequately is to open the window.

iii)   Non-touch techniques should be revived where possible and greater care taken when handling instruments.

iv)   Clothing should be reviewed; trousers should have cuffs and consideration given to entirely disposable suits.

v)   Instruments should be washed in an area specially designed, so that the practice of scrubbing dirty instruments with a scrubbing brush is avoided, a certain method of droplet dissemination.

vi)   Staff must be educated to be more careful with sharps. Needle stick injuries are on the increase.

vii)   Staff should not be in theatre if they have cuts or are subject to weeping eczema.

EQUIPMENT
A great deal of attention has been paid to disposables and there has been a plethora of disposable suits and gowns. Companies are now producing disposable

instruments more frequently; in our field a disposable laparoscopic trocar and cannula and a disposable Verres' needle look quite interesting, but of course are expensive.

NURSING CARE

Insensitivity of staff towards HIV positive or AIDS patients is thankfully rare, but not unheard of. The main problem will be one of attitude, specifically those who stand in judgement on patients who have HIV or AIDS. Many of the patients coming to a gynaecological theatre will be having terminations. Some staff already have a degree of difficulty coming to terms with this procedure without the additional consideration of "risk". Some staff judge patients unfavourably on so-called moral grounds, although it could be argued that nursing has no place for such people. Furthermore, such cases often occur at the end of the day when staff are tired; the high-risk procedures are time-consuming and may be seen as a nuisance. Thus attitudes towards an already vulnerable group may be compounded by the presence of the HIV stigma, and there will occasionally be a real problem unless the situation is sensitively handled.

CONCLUSION

Staff who are unfamiliar with the procedures are likely to treat precautions and good technique with varying degrees of attention, and it is not until something happens that they take notice. Although senior medical staff do pay attention to "high risk" procedures and are usually involved in all such cases, this is less often the case with more junior medical staff. They must have the opportunity to learn good technique earlier, and of course regular updating of available information is always necessary. Infection control nurses are uniquely placed to help in this regard.

In theatre, constant attention to good technique is demanded and in Edinburgh it is felt that staff involved have had the opportunity to develop such techniques to a fine art.

REFERENCES
1. Jessop J. Advances in medicine. *Health Service Journal* 1988; 249.
2. Royal College of Nursing. *Guidelines for operating departments.* Second Report of the RCN AIDS Working Party, 1986.
3. Department of Health and Social Security. Acquired immune deficiency syndrome (AIDS); guidance for surgeons, anaesthetists, dentists and their teams in dealing with patients infected with HTLV-III *DHSS Publication CMO* (86)7, 1986.

AIDS and barriers

Dr A. Mills

INTRODUCTION

It is vital to understand the precise mechanisms by which human immuno-deficiency virus (HIV) transmission occurs to enable us to adopt measures to prevent its transmission. Prevention is at the moment the only weapon we have against AIDS. Our understanding of transmission by sexual activity which results in the exchange of body fluids and ways of preventing spread in this way is limited and oversimplistic.

IS THE HETEROSEXUAL POPULATION AT RISK OF CONTRACTING HIV?

The case for both homosexual and heterosexual transmission of HIV is convincing based on cases of sexual partners of infected people developing AIDS,[1,2,3,4] and women artificially inseminated from an infected donor.[5]

By 31st January 1988 only 17 women and 27 men had acquired AIDS by heterosexual spread in the UK. These numbers were small although they obviously represent only a proportion of those who are HIV positive and may well develop AIDS. In Central Africa the male to female ratio of AIDS cases is 1:1. The routes of transmission in Africa are believed to be sexual intercourse, contaminated blood and contaminated needles used for therapeutic purposes. It has also been suggested that sexually transmitted diseases which are common such as chancroid and herpes, cause open genital sores which could facilitate the passage of the virus into the blood stream.[6,7]

Although some of these factors do not apply in the UK there are 2 reasons why we should not be complacent about heterosexual spread of HIV. Firstly, we may follow the United States where the number of cases of AIDS contracted by heterosexual sex doubled in 10 months in 1986 compared with doubling in 14 months among homosexual and bisexual men and intravenous drug users.[8]

The other reason is a difficulty in defining an individual's sexuality. At the moment we neatly define the populations as either homosexual—the group with a higher prevalence of HIV infection; or heterosexual—a group in which the risk appears to be low. It is assumed that HIV is unlikely to spread between these two groups.

At a meeting in December 1987 sponsored by the Kinsey Institute and the National Institute of Allergy and Infections it was claimed that 80% of lesbians have had heterosexual intercourse, 15% of homosexual men have had hetero-sexual intercourse in the previous year and approximately one third of heterosexual men have had one or more homosexual experiences.[9] Another study of homosexual men in San Francisco found that 32% had had heterosexual intercourse in the previous 6 months.[10] These findings may not apply to the population of the UK. It is important to find out, however, to help predict the spread of the disease and direct health messages in an appropriate way.

HOW DO WE PREVENT SEXUAL SPREAD OF HIV?

One option to decrease the spread of the virus is celibacy or a faithful relationship with another uninfected person. Realistically however, the human sex drive is such that these options are often unacceptable and unattainable. An alternative must be to reduce the number of sexual partners. It has been estimated that anyone who has six sexual partners in a lifetime will have indirectly had sexual contact with 56,656 people. This must give a reasonable chance of contracting a sexually transmitted disease.

For HIV positive women it must also be important to use effective contraception to prevent vertical spread of the disease to her children.

For many, the only acceptable option to reduce the risk of infection is to practice "Safer Sex". This often includes the use of the condom.

THE CONDOM

Condoms will only prevent the transfer of semen between partners. Other body fluids from which HIV has been isolated are also transferred during coitus (e.g. saliva, vaginal secretions and blood) or exchanged during orogenital sex or "French Kissing." Other sexually transmitted diseases are known to be con-tracted in this way and whilst theoretically the risk of contracting HIV in this way is small, the case is not proven.[11] Some limited data come from work on chimpanzees with LAV-1. One ml of virus stock containing approximately 10^4 TCID was applied directly to the oral mucosa of a chimpanzee. Nine months later the chimpanzee was uninfected.[12] These data are not adequate to make confident statements about the risks from exchange of saliva during close sexual contact.

Even if we assume that semen and vaginal secretions are the only source of infection during sexual intercourse, we need to look critically at how effective the condom is likely to be. It has been designed to prevent the passage of sperm. Sperm are 30 times greater in diameter than HIV (0.1mm).

Conant and his co-workers[13] tested *in vitro* 3 types of latex condom, 1 of natural lambskin and 1 synthetic skin. Four ml of a solution containing 10^6 "AIDS associated retro virus particles" (ARV-2) per ml were placed inside the condom. This was placed in a syringe and a plunger inserted into the condom 15 times. The side of the condom not in contact with ARV-2 was then placed in culture medium containing mink lung cells. Using various techniques no evidence of passage of viral particles across the condom membrane was detected. These data have been replicated by other workers.[14]

In vitro the condom prevents the passage of HIV provided there are no holes in it. The British Standards Institute allows an acceptable quality level of 0.5% for holes in condoms in continuous production i.e. up to 5/1000 are allowed to have holes. Undoubtedly the stress of intercourse could cause more holes.

We have little data on whether stronger condoms are required for anal intercourse. When 17 homosexual couples tested 5 different brands of condoms they found—depending on the brand used—that between 0% and 22% ruptured and between 0% and 33% slipped off.[15]

When advising the use of condoms for birth control we have to appreciate that there are both method and user failures. It is reasonable to assume a woman is fertile for only 5 days a month i.e. 60 days per year. Despite this, in a highly motivated group of couples in the Oxford/Family Planning Association Study, the failure rate varied between 0.7% and 6% depending on the age of the couple and past experience of using condoms.[16] The National Survey of Family Growth in the US found that between 6% and 22% of couples relying on condoms experienced an unplanned pregnancy within 1 year.[17] It is unrealistic to expect condoms to be 100% effective in preventing the spread of HIV from infected semen when they are not 100% able to prevent the 30 times larger sperm escaping.

Fischl and co-workers in a study on heterosexual partners, children and household contacts of adults with AIDS reported that of 45 partners of adults with AIDS, 32 were HIV negative at the start of the study.[1] They were followed up after a median period of 24 months, ranging from 12 to 36 months. Eight who practiced abstinence remained uninfected. Twelve out of 14 who continued to have sexual intercourse without using a condom seroconverted and 3 out of 10 partners who continued to have sexual intercourse but used condoms seroconverted.[18]

In summary, there is evidence that condoms have the physical properties necessary to prevent transmission of HIV in semen. In use however, they are not 100% effective in this role. The British Standards Institute is revising the standard for condoms, and manufacturers are making efforts to improve condom design. They are the only method of contraception for which there is *in vivo* evidence of helping to reduce the risk of HIV transmission from semen.

FEMALE BARRIER CONTRACEPTION

The physical properties of caps and diaphragms are similar to those of condoms. To be effective in preventing the spread of HIV they would need to prevent the male partner having contact with vaginal secretions and prove an absolute barrier to semen. We need to understand whether the virus infects the female by crossing the vaginal wall or ascending the genital tract. We also need to know whether the virus is attached to sperm or present in sperm coagulum.

The effectiveness of these female barrier methods in inhibiting the transmission of HIV is questionable. Johnson, Masters and Cramer Lewis[19] demonstrated loss of contact between a diaphragm and the sides of the vagina during sexual arousal. Moreover, in chimpanzee studies when LAV-1 strain of HIV was applied to the vaginal mucosa it became infected.[13] Obviously it was not possible to exclude contact of the swab with the cervix, but if the portal entry of HIV is across vaginal mucosa a diaphragm will be ineffective in providing protection. New developments must take these points into consideration. The Margaret Pyke

Institute is undertaking clinical trials into the acceptability of a female condom. This is a rather lax condom which entirely lines the vagina and is held in position by a soft ring which sits on the vulva. It should theoretically provide good protection against infection.

SPERMICIDES

Spermicides such as nonoxynol-9[20] and benzalkonium chloride have been shown to inactivate HIV *in vitro*. We need more information before assuming they will be equally effective *in vivo* and to know whether HIV is carried by sperm. Sperm can enter cervical mucus within 90 seconds of ejaculation, but animal experimental work suggests that nonoxynol-9 does not enter cervical mucus;[21] it may however coat the cervix and form a physical barrier. Is there enough time therefore for these spermicides to inactivate HIV? What dose of spermicidal agent is needed to inactivate HIV? Are spermicides safe for use in the rectum? Will the carrier interfere with the action of nonoxynol-9?

Until we have the answers to these questions we cannot be certain that HIV will be inactivated *in vivo* by spermicides and it is not possible to recommend the use of spermicide alone for reducing the risk of infection with HIV. In view of the *in vitro* data however, some couples may choose to use spermicides in conjunction with condoms. It is important that the spermicide used is not in an organic base which could have a deleterious effect on condom strength.

CONTRACEPTION POST AIDS

The Family Planning Association and National Association of Family Planning Doctors believe that it is important to separate discussion on contraception from advice about using condoms for prophylaxis against HIV.[22] They believe that the risk of contracting HIV during intercourse is best dealt with as a separate issue from the risk of getting pregnant. They recommend that women continue to use their chosen method of birth control, and use the condom as an additional measure to help protect against the possible transmission of HIV. If the chosen method is the condom, then no additional measure need be used.

Family planning clinics are the only source of free condoms to the general public. Family Planning has now become an important source of health education on cytology, smoking, obesity etc. It is important that this is extended to include health education on AIDS. A Mori poll concluded that the public saw family planning clinics as the second most important source of information on AIDS.

CONTRACEPTION FOR HIV POSITIVE WOMEN

HIV positive women should be strongly advised to discuss their HIV status with their sexual partner. Many HIV positive women believe it is important to avoid pregnancy. There are no data as to whether any specific methods of contraception are contraindicated for these women. On theoretical grounds the IUCD is not ideal as it provides no protection against pelvic infection. Condoms should always be used in conjunction with their chosen method.

If both partners are HIV positive it may be reasonable for them to use condoms as well as their chosen method of contraception. This is because of their need to avoid infections from exposure to other sexually transmitted diseases and also because semen may be immunosuppressive.[23,24,25]

CONCLUSION

The interrelationship between HIV and contraception is complex. The only contraceptive method available which has been shown *in vivo* to reduce the spread of HIV is the condom, but this is unlikely to be 100% effective. It is advisable that condoms should have attained the standards laid down by the British Standards Institute. Health Education messages should be adjusted so that they do not overstate the effectiveness of condoms in protecting against HIV.

Doctors and nurses providing family planning services are ideally placed to provide information and guidance to clients who wish to discuss AIDS. They should ensure that their knowledge and understanding of this subject is as full as possible.

ACKNOWLEDGEMENTS

I would like to thank the FPA for all the data supplied. This paper has not been submitted to the FPA medical advisory panel. It therefore represents my personal view unless otherwise stated.

I should like to thank Amanda Lob for her patience in typing this script.

REFERENCES

1. Fischl MA, Dickinson GM, Scott GB, Klimas N, Fletcher MA, Parks W. Evaluation of heterosexual partners, children and household contacts of adults with AIDS. *JAMA* 1987; **257**: 640.
2. Groopman JE, Sarngadharan MA, Salahuddin SZ, Buxbaum R, Huberman MS, Kinniburgh J, Sliski A, McLane MF, Essex M, Gallo RC. Apparent transmission of human-T-cell leukaemia virus type-III to a heterosexual woman with the acquired immunodeficiency syndrome. *Ann Intern Med* 1985; **102**: 63-66.
3. Harris C, Small CB, Klein RS, Friedland GH, Moll B, Emeson EE, Spigland I, Steigbigel WH. Immunodeficiency in female sexual partners of men with the acquired immunodeficiency syndrome. *N Engl J Med* 1983; **308**: 1181-1184.
4. Peterman TA, Rand L, Stoneburner MD, Allen JR, Jaffe HW, Curran JW. Risk of human immunodeficiency virus transmission from heterosexual adults with trans-fusion-associated infections. *JAMA* 1988; **259**: 55-58.
5. Stewart GJ, Tyler JPP, Cunningham AL, Barr JA, Driscoll GL, Gold J, Lamont BJ. Transmission of human T-cell lymphotropic virus type III (HTLV-III) by artificial insemination by donor *Lancet* 1985; **2**: 581-585.
6. Wofsy CB, Cohen JB, Hauer LB, Padian NS, Michaelis BA, Evans LA, Levy JA. Isolation of AIDS-associated retrovirus from genital secretions of women with antibodies to the virus. *Lancet* 1986; **1**: 527-529.
7. Biggar RJ. The AIDS problem in Africa. *Lancet* 1986; **1**: 79-83.
8. Chamberland M, White C, Lifson A, Danders TJ. AIDS in heterosexual contacts, a small but increasing number of cases. Paper presented at the Third International Conference on AIDS, Washington, 1987.
9. Editorial. AIDS and sex. *Lancet* 1988; **1**: 31.
10. Winkelstein W, Samuel M, Padian NS, Wiley JA. Selected practices of San Francisco heterosexual men and the risk of infection by the human immunodeficiency virus. *JAMA* 1987; **257**: 11.
11. Goedert JJ, Biggar RJ, Winn DM, Mann DL, Byar DP, Strong DM, DiGioia RA, Grossman RJ, Sanchez WC, Kase RG, *et al.* Decreased helper T-lymphocytes in homosexual men: sexual practices. *Am J Epidemiol* 1985; **122**: 637-644.
12. Fultz PN, McClure HM, Daugharty H, Brodie A, McGrath CR, Swenson B, Francis DP. Vaginal transmission of human immunodeficiency virus (HIV) to a chimpanzee. *J Infect Dis* 1986; **154**: 896-900.

13. Conant M, Hardy D, Sernatinger J, Spicer D, Levy JA. Condoms prevent transmission of AIDS-associated retroviruses. *JAMA* 1986; **255:** 1706.
14. Eglin RP. Nonoxynol-9 pessaries and condoms prevent transmission of HIV in vitro. *B J Sexual Med;* In press.
15. Wigersma L, Oud R. Safety and acceptability of condoms for use by homosexual men as a prophylactic against transmission of HIV during anogenital sexual intercourse. *Br Med J* 1987; **295:** 94.
16. Glass R, Vessey M, Wiggins P. Use-effectivemess of the condom in a selected family planning clinic population in the United Kingdom. *Contraception* 1974; **10:** 591-598.
17. Grady WR, Hayward MD, Yagi J. Contraceptive failure in the United States: estimates for the 1982 National Survey of Family Planning Growth. *Fam Plann Perspect* 1986; **18:** 200-209.
18. Editorial. Sheaths no barrier. *New Scientist* 1987; **1548:** 12.
19. Johnson V, Masters W, Cramer Lewis K. In: *Manual of family planning and contraceptive practice.* Ed. ML Calderone. Baltimore: Williams and Wilkins, 1974; pp.237-238.
20. Hicks DR, Martin LS, Getchell JP, Heath JL, Francis DP, McDougal JS, Curran JW, Voeller B. Inactivation of HTLV-III/LAV-infected cultures of normal human lymphocytes by nonoxynol-9 in vitro. *Lancet* 1985; **2:** 1422.
21. Sharman D, Chantler E, Dukes M, Hutchinson FG, Elstein M. Comparison of the action of nonosynol-9 and chlorhexidine on sperm. *Fertil Steril* 1986; **45:** 259-264. ·
22. *AIDS (Acquired Immune Deficiency Syndrome) and family planning and well woman services.* Provisional guidelines from the Family Planning Association and the National Association of Family Planning Doctors. London: Family Planning Association, 1987: pp.1-9.
23. Soutter W, Turner MJ, White JO. Effects of human seminal plasma on the lymphocyte response to viral infection. In: *AIDS and obstetrics and gynaecology.* Proceedings of the 19th RCOG Study Group. London: Royal College of Obstetricians and Gynaecologists/Springer-Verlag, 1988. pp.49-57.
24. Alexander NJ, Anderson DJ. Immunology of semen. *Fertil Steril* 1987; **47:** 192-205.
25. James K, Hargreave JR. Immunosuppression by seminal plasma and its possible clinical significance. *Immunology Today* 1984; **5:** 357-363.

Infertility and AIDS

Dr J. P. P. Tyler and Dr J. A. Crittenden

INTRODUCTION

Until April 1985, when a recipient of donor semen presented with symptomless lymphadenopathy at the Westmead Hospital in Sydney, AIDS and infertility were regarded as separate fields in the medical and scientific world. Subsequently 4 out of 8 women receiving semen from an infected donor were found to have antibodies to the human immunodeficiency virus (HIV). This was the first report of HIV transmission within a fertility clinic.[1]

ACQUISITION OF HIV BY DONOR INSEMINATION

This incident provided convincing evidence for transmission of HIV via donor insemination of cryopreserved semen, but it also established several other points. The first of these was that HIV could be transmitted by infected persons who are clinically asymptomatic. Currently there are few data on whether an individual becomes less infectious with the passage of time, but it was noted that women receiving semen donated by the infected donor 2 years after his initial infection failed to seroconvert. Second, there appeared to be no correlation between the number of inseminations with HIV-infected semen and the development of antibodies. Third, of the 4 antibody positive women who received HIV-infected semen none passed the virus on to their husbands who remain antibody negative despite unprotected intercourse. Three of these women, who eventually conceived using semen from other donors, did not pass the virus on to their children despite being exposed to HIV before conception. All 3 children are now over 4 years of age and are antibody negative. Fourth, the 4 antibody positive women did not develop the acute 'mononucleosis-like' syndrome which has been reported following homosexual or blood transmission of HIV. Finally, in each case, the semen was inseminated atraumatically into the posterior fornix from a 0.5ml 'straw' and in each case the cervix was visualised and "erosions" were not seen.

Effects on donor insemination programmes

Until preventive measures could be considered all Donor Insemination clinics in Australia were closed, even though a survey of all semen donors from all 14 clinics in Australia, showed that only 1 donor (out of a total of 1082) had violated the screening procedures used at that time. However, the Fertility Society of Australia later published guidelines for the screening of semen donors, which included a quarantine period of storage in liquid nitrogen for at least a 3-month period following 2 negative HIV antibody tests 3 months apart. This attempted to cover the 'window' period for seroconversion thought to occur in most infected people.[2] The use of fresh semen for use in donor insemination programmes has been banned in Australia. Apart from this single instance the authors are not aware of any other transmission of HIV by any form of infertility treatment.

i)   Effect on recipients
The report of transmission of HIV by donor insemination produced great anxiety amongst past recipients which was subsequently removed by the demonstration of a negative antibody test. The infected women suffered greatly, similar to those infected by blood transfusion, but this was compounded in some by the inability to confide in close friends and relatives from whom they had concealed their involvement with a donor insemination programme. The inadvisability of further pregnancies has also added to the usual burden of HIV carriage. Interestingly none of the infected recipients bears a grudge against the donor who has also suffered greatly.

ii)   Counselling of recipients
Couples awaiting donor insemination need to be reassured that their donor has been reliably screened but, in Australia at least, the current anxiety over HIV seems to emanate more from the professionals in control of programmes than from patients on a waiting list. It is necessary to inform couples that the possibility of HIV infection cannot be totally ruled out, but the risk is very low given the extremely low frequency world-wide of this problem and current screening methods. It is also felt that it is prudent to test with consent all prospective recipients and their husbands for HIV antibodies in order to avoid the problems of pregnancy in an already infected woman (although this may not be so great as was previously thought), and to remove the possibility of false implication of the donor insemination programme in subsequent HIV-related health problems.

iii)   Effect on donor recruitment
The HIV screening programme has further increased the difficulties of providing sufficient donor semen, and consequently increased waiting list times for recipients on programmes. Ill informed publicity and the acronym AIDS has been unfortunate and led, in Australia, to the change of name to Donor Insemination—with no abbreviation. Other components which may have deterred donors appear to be the knowledge that their records will be maintained permanently by clinics, and that being positive for HIV antibodies is notifiable to the Health Department.

iv)   Effect of mandatory use of cryopreserved semen
There is conflicting evidence on the fertilization rate achieved by the use of fresh and frozen semen although in properly controlled trials no differences can be shown.

Effects on the practice of infertility
Proper laboratory and surgical procedures for handling blood, serum and semen which presume all specimens to be potentially infected, do not place the

personnel at high risk. It is when "high tech" procedures such as intrauterine artificial insemination by husband, and *in vitro* fertilisation (IVF) and its related techniques are practiced that problems may arise. Similarly if treatments used to obtain pregnancy are successful and transmit HIV then the resultant child may become infected and emotional and legal liabilities of the fertility clinic are obvious.

An embryo can be created from its genetic parents, be donated, or depend on the provision of donor gametes either as spermatozoa or egg with the parental opposite (Figure I). The use of donor serum in culture media used for the preparation of spermatozoa when antispermatozoal antibodies are present is a further complicating matter. This medium would also be used for embryo growth.

Naturally serum can be screened beforehand, as can donors of eggs or spermatozoa, although more care would be needed with the former since oocytes cannot be successfully cryopreserved. Similarly, the routine heating to 56°C to inactivate compliment is also effective against HIV, and commercial preparations of albumen, sometimes used as a substitute, are now guaranteed free of HIV and Hepatitis B. However, if a couple do not want donor gametes, and one or both of them have antibodies to HIV, the potential for infection occurs at the earliest stages of embryo development. A problem for the future will be couples proven to have antibodies to HIV but who are otherwise healthy and at present condemned to a lifetime of wearing condoms because of the risk of infecting their partner. While surrogacy is generally banned in most countries it is interesting to speculate on its possible use as a means of avoiding potentially infecting the fetus when the genetic mother is HIV positive.

Figure I

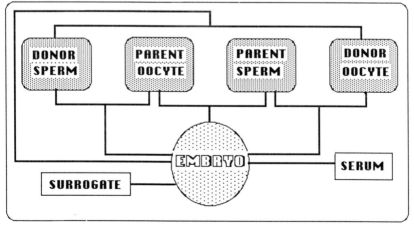

The interrelationships between potential carriers of HIV and the formation of a human embryo.

SEMEN

HIV has been isolated from semen, but only from the mononuclear cell fraction, particularly lymphocytes.[3,4] It has not been conclusively demonstrated that the virus can be incorporated on, or into, spermatozoa as Ho et al[3] could not culture virus from spermatozoa despite attempts on 11 infected individuals. Because of the toxic effects of seminal plasma on target cells used for virus isolation in culture, it has also not been possible to determine whether there is cell-free HIV in the seminal plasma.

In 1987, Ashida and Schofield[5] demonstrated that spermatozoa can bind and penetrate lymphocytes because of HLA-DR structures on lymphocytes and T4-like molecules on spermatozoa. They proposed that HIV might be transmitted by the virus binding to the T4-like receptor on spermatozoal surfaces. These virus-bearing spermatozoa could then bind peripheral blood lymphocytes or macrophages, thereby infecting them. The sharing of antigenic determinants between spermatozoa and lymphoid cells[6] also suggests that HIV may be carried by spermatozoa. Even so it is evident that the route for transmission of seminal HIV has not been clearly established. Since it is apparent that the immunosuppressive factors in seminal plasma may act as co-factors in transmission the first step in preparing samples in reproductive procedures is to remove seminal plasma.

CURRENT RESEARCH

Preparation of "HIV-free" spermatozoa

Preliminary studies have aimed at separating motile spermatozoa from seminal plasma and its other cellular components, before freezing. Since methods for the isolation of white blood cells from blood already exist, and procedures for isolating motile spermatozoa have been developed in IVF programmes, experiments to link the two techniques and provide spermatozoa uncontaminated by other seminal components have been carried out. Confirmation that such isolates are HIV-free will involve contamination and recovery experiments using the Flow Activated Cell Sorter which to date has been shown capable of detecting lymphocyte contamination at a level less than 1%. The development of such a technique and the possibility of freezing such preparations of spermatozoa, would not only markedly reduce the potential risk of virus transmission, but would also offer haemophiliacs infected by blood transfusions the possibility of fathering children. However, current technqiues for freezing whole semen are not directly applicable to seminal plasma-free spermatozoa and more research is needed in this area.

Cryopreservation

Transmission of HIV through donor insemination also established that the virus was able to survive in cryopreserved semen. Among women given semen from the seropositive donor, seroconversion only occurred in the 4 who were given semen stored for 1 to 4 months, and in none of the 4 who were given semen frozen for 16-17 months. It is possible, therefore, that the seminal lymphocytes, and more importantly the virus within them, can only survive for short periods of time when cryopreserved in the glycerol-based medium specifically developed for storage of spermatozoa. In contrast to spermatozoa, leukocytes have a large cytoplasmic to nuclear ratio and DMSO is a more effective cryoprotectant. In the light of this disparity a long term experiment has begun where a semen sample from a 'normal' donor has been contaminated with a known number of lymphocytes and subsequently frozen. It is intended that these samples be thawed after defined periods in order to determine if the glycerol-based cryoprotectant affords protection to leukocytes, particularly T-cells, over long as well as short time periods. Currently 6 months into the trial no difference in lymphocyte numbers has been seen.

Seminal quality in infected men

The quality of semen from asymptomatic HIV-infected men is unknown. Thus studies are being conducted to determine whether:

i)   spermatozoal profiles of HIV-infected men are significantly different from those of healthy males (in terms of spermatozoal counts),

ii)   other non-spermatozoal cellular components (including lymphocyte subsets) differ significantly in HIV-infected men compared with the normal,

iii)   HIV does have an effect on testicular function with time (as reflected in seminal output) and whether it is related to the clinical stage,

iv)   the drugs currently used to treat HIV patients (specifically AZT) interfere with testicular function as reflected in seminal output.

CONCLUSIONS

If the infected heterosexual population continues to increase it is imperative that infertility clinics abide by stringent rules regarding all donor selection and screening, in order to ensure that any sexually transmitted disease, including HIV, is not transmitted. However, preparative techniques for isolating spermatozoa free of seminal plasma and its infective components, and its further quarantine by cryopreservation may provide hope for couples who are asymptomatic carriers of HIV and wish to start a family. Research on the pathophysiology of seminal infection in males must continue.

REFERENCES

1.   Stewart GJ, Tyler JPP, Cunningham AL, Barr JA, Driscoll GL, Gold J, Lamont BJ. Transmission of human T-cell lymphotropic virus type III (HTLV-III) by artificial insemination by donor. *Lancet* 1985; **2**: 581-585.
2.   Fertility Society of Australia Newsletter. Volume 9, March 1987.
3.   Ho DD, Schooley RT, Rota TR, Kaplan JC, Flynn T. HTLV-III in the semen and blood of a healthy homosexual man. *Science* 1984; **226**: 451-453.
4.   Zagury D, Bernard J, Liebowitch J. HTLV-III in cells cultured from semen of two patients with AIDS. *Science* 1985. **226**: 449-456.
5.   Ashida ER, Schofield VL. Lymphocyte major histocompatibility complex-encoded class II structures may act as sperm receptors. *Proc Natl Acad Sci* 1987. **84**: 3395-3399.
6.   Witkin SS. Suppressor T-lymphocytes and cross-reactive sperm antigens in human semen. *AIDS Research* 1984; **1**: 339-345.

Discussion

Chairman: Professor W. Thompson

THOMPSON: The report (see Appendix) and the guidelines which have been published have covered most of the areas that we have mentioned. Some of these perhaps need to be modified in the light of what has happened in the intervening period. We have identified the problems of managing these patients and the question of one-tier and two-tier systems.

JOHNSTONE: May I comment on numbers. I can think of patients that I know personally in the last 6 months: 4 Caesarean sections, 4 evacuations, 1 set of twins, 4 suction terminations, 2 laparoscopic sterilisations. You suggest examples of insensitivity to patients and prejudice in the theatre. I think that the nurses who have been looking after these patients have not been displaying the attitudes that you have attributed to them. I think that we should be very careful before being critical of those who are doing the very best they can, often in quite difficult situations.

CAMPBELL: I take your point completely. The statistics are based on data supplied by theatre staff. I am not talking about the number of patients actually with HIV; I am talking about the ones that they knew to be "high risk". But I take your point that we do need to be much more specific about what we are saying.

In relation to sensitivity, I stand by my comments. They are based on my own experiences as well as those of other people who I feel are well qualified to speak. Senior people are much more aware of the problem because they know now what they are dealing with.

THOMPSON: We are talking about two different things. We are talking about high risk cases where you have experienced staff. But there is going to be the occasional case coming through in low risk areas.

JOHNSTONE: Nursing staff, particularly midwifery staff, have had to do a lot with high risk patients. I think that they have done it excellently.

CAMPBELL: I stand corrected for the sweeping statement.

SCRIMGEOUR: Surely we should know how many high risk patients are going through theatres. The fact is that Miss Campbell could not find this evidence in the theatres where she asked for the information.

THOMPSON: There is a lack of firm data. There is no mechanism for recording it as far as I know. As soon as central recording is started confidentiality is broken. Of course, the DHSS would want to get involved in that.

SCRIMGEOUR: We have a good case for quoting the figures from the hospital where I work. They can be recorded here.

McQUEEN: One aspect that did worry me was leaving the theatre for an hour after an HIV positive patient in order to clean it. I think that this is quite unnecessary. It irritates the surgeons because of the long wait. If we really think that HIV is airborne I suggest that the air changes in the theatre should be increased. The other issue is the labelling of specimens or notes. HIV is not the only worry; MRSA is an increasing worry especially in London. Why can we not put "infection risk" or "please inform the infection control team" on the records? When it comes to blood spillage, using glutaraldehyde on blood spillage does make it very gelatinous and if you soak certain instruments in glutaraldehyde it is very difficult to clean them afterwards. My suggestion is that spillages be cleaned up and then the surface treated afterwards either with glutaraldehyde or a hypochlorite solution. When it comes to anaesthetic equipment there was a question about whether it was necessary to clean the laparoscopes between patients. I think that we should do this between all patients, not just the high risk or HIV positive ones. This is where we really need to tighten up our infection control procedures.

JEFFRIES: The British Society for Gastroenterology has done a survey of endoscopy nurses and about 30% are hypersensitive to glutaraldehyde. I think that it is not a disinfectant to leave to evaporate in the air. In that situation if one needs to use a liquid disinfectant it should be hypochlorite.

One other point which I wish to raise is the question of whether surgery enhances the effects of HIV. In other words does surgery precipitate active disease in HIV positive patients? That is a question which we very much wanted to answer at the meeting on AIDS and surgery in London last November. We thought that one of the ways that we could get close to an answer was to bring surgeons out from other parts of the world who had a great deal of experience of surgery on HIV positive individuals. The best we could get was a surgeon from the Bronx who very commendably had been doing open heart surgery on HIV positive patients. From memory, it involved 20-24 cases and there was in that situation evidence of a stormy postoperative period in terms of bacterial infections. It is only a small series, but covers very major surgery. For minor and intermediate surgery; I know of no data suggesting that HIV and surgery together leads to a precipitation of HIV-related disease. It can often be used as an excuse for people not operating. I have evidence of that.

THOMPSON: One wonders whether the indications for operation were correct if when they discover a patient is HIV positive they suddenly decide not to operate.

SCHOENBAUM: We have epidemiological and population-based studies that have shown no transmission from casual contact and other studies that have shown no transmission to people who are working in the San Francisco AIDS wards who do not have other risk factors. There has been discussion about trying to ascertain how the HIV positive people come through surgery. Given the amount of fear and elaborate precautionary measures that have been suggested including surreptitious testing of patients, there is a need for a study similar to the one that was done among dentists to be done among surgeons who are operating in high risk areas. This would provide data and help us to understand what the risk is in the operating room.

THOMPSON: Could we now move on the discussion to the area of family planning.

GREEN: With regard to the issue of condoms and dual contraception, we have always advised our HIV patients to use dual contraception, usually a condom plus another contraceptive method. What worries me is that a great deal of material, including the Government's health education campaign and indeed the RCOG Sub-Committee report does not mention another method of contraception. The average heterosexual woman starting out in a relationship will want to use a condom, but at some point she will probably want to give it up, either because she is going to get pregnant or she will just want to give it up as the relationship develops. That issue is not being addressed. It is never stated how long you have to be in a relationship before you can not use a condom.

MILLS: I have no more information than anybody else on that. I think that it is going to depend on the woman and whether she feels that it is a permanent relationship, how she feels that this will affect her partner, what her partner feels about it. It is a very complex issue and it is really up to the individuals, rather than the woman and her doctor. Every method of birth control has a failure rate and at the Family Planning Association we try to be very fair in saying what that failure rate is. It is then up to the couple to decide how acceptable that failure rate is to them. They can then find the condom which suits them. It has been shown that with different groups different condoms have different effectiveness depending on age and experience. I would not be very happy to say that condoms provide absolute contraception. They have failure rates the same as any other method.

JEFFRIES: One gets many enquiries about the use of spermicidal cream, and I agree that it would inactivate the virus *in vitro*. It is very difficult to assess the dynamics of infection *in vivo*. We know that a latex condom is affected by a spermicide, but you were worried about its effect on the rectum. Do we really know what it is doing to the vaginal epithelium or to the cervix. In other words, if used in combination with a condom could it, in fact, make the genital tract wall permeable if the condom failed? What is its effect on normal genital tract epithelium?

MILLS: We have got some answers to the reaction of the vagina. It might unfortunately increase the permeability of the vagina, and that is a new question.

JEFFRIES: It is a worry in my mind that it might just make matters worse rather than better.

MILLS: I do not think that anyone has looked at the permeability of the vagina.

HOWIE: How good is a condom at protecting a female who is having sexual intercourse with an HIV positive subject? You mentioned that 3 out of 10 sero-convert. You cannot rely on its protecting all those individuals. Method failure may be an explanation for at least some of these failures. The question at the other end of the equation is that if a woman says, "If I use a condom all the time, and provided that I am extremely conscientious about it, what sort of reliability can I expect if I do not allow method failures to occur?"

MILLS: We have conflicting data on that.

HOWIE: If you look at a group of women who are using condoms, a proportion will seroconvert despite apparent use of condoms. Some of the explanation will be user failure. What I am asking is that if an individual comes to the clinic and says, "If I reliably use a condom all the time, will I seroconvert irrespective of that? Will the condom give me a high degree of protection?"

MILLS: I cannot give you an answer because in the particular study we did not actually comment on the problem of the condom bursting or slipping off, and obviously these are important data. One of the 3 women was also involved in having oral sex and we do not know if that was a factor. If we are looking at the population as a whole this is a highly motivated population which uses condoms very effectively. I find it very worrying that despite the fact that they were highly motivitated 3 out of 10 seroconverted. Not many other people are going to have quite such a high degree of motivitation because they are not going to know if their partner is HIV positive. I should very much like to say that if they use it all the time, if it does not burst, if it does not slip off then it will give 100% protection. If you look at the experimental work that would be a reasonable assumption, but if you look at the way people use condoms, they are unfortunately not that effective.

THOMPSON: Perhaps I could summarise the differences in policy regarding infertility practice that we have adopted here in the UK as opposed to Australia. For example, we do not have a mandatory policy for the screening of donors. A recent survey carried out by this College showed that 100% of donors are screened. You do not have the same difficulty asking donors whether they are homosexuals. We have got round that in a sense by giving them a leaflet. They read it and then sign a consent form stating that they have read the leaflet and that they do not belong to a high risk group. We have had no adverse response to that. As far as the quarantine figures for semen are concerned, my latest figures are up to 80%. However, the introduction of classes of semen has presented many problems in this country where semen, believe it or or not, is a very scarce commodity. The result is that we have lost 3 or 4 clinics in the past year because of the quarantine policy.

TYLER: Most of the clinics, in fact, screen regularly and routinely screen the recipient in the IV programme before they receive any donated semen.

THOMPSON: There is also the question of whether any donated material including embryos and eggs should be carefully screened for HIV before they are used. They seem to have been left out of this programme.

HARE: I feel that your policy of offering a leaflet to your donors is very unlikely to identify the high risk group. For example, I recently had a discussion with a genito-urinary physician about a patient of his who was a monogamous, faithful husband for 51 weeks of the year. But once a year he went on a homosexual "bender". That kind of person is not going to recognise himself in the leaflet. He is going to identify himself as heterosexual and monogamous. I think that questioning by a skilled person who knows how to put the questions in such a way as to get positive answers is the only solution to this.

THOMPSON: It would be interesting to discuss laser treatment.

SHARP: A few years ago we held a Study Group in the College which addressed the question of gynaecological laser surgery. Within the recommendations from that Study Group was the positive recommendation that appropriate scavenging systems with effective and appropriate filters should be used in all gynaecological laser surgery using the CO_2 laser. Laser smoke is toxic when it gets out. This is now becoming such a large part of gynaecological practice that there are health care personnel at all levels who conceivably could be exposed to this smoke in the long term.

Originally some of the studies looking for viable material in what our North American colleagues euphemistically call the "plume" suggested that there was possibly some viral DNA floating around. The better scavenging apparatus available now has focussed on the possibility and we are down to less than a micron pore size in filters. Some of these machines will recirculate the air back into the room. I think that when you are working on the vagina or on the cervix with a laser with the currently available specula it is a very efficient way of removing the smoke. A more important situation is when you are using the laser on the open exposed skin of the vulva. There may be an amount of splattering, in which case the use of a mask is essential just to catch the larger bits of charred tissue which come off. Also, in that particular situation we need a very efficient sucker effectively to collect the smoke.

McMANUS: When we are involved in the long term care of HIV positive patients what we look for are other infections which we try to treat promptly. We have also had about 20 people who are HIV positive and they all had abnormal smears. These are immunocompromised women. As such it has been long understood that HIV will be found more readily in that group as will CIN, presumably by reason of their immune system.

Counselling on safer sex

Miss M. McElwee

INTRODUCTION

The advent of HIV and AIDS has made us face topics that were regarded as taboo and is making us re-evaluate centuries of sexual and social conditioning. Therefore the challenge of AIDS is not only medical but also personal and professional.

THE ISSUES

The issues surrounding safer sex are contentious, not least because they challenge our preconceptions about what "real" sex should be. Before AIDS, the commonly held view was that real sex meant penetration, be it for pleasure or procreation, the only difference being was that for the former a condom was an optional extra! Now, in the face of AIDS, we are being told that a condom is no longer an optional extra, but a necessity. The concept of safer sex undermines this belief and offers opportunities for pleasurable and meaningful sex, without penetration.

AIDS is not shutting doors to sex, but opening new ones, encouraging exploration in areas that were previously just considered the realms of foreplay. Before, foreplay was an overture to the main event. Now, with imagination and thought, it can be the main event in its own right.

COUNSELLING ON SAFER SEX

The main aim of counselling should be the dissemination of information on the practical aspects of safer sex, and to distinguish those activities which constitute high and low risk. A second, but equally important aim, should be to allow the clients space and time to explore the wider implications of what safer sex may have for them.

In the light of the AIDS crisis, counselling has acquired an aura of mystique. We all have some ability to counsel, given the right conditions, and these latent skills can be improved and extended. Counsellors should try to avoid, or at least be aware of, the social conditioning that we all carry, and how that might allow for value judgements to be made. These factors may include age, gender, culture and religion, but permeating all of these is the force of how we view sex and sexuality. If our perceived notions of sexuality are carried into the counselling session, then so are our notions on age. Sex is often seen as the prerogative of those aged

315

between 20 and 40. To have sexual feelings at 16 or 60 is seen as immoral in the former, and disgusting in the latter. Clear instruction on safer sex might be overlooked if one was not prepared to deal with an "amorous adolescent" or a "passionate pensioner".

Culture and religion may be less of a barrier if they are common to both counsellor and client, but problems may arise if they vary, especially if the culture is completely unfamiliar. As far as counselling goes, we have to establish what role sex already plays in that culture. Once that has been done, a counsellor will be more able to assess how safer sex can be tailored to meet the demands of their culture and religion, without undermining their belief system. It might be that a client is subject to 2 conflicting cultures and is unable to work out where he, and his sex life, fits into either of them.

All of these factors need to be recognised when counselling for safer sex and gynaecologists may well be more accessible to this patient group than other sources of information. As women tend to be rather reluctant about visiting STD clinics, they may feel more comfortable asking about safer sex in the context of a gynaecological or obstetric setting. Some gynaecologists and midwives may feel they are ill equipped to cope with the extra professional and personal pressures that counselling on safer sex and AIDS in general will undoubtedly cause. To combat this, gynaecologists and midwives should have recourse to support systems. Without them, they may feel isolated and as unprepared for AIDS and safer sex counselling as their patients.

Preconceptional counselling

Mr S. J. Steele

AIDS was not a significant problem in 1980 when Chamberlain described a pre-pregnancy clinic.[1] Now there is widespread public awareness of the disease, and inevitably young couples, spouses and partners will worry about the possibility of infection and the risk to any child they may have. The responsibilities of parenthood are not always accepted and there are still too many unplanned and even unwanted children, but many couples thinking of parenthood and aware of infection or the risk of it will wish to act responsibly and to acquire the information to enable them to do so.

Preconceptional counselling in relation to AIDS and human immunodeficiency virus (HIV) might cover the following. At present, health education relating to AIDS does not include reference to pregnancy, though the advocacy of condoms by implication excludes it. Women or couples may be motivated to seek counselling through anxiety or primarily as a means of obtaining a test to exclude infection. Alternatively, they may be advised to seek preconceptional counselling by professional advisers or counsellors. Counselling in relation to AIDS generally may also include preconceptional counselling where individuals or couples wish it; this raises the question of who should provide counselling.

Women in the high risk groups considering pregnancy should logically be tested then (and retested after an interval) if they wish to know the risk to which they and any child born to them might be exposed. Counselling would follow according to the result. Those women who are known to be infected can be counselled taking relevant account of whether they have had a child or not, and if so, whether any child is, or was HIV positive.

TESTING

The consensus view is that the patient must give informed consent for testing, and this presents no especial problem in the context of preconceptional counselling. The information which patients and we, their advisers need, is not yet fully available, and is unlikely to be so for some time. Meanwhile, to fail to encourage those who may be at risk to be tested, and to face up to the implications of unprotected sexual activity, must surely be irresponsible.

If patients who have no risk factor enquire about testing they may either go ahead or accept reassurance that the risk is low. There are, however, women known to be HIV positive where the means or source of infection is unknown, and furthermore, a woman may be unaware of a risk factor relevant to her partner or vice versa.

Preconceptional counselling may be sought primarily because of fear, justified or unjustified, of AIDS. It may be urged on women or couples when infection is diagnosed or the risk identified by professionals working in other areas of medicine e.g. genito-urinary medicine. Finally, it is logical at least to exclude high risk factors for HIV infection where people seek general preconceptional counselling simply as a prudent measure before contemplating pregnancy against a background of other disease or potential complication. Some of those seeking advice in relation to HIV will have other medical or social problems which are highly relevant to pregnancy and the future of any child born as a result. Drug abuse is an example both for its high risk relevance to AIDS and for its own implications for pregnancy and the subsequent health and welfare of parents and children.

Since counselling is not just about AIDS or HIV infection but may include related disorders (for example, hepatitis, drug abuse and drug therapy) medical knowledge must be reasonably broad and must include some expertise in obstetrics.

There is no doubt that obstetricians do not as yet have much experience of seeing or treating people suffering from the effects of HIV. Rather than set up special clinics which may be intimidating as well as expensive it would be better to train staff, including midwives and health visitors, who may be faced with the necessity of providing counselling. Furthermore, the consequences of infection with HIV must not be treated as an isolated problem. Those in need of expert counselling can be referred on appropriately, if this is required, after preliminary discussion and perhaps testing.

INFORMATION REQUIRED ABOUT INFECTION TO ENABLE SOMEONE TO MAKE AN INFORMED DECISION

1. The risk of HIV infection, either lately or subsequently, if the woman is HIV negative.
2. The risk of coitus resulting in infection.
3. The risk of pregnancy to the mother's health.
4. The risk of infection of the fetus and of the baby developing AIDS; and the reliability of tests.

In addition to the medical information individuals should be encouraged to consider other implications:

1. Mother and baby may be subject to special precautions while in hospital, which can cause considerable distress if not anticipated.
2. Adopting and fostering may be difficult particularly if the child is HIV positive and there may also be implications for school and other activities given the unsympathetic and fearful reactions which this infection can provoke.
3. The possible consequences of being HIV positive for a woman: loss of partner; loss of opportunity to become a parent; decreased chance of further relationship and marriage; uncertainty about prognosis, treatment, vaccine prophylaxis and any prospect of cure in the future.
4. A special consideration is the desire of some lesbians to have children and the risk that a few may run in resorting to "do it yourself" donor insemination.

Figure I

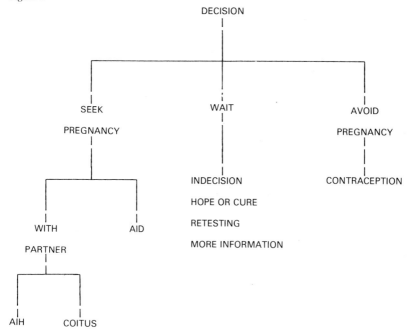

THE DECISION

The couple has three choices: seek pregnancy; wait i.e. not to make a final decision; or to avoid pregnancy.

It is salutary to remember that in adversity some people see pregnancy as an achievement. This is a factor in the face of unemployment, deprivation and similar situations and the concept may appeal to some who are HIV positive; the consolation and company of a child seem to the parent or parents to outweigh the risks and disadvantages so obvious to others, particularly those who view the prospect as totally without hope. The possible implications of the decision are shown in the flow diagram in Figure I. They may imply further counselling about infection, AIDS, further testing, treatment to aid conception and many other issues. Any advice on such matters as contraception and artificial insemination must be authoritative, practical and clear.

REFERENCES
1. Chamberlain GVP. The pregnancy clinic. *Br Med J* 1980 **281**: 29-30.

Discussion

Chairman: Mr C. Hudson

McMANUS: May I ask Miss McElwee how she suggests that we should train our young doctors so that they will be able and competent to talk about safer sex. I find that talking about safer sex with gay men is easy; talking about it to heterosexual people is very difficult.

McELWEE: I have a way of doing training which is quite different to the lecture type of scenario. The thing that you have to do first is to acknowledge that we have our own personal feelings and difficulties with sex. If a safe enough environment can be built up, when it is felt that the environment is confidential and safe and when our own value judgements are passed on as people about how we feel, then we may get to a place where we are aware that sex is difficult and start to work on why it is difficult for us and be aware of that so that we are not in a position where the worst possible impression is given to the patient.

HUDSON: When do you think this training should begin?

McELWEE: As soon as they enter medical school, because it is one of life's skills.

McMANUS: Do you think that doctors are well equipped?

McELWEE: I do not think that any of us do it that well.

HUDSON: You did not specifically address the particular problems of haemophiliacs who may have acquired their HIV infection at a young age and their later problems of contraception. Do you have any specific thoughts about them as a group?

STEELE: It is very difficult to say, I think that we have to look at each case on its individual merits.

SCRIMGEOUR: May I take up the point of teaching successors as professionals. Do either of the speakers, or anyone here have one of the junior medical staff or medical students or nursing staff with them when they counsel? That is the way to teach them.

McELWEE: When I worked at the clinic, with patients' permission we did have students in for observation during interviews. But that does break up the relationship.

STEELE: The tendency that doctors have to usher the student out when they see a difficult consultation coming should be the other way round. That is precisely when they should be there.

321

CONCLUSIONS

Conclusions

EPIDEMIOLOGICAL STUDIES:

1. There is an urgent need for carefully designed epidemiological studies to determine the prevalence of HIV and the patterns of spread within the population.
   In Europe there is an increasing prevalence of HIV among injecting drug users. There is a need to know whether infection has spread heterosexually to women outside this group.

2. The pregnant population is a suitable group for epidemiological studies because they are a representative sample of the female population in the "at risk" age group.

3. Difficult issues arise in relation to the strategy of antenatal population screening. The most controversial of these is the question of testing with or without informed consent.
   It was unanimously agreed that individually attributable testing without consent was unacceptable. It was also agreed that population screening with consent, whether individually attributable or not, was acceptable.
   Because population screening with consent might be unrepresentative, a considerable body of opinion was supportive of blind, non-attributable testing of historical blood samples without specific consent. There was, however, no consensus on this point. The Study Group recommends that the Royal College of Obstetricians and Gynaecologists and other professional organisations re-examine their previous stance on this issue.

CASE FINDING FOR CLINICAL MANAGEMENT

4. There is an established need to offer HIV testing to pregnant women in identified "high risk" groups so that mothers and their babies can be given appropriate treatment with counselling for the family. Early recognition of the child at risk is of great importance to optimum management, and may improve prognosis.

5. In areas with a high known prevalence of the disease in the general population, universal individually attributable antenatal testing should now be made available. In order to assess the need for universal screening, low risk areas also should consider periodic sampling of their populations.

NATURAL HISTORY

6. Existing literature on the immune effects of pregnancy in infectious diseases provided a theoretical basis for concern that pregnancy may adversely affect

progression of HIV-related disease. There is presently no conclusive evidence that pregnancy has an adverse effect on the natural history of HIV infection. Studies to clarify these issues are required.

7. The present WHO criteria for case definition designed specifically for countries with limited access to laboratory facilities are not good predictors or discriminators of children with AIDS.

8. In view of the lack of data on perinatal transmission of HIV, there is an urgent need for prospective studies to:
   (i)   define the risk of HIV transmission from mother to child;
   (ii) identify factors which might affect this risk;
   (iii) gain knowledge about the natural history of paediatric HIV disease.

9. Diagnosis of HIV infection in the newborn infant is difficult because of passive transfer of maternal antibody which may persist up to 18 months of age.

10. Diagnosis of infection in the child less than 18 months of age can be made by: positive HIV culture; positive p24 antigen; development of a new antibody or increasing titres of existing antibody; development of clinical symptoms.

11. Preliminary data from prospective studies suggest that about 25% of infants born to HIV-infected women are infected with the virus.

OBSTETRIC AND MIDWIFERY MANAGEMENT

12. In all situations the patient's best interest is paramount.

13. Although the transmission risk to staff is very small, there should be no reasonably avoidable contact with blood.

14. At present, the two-tier hygienic measures indicated in the Sub-Committee Report remain adequate for the UK. The Study Group recognises, however, that in some areas one-tier safety precautions may eventually become necessary, as is currrently the case in some overseas centres.

15. There is an outstanding need for continuing education of medical and midwifery staff both in the standards of clinical hygiene in the delivery suite and elsewhere, and in the development of counselling skills and a sensitive attitude to consumer concerns in all risk categories.

16. Techniques and items of resuscitation equipment were reviewed, many of which where unsatisfactory, and some downright dangerous. Resuscitation devices should only be employed by those with appropriate training. Further research and development in this area is required.

NEONATAL PROBLEMS

17. The absolute priority is the highest possible level of care to the newborn. The standard and availability of care should in no way be influenced by the HIV status of the mother or infant.

18. There should be a single tier of infection control measures for all newborn.

19. To limit the risk of transmission, a minimum standard of staff protection is thus needed for resuscitation and invasive procedures, ie, latex gloves, spectacles and mask. Detailed procedures for various aspects of general, special and intensive care as given in the Royal College of Obstetricians and

Gynaecologists' Sub-Committee Report should be revised to encompass the routine care of all neonates.

20. Each neonatal unit should conduct detailed, regular and reviewable consultations within the unit and with others, such as obstetric, midwifery and laboratory staff, and those who work in the community to develop working protocols.

21. In developed countries it may be wise to advise against breastfeeding by high risk mothers, at least until more is known about the infectivity of the breast milk of HIV positive women. In developing countries, against the background that vertical transmission may have already occurred, the over-riding concern should be to promote breastfeeding because of the risk of intestinal infection.

22. "Donated human milk is associated with a theoretical risk of HIV infection to infants receiving milk, either as individually donated samples, or from human milk banks. The general use of donated human milk for pre-term infant feeding is debatable. Certainly, for a small number of extremely immature babies, human milk is valuable especially when the baby is being weaned off parenteral nutrition. Infants recovering from necrotising entercolitis and other neonatal bowel disorders also benefit from donated human milk.

    Specific steps should now . . . be taken to safeguard babies from the accidental transmission of HIV in donated human milk . . .

    (i)   Mothers selected for milk donation should answer a questionnaire to exclude those at high risk of HIV infection.

    (ii) Donors should also be known to be HIV antibody negative.

    (iii) Heat treatment of milk by the Holder method is essential to safe-guard against HIV infectivity (except in the situation described below). Proper practices in pasteurisation are very important.

    (iv) Human milk banks should maintain records about the donors and the recipients of milk.

    (v) Wetnursing by any mother, whatever her risk status, should be discouraged.

    If, in exceptional circumstances, a clinician wishes to give unpasteurised donated human milk, adoption of the following procedure is acceptable. Milk intended for raw consumption should come only from mothers who are at low risk for HIV infection and who are prepared to be subjected to re-peated serotesting. After an initial negative test for HIV antibody, the unpooled donated milk should be frozen and stored for three months. After that time the mother should be retested for HIV antibody and if the test is negative, the milk she gave three months before may be used. The mother should continue to be HIV serotested monthly while she donates milk."[1]

COUNSELLING: CONSUMER CONCERNS

23. Clear, consistent and confidential counselling is of the utmost importance.

24. The data on consumer concerns illustrate a clear need for continuing education.

LEGAL TERMINATION

25. The data on progression of maternal HIV do not support the concept of a significant risk of enhanced progression during pregnancy. The advice regarding the place of legal termination contained in the Royal College of Obstetricians and Gynaecologists' Sub-Committee Report should stand unaltered.

GYNAECOLOGICAL SURGERY

26. Although two-tier precautions in operating suites remain in use, the lack of precision in pre-operative HIV diagnosis means that the level of safe practice in handling patients generally should be elevated. The use of spectacles by all personnel in close contact with surgery is recommended, and meticulous care in the containment and handling of blood spills is required. Glutaraldehyde is not recommended for blood spills, and the DHSS Guidelines[2] on sterilisation procedures are commended. It is essential that good communication be maintained between clinicians and operating suite staff.

27. Gynaecological outpatient practice encompasses not only pelvic examination, but invasive procedures such as those used in infertility and family planning clinics.

28. Disposable plastic gloves at present in wide use are totally inadequate and should be replaced by latex gloves of adequate strength. Both hands must be gloved prior to gynaecological procedures if adequate protection is expected, and staff must be advised to adhere to these practices.

29. Donor insemination has been shown to be associated with HIV transmission. It is advised that all donors of gametes should be carefully counselled to exclude high risk groups, and should have HIV tests at regular intervals. Quarantined stored semen offers the best treatment option.

30. The smoke generated by CO_2 laser vapourisation treatment of lesions in the lower genital tract has been recognised generally as potentially hazardous for the health care personnel; this *may* contain viral material of uncertain infectivity.

SAFER SEX EDUCATION

31. An important preventive health care measure is to reduce the spread of HIV by sexual contact. Condoms may reduce the risk of transmission of HIV from infected semen or vaginal secretions. Data indicate that this protection cannot be guaranteed. A couple's choice of contraception should be considered as a separate issue from their need to reduce the risk of contracting HIV.

32. Safer sex education is perhaps the most important long term measure discussed at this Study Group. It is very important that all health professionals receive early education about safer sex to allow them to advise their patients.

PRECONCEPTIONAL COUNSELLING FOR HIV POSITIVE INDIVIDUALS

33. Preconceptional counselling should take place in ordinary preconceptional clinics rather than genito-urinary medicine clinics. The long term prognosis of asymptomatic individuals is sufficiently uncertain that a cautious attitude to preconceptional counselling is required. Of particular importance is discussion of the long term effects on the family unit.

REFERENCES
1. Anon. HIV infection, breastfeeding and human milk banking. *DHSS Publication PL/CMO(88)13, PL/CNO(88)/7*, 1988. London: DHSS, 1988.
2. Anon. Decontamination of Equipment, Linen or Other Surfaces Contaminated with Hepatitis B or Human Immunodeficiency Virus. *DHSS Publication HN(87)1*. DHSS, 1987.

APPENDIX

Report of the RCOG Sub-Committee on problems associated with AIDS in relation to obstetrics and gynaecology

Published by the Royal College of Obstetricians and Gynaecologists, London, October 1987

Membership of the Sub-Committee:

Mr C. N. Hudson Chairman	Royal College of Obstetricians and Gynaecologists
Dr D. Jeffries	Clinical Virologist invited by the Royal College of Obstetricians and Gynaecologists
Ms E. McAnulty	nominated by the Royal College of Midwives
Professor W. Thompson	Royal College of Obstetricians and Gynaecologists
Professor C. B. S. Wood	nominated by the British Paediatric Association including the British Association of Perinatal Medicine
Miss C. E. Beech	Secretary

The co-opted membership included official representation from the Family Planning Association and National Association of Family Planning Doctors (Dr A. Mills) and the Royal College of Nursing (Paediatric Forum) (Ms S. McQueen).

The views of anaesthetists were sought by co-opting Dr David Zideman, who also communicated opinions on behalf of the Resuscitation Council.

Professor C. Peckham was co-opted personally as Clinical Epidemiologist.

Dr R. G. Penn from the DHSS attended as an observer. Additional assistance was received from Dr J. Davies (Public Health Laboratory Service), and Dr T. McManus (Consultant in Genito-Urinary Medicine).

CONTENTS

Membership of the Sub-Committee

Terms of Reference

TERMS OF REFERENCE

To consider and advise on the impact of AIDS and AIDS-related conditions on obstetrics, gynaecology, neonatal infant care and family planning; to produce guidelines for management in clinical practice.

This Report has not addressed the philosophical issues involved, and does not represent the views of the College or sponsoring bodies on such issues.

1. INTRODUCTION

1.1 This report, prepared by a multidisciplinary Sub-Committee established by the Scientific Advisory Committee of the Royal College of Obstetricians and Gynaecologists, must be regarded as interim. Data on all aspects of HIV infection are continually being collected and the basis for interim recommendations may change as knowledge increases.

1.2 **Resource material:**

(1) Bulletins from the Centre for Communicable Diseases, Colindale and Centers for Disease Control, USA; (2) Guidance from the AIDS Unit, Department of Health and Social Security; (3) Bulletins from the District Control of Infection Committee, St Mary's Hospital, Paddington; (4) Code of Practice in Delivery Suites, Department of Health, New South Wales; (5) Review commissioned by the Scientific Advisory Committee (Pinching and Jeffries 1985); (6) Verbal and written assistance from Dr Jacqueline Mok and Mr Frank Johnstone in Edinburgh and Dr Anthony Pinching in London is acknowledged. Relevant bibliography is attached (Appendix IV).

2. GENERAL FEATURES OF THE PRACTICE OF OBSTETRICS AND GYNAECOLOGY

2.1 Obstetrics and gynaecology, and family plannning, together with neonatal paediatrics, are areas of clinical practice in which the special implications of HIV infection now merit urgent and serious consideration.

2.2 HIV infection is but part of a spectrum of transmissible viral disorders of special relevance to obstetrics and gynaecology. Some of these (e.g. Hepatitis B) have a greater infectivity than HIV.

2.3 HIV infection is unique in that (a) there is as yet no prophylactic vaccine, (b) there is no curative treatment and (c) infection is followed by high longterm morbidity and mortality. Under these circumstances even a small but avoidable risk of transmission may not be acceptable.

2.4 The guidelines and general principles already issued for clinical practice in AIDS-related conditions are widely but not universally applicable (CDC Recommendations, 1986; Pinching and Jeffries, 1985; Rogers, 1985; Rubinstein, 1986; Infectious Diseases Society of America, 1986). Other features and considerations are virtually peculiar to obstetrics and gynaecology and suggest the need for modification of existing guidelines.

2.5 Those features of obstetrics, gynaecology and neonatal paediatrics of particular relevance to AIDS are:—

a) Pregnancy may accelerate the clinical progress of AIDS-related conditions.

b) It is estimated that at least 50% of babies born to HIV-positive mothers will themselves remain HIV seropositive and that up to 50% of seropositive infants will go on to develop AIDS. There is evidence that transplacental infection occurs, although the proportion of babies infected from their mothers by this route has not yet been determined (Mok *et al* 1987).

c) The HIV virus has been isolated in female genital secretions (Vogt, Witt and Craven, 1986; Wofsy *et al* 1986). In gynaecological practice, especially in fertility work and family planning there is the added risk of exposure to semen. In obstetrics in relation to abortion or delivery, amniotic fluid, blood and lochia are shed in variable, sometimes large, amounts. These body fluids may be shed unexpectedly and explosively (CDC, 1987).

d) In the puerperium, blood loss as lochia is a normal physiological feature.. At the same time, freshly repaired lacerations or surgical incisions in the perineum are relatively common, even following normal delivery. This has important implications for the use of communal toilet facilities in postnatal wards (see Appendix II(k)).

e) There is presumptive evidence that on one occasion HIV infection may have been transmitted in breast milk (Ziegler *et al* 1985). In the UK, artificial feeding is safe and preferred for the known HIV seropositive woman. However, any recommendation concerning autologous breastfeeding needs to be carefully weighed against other neonatal hazards which may be introduced by abandonment of breastfeeding in an environment where bottlefeeding may not be easily and safely achieved.

2.6 HIV infection is a problem to be faced in all obstetric and gynaecological units and during associated care in the community. The principles in this document apply in all these situations. The Sub-Committee dismissed the concept that HIV-positive status in women will be very rare and can be identified promptly and effectively, so that sufferers may be segregated in special units designated for the purpose, as being totally unrealisitic.

2.7 Universal screening applied to all antenatal patients cannot yet provide quite 100% detection of asymptomatic carriers in the obstetric population. This is because of the timelag before seroconversion (normal range 6-16 weeks; occasionally much longer) and the fact that false negatives have sometimes been known to occur with exisiting tests (Allain *et al* 1986). It may be that a policy of antenatal population screening will be recommended at some future date if the scientific and economic considerations change. Accordingly, the main thrust of the Sub-Committee's recommendations will be towards some modification of obstetric, midwifery, gynaecological and neonatal practice, as well as support for preventive health measures, irrespective of whether or not the patient is identified as being HIV antibody positive. If these sensible steps are taken, local proposals for isolation and barrier nursing may now be modified without detriment to staff and others in contact with HIV sufferers, and with great improvement in the humanity with which these individuals are treated.

OBSTETRICS

3. HIV AND PREGNANCY

3.1 Prevalence

Reliable data on the prevalence of HIV seropositive mothers in the UK are not yet available. Over a two-and-a-half year period up to 30th June 1987, 5110 HIV antibody positive individuals in England, Wales and Northern Ireland have been reported to CDSC; 13 were children of HIV positive mothers (PHLS, CDSC unpublished data). Acquisition of such data should be regarded as a matter of prime importance.

3.2 Maternal risk of progression of HIV disease in pregnancy

The view that pregnancy itself can accelerate HIV disease is still unsubstantiated and is based on a series of case reports of severe infections in pregnancy or the development of AIDS during pregnancy in previously asymptomatic women who have already had one child with AIDS. This urgently needs further research and requires follow-up of both pregnant and non-pregnant seropositive women.

3.3 Recommendations

(1) *Universal antenatal screening for HIV:* This is not recommended at present (see Section 2.7). However, careful **selective** testing (or "case finding") is recommended according to the risk groups as defined from time to time by the Department of Health (see Appendix I). Subsequent testing of negative cases in high risk groups may be advisable if the first test was performed within the first trimester.

(2) *Consent:* The DHSS recommendation that information on the nature and specific implications of all tests performed in pregnancy should be given to the woman concerned should apply no less to HIV testing. All antenatal patients should therefore be given information on the current categories of HIV risk groups and thus invited to declare themselves if they are in a high risk group. Some women, however, will be identified in ordinary clinical practice as being in a high risk category. They should be encouraged to have the HIV test along with certain others (e.g. Hepatitis B) after being given the appropriate explanation and information and, as for any other test in pregnancy, being given the option to refuse.

(3) *Counselling:* The basic counselling of pregnant women must devolve upon the medical and midwifery staff involved and appropriate staff education on a continuing basis is essential. This should include knowledge of the need and means of obtaining further expert guidance. It is considered that additional counselling should be offered to pregnant women for whom a positive result is obtained (see below). Some women in high risk groups with a negative result may also benefit from additional counselling. Such counselling must include advice on safe sexual practice during pregnancy and thereafter.

It is essential, therefore, to ensure that positive results are not communicated to patients in a haphazard or routine fashion. It is envisaged that a positive result reported to an obstetric unit should be kept confidential to a senior obstetrician or a senior midwife and a trained AIDS counsellor until it has been fully discussed with the woman concerned. Thereafter the information should be kept confidential to staff on a "need to know" basis, including those involved in emergency care. The propriety of communication of a positive result to a woman's General Practitioner is a matter for debate; her views on this should be sought and respected, even though such communication may be considered desirable.

(4) *Termination of pregnancy:* Based on the serious consequences of intra-uterine transmission, it is considered that HIV seropositive status is adequate grounds to comply with the requirements of the 1967 Abortion Act. Accordingly it is recommended that the knowledge of seropositive status should be made rapidly available, with appropriate counselling, to any pregnant woman for whom a positive result is obtained. It is recognised that at present confirmation of a positive result involves more complex and time-consuming procedures. There are particular time constraints in this situation because the techniques and hazards of abortion vary with the duration of pregnancy. Accordingly, after repetition, failure to obtain a negative result on a fresh sample may need to be communicated **without final confirmation but with appropriate counselling** to the woman when this result becomes available. She should be given the right to decide whether to opt for termination at that stage or to wait for confirmation later. Full consultation between the microbiological and obstetric specialists on the use and interpretation of the tests is essential at all times.

(5) *Antenatal diagnostic tests:* Invasive procedures for diagnosis not only produce body fluids (amniotic fluid, blood) which require appropriate handling precautions, but also pose an as yet undefined risk of transmitting HIV to the fetus.

(6) *Untested individuals:* It is recommended that a woman in a known high risk group who declines HIV testing should be treated as though she were HIV positive for the remainder of that pregnancy (e.g. special precautions with blood testing and in labour; see Sections 4.2 and 5). This may also apply to a woman who continues to engage in a high risk activity even though negative at testing. However, if sensible modifications to existing standards of obstetric and gynaecological practice are accepted (see Appendix II), the need for segregation should prove to be minimal, except for labour, delivery and the immediate early puerperium (see Appendix III) or haemorrhage at any time. At other times, ordinary social contact carries no definable risk of HIV transmission.

4. ANTENATAL CARE OF IDENTIFIED HIV SEROPOSITIVE WOMEN AND UNTESTED WOMEN IN HIGH RISK GROUPS [See Section 3.3(6)]

4.1 It is not considered necessary to advise segregation in the antenaal period unless haemorrhage has occured, although local policy must determine the need for single accommodation.

4.2 All blood samples should be taken by appropriately trained staff wearing gloves with maximum precautions against inadvertent needle stick injury [see

Section 12.3 (c) and Appendix II (g)]. At present, surgical rubber gloves are the only single-use medical gloves for which there is a standard specifying strength and freedom from perforations.

5. LABOUR AND DELIVERY IN IDENTIFIED HIV SEROPOSITIVE WOMEN AND UNTESTED WOMEN IN HIGH-RISK GROUPS
[See Section 3.3(6)]

5.1 Method of delivery
Transplacental infection is known to have occurred but the importance of this route relative to others is unknown (Chiodo, Ricchi and Costigliola, 1981). HIV has been isolated from cervical secretions, suggesting that these could be a potential route for the transmission of infection. Nevertheless, there are insufficient grounds to indicate a policy of elective Caesarean section on the grounds of HIV infection. Caesarean section carries some maternal hazard and it is not known whether this operative procedure may be prejudicial to the health of a carrier of HIV.

Operative vaginal procedures: If operative vaginal delivery is required, it may be considered that obstetric forceps will produce less risk of fetal skin trauma than the vacuum extractor. If intrauterine manipulation, such as manual removal of the placenta, is required, impermeable forearm protection will be necessary.

5.2 Control of infection
Labour and delivery constitute an obvious risk because of the occasional uncontrolled dissemination of body fluids, especially blood. As it is known that under experimental conditions the virus can survive in dried blood (Barré-Sinoussi, Nugeyre and Cherman, 1985) it is important that all guidelines for safe practice in delivery should take cognizance of this fact. The fine detail of control of infection arrangements is a matter for local decision. This Report is concerned with outlining the principles which should be observed.

5.3 Management
Procedures will usually closely follow those used for Hepatitis B patients. The details of such protocols should be a matter for local decision. Architectural features, for instance, may influence local policy. The principles in Appendix III may help establish such guidelines.

5.4 Maternal resuscitation
It is essential that maternal resuscitation be carried out immediately according to the current recommended practice and standards. Direct contact with blood or other body fluids should be avoided, if possible, by the wearing of protective clothing as described in Appendix III. All resuscitation equipment should be treated as infected and either disposed of or resterilized as appropriate. It must be emphasised that maternal resuscitation should not be delayed whilst awaiting the appropriate equipment.

6. POSTNATAL CARE OF IDENTIFIED HIV SEROPOSITIVE WOMEN AND UNTESTED WOMEN IN HIGH RISK GROUPS [See Section 3.3(6)]

6.1 Although postnatal isolation may not be essential, **dedicated toilet facilities** are desirable.

6.2 It is considered that there would be a high level of anxiety were a known seropositive woman to handle **the baby of another woman** and appropriate counselling should be given in this respect and on related matters, preferably during the antenatal period.

6.3 It is appreciated that women who are both HIV positive and **drug users** may have additional problems and it will be necessary to seek expert advice. The general problems associated with caring for drug users also need to be anticipated, with especial vigilance on the security of needles, drugs and syringes.

6.4 **Women with AIDS-related symptoms** will require appropriate special nursing attention (Royal College of Nursing Guidelines on Management of Patients in Hospital and the Community Suffering from AIDS, 1986).

6.5 **Postnatal care and counselling** are essential for both the mother and her partner, whether in the maternity unit or at home, and this should include advice on safe sexual practice.

PAEDIATRIC CONSIDERATIONS

7. IMMEDIATE CARE OF THE NEONATE BORN TO AN IDENTIFIED HIV SEROPOSITIVE WOMAN OR TO A WOMAN IN A HIGH RISK GROUP WHO HAS NOT BEEN TESTED [See Section 3.3(6)]

7.1 Neonatal resuscitation

Neonatal resuscitation must be available wherever deliveries occur and these will include those at high risk for HIV. In all these cases the use of mouth-operated suction should be abandoned [see Appendix II (d)]. The doctor or midwife should wear surgical gloves (see Section 4.2) and a visor and be gowned over a plastic apron. Bag and mask apparatus will require sterilization, as will laryngoscopes. Most endotracheal tubes and suction tubes are for single use, but the mattress of the Resuscitaire and the Venturi suction apparatus will need to be disinfected with sodium hypochlorite.

7.2 Management of the cord and washing of the infant

After standard management of the cord, the infant should be washed with soap and water without any anti-microbial agent in the delivery room to remove all traces of maternal blood and amniotic fluid and, until this has been achieved, the attendant should wear full protective clothing, including a visor. Care should be taken to prevent the infant from becoming chilled and also to prevent contamination of the cut cord by maternal blood or secretions during cleaning.

8.   CARE OF THE NEONATE OF AN IDENTIFIED HIV SEROPOSITIVE WOMAN OR A WOMAN IN A HIGH RISK GROUP WHO HAS NOT BEEN TESTED [See Section 3.3(6)]

8.1   Routine care of the apparently normal neonate

The infant should be cared for in the same room as the mother. Surgical gloves should be worn when attending to the cord, when performing heel pricks, or when dealing with nappy changing or vomit; otherwise no further precautions need be taken (see Section 4.2). Alcohol swabs should be used on the cord stump.

Only disposable napkins should be used and they should be placed in yellow plastic bags and incinerated. Particular care should be taken with infants who have temporary vaginal discharge, whose napkins may be bloodstained.

A disposable paper tape measure should be used to measure length and head circumference of the infant.

8.2   Tests and equipment

Blood samples and Guthrie test cards should be labelled with Biohazard labels and placed in individual plastic bags.

Bilirubin should not be estimated on a communal ward bilirubinometer, nor should the samples be centrifuged [see Appendix II (g)].

After discharge, the baby's glass thermometer should be cleaned and then soaked in a solution of 0.5% chlorhexidine and 70% ethanol for 30 minutes. The ethanol should be allowed to evaporate and the thermometer should be stored dry.

Scales for weighing the infant should be cleaned using 0.1% sodium hypochlorite (1,000 ppm available chlorine) or 70% alcohol and then wiped with detergent. Stethoscopes should be cleaned using 0.1% sodium hypochlorite and then wiped with detergent.

8.3   Special problems of resuscitation and management and precautions appropriate to the care of the sick neonate of an HIV seropositive mother in a neonatal intensive care surround

In the neonatal intensive care room, the principles in 8.1 apply, but all handling should be done with surgical gloves (see Section 4.2), especially because long intravenous lines and infusions frequently need attention and re-siting; they are potential sources of blood escape.

8.4   AIDS in the newborn

The majority of children do not present with symptoms related to their infection in the newborn period but may have other problems relating to maternal risk factors such as drug addiction.

9.   TESTS AVAILABLE ON THE NEONATE

The time required for elimination of passively transmitted IgG will affect the significance of the results. It is important to collect as much cord blood as possible at the time of delivery so that this can be used for tests to assess the possibility of the infection of the newborn. This will enable the virology laboratory to compare antibodies present in the baby with those in a blood sample obtained from the mother. Of particular value in these paired samples is Western blotting. The cord blood sample should be collected into a container with preservative-free heparin (20 IU/ml) and it may be possible to isolate virus from the lymphocytes in the sample, although this test is not yet generally available. Sequential antibody testing on the newborn child may indicate infection if the antibody levels remain static or increase in titre. A further development is a test for antigen which should contribute to the neonatal diagnosis of HIV infection (Borkowsky *et al.* 1987).

10. BREASTFEEDING

It is not yet possible to determine at birth whether an infant born to an HIV positive mother is affected. This is because passive transplacental transfer of IgG antibodies will have occurred and these take some months to be eliminated. Breastfeeding recommendations should therefore follow the guidelines in Section 2.5(e) (for Milk Banks, see Section 11.1). No specific measures outside those in section 2.5(e) are required.

Further advice may be forthcoming from the DHSS in the near future.

11. TISSUE DONATION [see DHSS Guidelines CMO (87)5]

11.1 Milk banks

(a) The same general precautions now applying to any tissue donation should apply to breast milk banking. Unplanned donation is probably not feasible and milk banks organized on this basis should be discontinued.

However, with regard to HIV infection, planned donation after appropriate donor screening may be acceptable, either with pasteurization or with cryo-preservation for three months [see Section 11.1(b)]. No donation from any individual in a designated high risk group should be accepted. Low risk individuals would need to volunteer to be tested before donation of breast milk.

(b) One study (Eglin and Wilkinson, 1987) suggests that pasteurization may achieve inactivation of the virus in breast milk, using a temperature of 56°C for 30 minutes. Studies on freeze storage of breast milk for donation are required. This is an area in which guidelines for clinical practice may be expected to change rapidly as more data become available. In the interim, a cautious approach is indicated.

11.2 Amnion donation for temporary skin graft cover

Obstetricians should not provide amnion except from screened donors outside the high risk groups. Similar considerations apply to the establishment of a frozen amnion bank.

11.3 Placenta

The placenta should always be handled according to the principles of safe practice in handling blood. The collection of placentae for research purposes or for commercial use in preparing products for therapeutic purposes is a long established practice. Pending transport, placentae should be stored in boxes in a freezer cleaned with hypochlorite solution. Placentae from women who are HIV positive, or from those in a high risk group, should not be collected for this purpose. Whether it is reasonable to continue the practice of collecting placentae for commercial use from other untested women is currently under consideration by the DHSS (Hill *et al*, 1987).

GYNAECOLOGY AND FAMILY PLANNING

12. GYNAECOLOGY

The implications of HIV for gynaecological practice fall into three main categories:

    a) Pelvic examination
    b) Infertility practices
    c) Gynaecological surgery, including termination of pregnancy

12.1 **Pelvic examination**

The following features apply both to gynaecological and family planning practice.

(a) *Gynaecological examination* inevitably exposes health professionals to genital secretions which may include semen (and at times blood) in an unscreened population. Some measures to minimise the risk to the examiner and also to eliminate the risk of transmission to other individuals are required [see Appendix II(1)].

(b) *Gloves:* Thin disposable plastic gloves are widely available but suffer from an unacceptable tendency for the seams to dehisce and so are unsatisfactory. The use of gloves of adequate strength and good fit is to be preferred. The question of a standard for general use procedure gloves is currently being examined by the DHSS.

(c) *Specula:* For specula, vulsella and other instruments which are unaffected by heat treatment, central decontamination by autoclaving is the preferred practice.

In institutions where a central decontamination service is not available, and there is no autoclave on site, boiling, if properly controlled, is an acceptable means of disinfection. Only autoclaving will destroy bacterial spores but HIV is susceptible to boiling temperatures.

Instruments to be boiled must be totally immersed and adequate time allowed for items to heat up before a hold-time of not less than 5 minutes is maintained at boiling temperature.

The use of chemical disinfectants for decontaminating instruments used for invasive procedures is strongly discouraged. None is entirely reliable and glutaraldehyde in particular can raise problems of sensitisation. (In some exceptional cases such as endoscopes and thermometers, chemical disinfection is the only current means of decontamination.)

Several models of low cost pressure sterilizers are under evaluation and information on them may be available at a later date.

(d) *Single-use disposable specula* are a more expensive alternative but are appropriate to low demand areas e.g. isolated General Practitioner surgeries. Both used disposable specula and gloves and also spent spatulae used for taking cervical smears must be regarded as contaminated waste and disposed of accordingly. This point may require special attention in areas where such examinations are infrequently performed.

12.2 Infertility practices

(a) *Post-coital tests* involve exposure to semen and need to be handled with appropriate care, including the correct disposal of spent material, e.g. glass slides etc.

(b) *In vitro fertilization:* The various techniques involve invasive procedures for oocyte retrieval and embryo replacement, and contact with or handling of semen. Precautions will be required at all stages.

(c) *Donor insemination (semen):* A report from Australia has highlighted the dangers of HIV transmission via cryopreserved semen from a symptomless carrier of the HIV virus (Stewart *et al.*, 1985). All donors must be carefully counselled to exclude high risk groups and regularly tested for HIV antibodies. Clinics using fresh or frozen semen are advised to consult the DHSS Guidelines [CMO(86)12] and strictly adhere to the policies contained therein. Quarantined stored semen offers the best treatment option as regards prevention of HIV infection and it is recommended that all clinics should aim to provide such a service as soon as possible.

(d) *Gamete intra-fallopian transfer (GIFT); oocyte donation; embryo donation:* It is recommended that similar precautions to those pertaining to donor insemination be introduced [see DHSS Publication CMO (87)5].

12.3 Gynaecological surgery

The general guidelines applicable to surgical operations in HIV positive patients apply [DHSS Publication CMO(86)7], which should include prior notification of anaesthetic and operating suite staff, with due regard to confidentiality.

(a) *Nursing Care:* The special features of nursing gynaecological patients will reflect those outlined in the obstetric section when vaginal bleeding occurs (see Appendices II and III).

(b) *Sterilization of endoscopes:* It is noted that there is very variable and inconsistent use of glutaraldehyde in the sterilization of non-autoclavable endoscopes. It is recommended that logical central guidelines, applicable to all patients, not just those who are HIV or Hepatitis B positive, be urgently prepared [see DHSS Publication CMO (86)7, 1986].

(c) *Needle stick injury*
i) Pelvic surgery, because of the poor visibility, relies extensively on digital exploration for instrumental and needle direction. Operators need to be aware of an enhanced risk of needle stick injury [DHSS Booklet CMO(86)7]. This can be so in even quite minor procedures and such surgery, for example repair of episiotomy, should not be left to inexperienced operators in the case of known or suspected HIV seropositive patients. Extra care would be required were an operator known to be HIV seropositve.
ii) All staff involved in venepuncture and intravenous cannulation must be familiar with safe practice and with the safe disposal of sharps (DHSS specification for sharps containers is TSS/S/330.015).

(d) *Termination of pregnancy*
Many abortions will be carried out on untested individuals. Special care in the

handling of blood and products of conception is required, including the preparation of material for pathological examination. These measures need to be drawn to the attention of institutions solely devoted to the termination of pregnancy.

13. FAMILY PLANNING

13.1   Guidelines have been produced by The Family Planning Association and National Association of Family Planning Doctors (British Journal of Family Planning, 1987). Attention is drawn to the importance of family planning and well women services in the extension of their traditional role of preventive health care to include the prevention of the spread of HIV infection. This will be achieved through health education and the nature of the services provided. The importance of an adequate relevant history is stressed.

13.2   **Additional instruments** such as vulsella are required which will need sterilization in like manner to specula. This may present a problem in isolated General Practitioner surgeries or clinics without autoclave facilities. [See also Section 12.1(c)].

13.3 Family planning clinics carry a small additional risk of exposure to **semen** which should not be overlooked.

13.4 **Care of diaphragms**—See guidelines (British Journal of Family Planning, 1987).

14. CONCLUSIONS

14.1   HIV is but part of a spectrum of transmissible micro-organisms which have considerable impact on the practice of obstetrics and gynaecology. AIDS is unique because the social stigma, lack of prophylactic vaccine and lack of effective therapy have combined to surround it with a highly-charged atmosphere. Over-reaction can result in the insensitive handling of HIV seropositive individuals. At present, population screening is not recommended although general testing may be worthwhile on an experimental basis in some localities. However, stringent selective testing (case finding) with appropriate pretest counselling is recommended throughout the country. The special considerations of pregnancy are the need to determine the risk to the infant and the need to determine the risk of progress of maternal disease and hence the need to offer legal termination. These and other recommendations may well require revision as more data become available, perhaps from local studies.

14.2   There is inadequate evidence to advocate a policy of elective Caesarean section, or to advise against breastfeeding by all HIV positive mothers.

14.3   Arrangements for the donation of breast milk, amnion, oocytes and embryos should be subject to the same stringent controls as apply to the donation of blood and semen.

14.4   The importance of in-service education for all medical, nursing and paramedical staff dealing with this problem is emphasised. It should include knowledge of access to expert information and counselling.

14.5 The most important message to get across is that some modification of certain existing obstetric and gynaecological practices may diminish the risk of inadvertent contamination from unidentified carriers and also reduce the need for stringent segregation processes which in themselves cannot be guaranteed to afford protection to staff and other patients.

14.6 Specific managerial implications of this recommendation include the need to provide alternative measures for mucus extraction and to supply protective gloves, clothing and other equipment in situations where they may not be used at present.

APPENDIX I
HIGH RISK GROUPS FOR SELECTIVE HIV TESTING IN PREGNANT WOMEN
(as defined by DHSS AIDS Unit, July 1987)

Not all these groups may readily be determined by direct questioning.

a)   Sexual partners of men who have had sex with other men at any time since 1977.

b)   Drug users or sexual partners of drug users who have injected themselves with drugs at any time since 1977.

c)   Women who have had sex at any time since 1977 with people living in African countries except those on the Mediterranean, or who have sexual partners who have done so.

d)   Sexual partners of haemophiliacs.

e)   Women who are prostitutes.

APPENDIX II
RECOMMENDED REVISION OF CURRENT CLINICAL PRACTICE

Serious consideration should be given to revision of the following practices:

(a)   The practice of conducting normal delivery, protected only by non-sterile plastic aprons and sterile gloves must now be regarded as inadequate. It is **strongly** recommended that the practice of wearing a gown over a plastic apron should be universally adopted for the conduct of a delivery and for procedures in which the membranes are intended or are likely to be ruptured. The objective is to avoid inadvertent and often unrecognized soiling of uniform or street clothes.

(b)   Owing to the frequent risk of contamination of clothing and footwear, it is recommended that protective footwear (boots or plastic overshoes) should be worn by those directly involved with delivery, especially for operative procedures when the patient is in the lithotomy position.

(c)   Protective clothing and contaminated footwear should be changed before staff move to other patients or areas.

(d)   It is recommended that the practice of **mouth-operated** mucus extraction should be rapidly phased out, as should **mouth-operated** aspiration of blood for fetal scalp sampling. Instead, for mucus extraction, aspiration should be by means of a syringe, preferably a bulb syringe fitted with a de Lee trap, or by mechanical suction apparatus attached to an 8 or 10 FG suction catheter, using pressure normally not exceeding minus 100 mm Hg (minus 136 cms water) (Standards and Guidelines for Cardiopulmonary Resuscitation and Emergency Cardiac Care, 1986).

(e)   The practice of bleeding the umbilical cord directly into a laboratory tube should be abandoned. The use of a disposable funnel to reduce contamination is a recommended alternative. If a needle and syringe must be used, great care must be taken to avoid needle stick injury.

(f)   Preservation of the placenta for commercial use or research will require appropriate safety precautions (see Section 11.3).

(g)   Clinicians performing laboratory tests on body fluids in a clinical area or ward laboratory should be aware of the potential hazards and conform to accepted laboratory standards of practice.

(h)   Gloves should be worn:

   i)   in any close physical contact if the obstetrician or midwife has any cuts or grazes on the hands; such abrasions should always be covered by a closed, unperforated waterproof plaster [see also Section 12.1(b)].

   ii)   whenever the hands of the obstetrician or midwife would otherwise be in contact with the blood of a patient.

(i)   Women may be encouraged to remove their own sanitary towels prior to any procedure or examination. Sanitary towels should always be disposed of in a safe manner (e.g. sealed in yellow plastic bags and incinerated).

(j)   Washing: Baths—The use of immersion baths should be discouraged and local consideration given to a policy for the provision of adequate showers with detachable heads. If used, adequate decontamination arrangements for baths are required (see Nursing Guidelines on the Management of Patients in Hospital and the Community Suffering from AIDS, Royal College of Nursing, 1986).

(k)   Lavatory and bidet facilities: The possibility of spread of transmissible infection via lavatory seats has always attracted public comment and speculation. There is no evidence that Hepatitis B or HIV has been spread in this way so for the population at large there should be no risk. However, puerperal women are a special case as they have lochial discharge and many have fresh perineal wounds. Consequently a change in routine toilet practice in postnatal wards is recommended, the details to be determined by local policy. It is considered that preliminary wiping of the lavatory seat with a suitable size of alcohol-impregnated wipe would be entirely adequate and appropriate because alcohol will inactivate the virus. Alcohol will evaporate and will not cause an adverse skin reaction as might follow the use of hypochlorite. The responsibility for wiping the lavatory seat should always be upon the woman about to use it, rather than the preceding user. It is recommended that this feature of postnatal hygiene be introduced into antenatal education.

(l) Care must be taken to prevent cross-contamination with body fluids in high turnover situations such as clinics. This applies especially to vaginal blood loss which can lead to soiling of drawsheets, modesty drapes or communal dressing gowns.

APPENDIX III
MANAGEMENT OF LABOUR AND DELIVERY IN HIV SEROPOSITIVE WOMEN AND THOSE IN HIGH RISK GROUPS WHO HAVE NOT BEEN TESTED

(a) The **need for segregation** is confined to the time of established labour, including spontaneous premature rupture of the membranes, and for a period of time which probably need not exceed that usual for an uneventful normal delivery. This general recommendation would clearly need modification in the light of any associated haemorrhage, whether antepartum or postpartum. Most cases of primary postpartum haemorrhage will have commenced within a six hour period after delivery. Clearly circumstances predisposing to secondary postpartum haemorrhage may call for a more cautious attitude.

(b) All staff in attendance on the woman normally require a disposable apron and gloves, but for those taking part in procedures in established labour and for delivery **full protective clothing,** including cap, eye protection, mask and boots, should be worn. Protective clothing and footwear should be changed before leaving the area and subsequently handled according to local Control of Infection procedure.

(c) Qualified **medical and midwifery staff** should provide the care. If any have exposed skin lesions, these should be covered by an impermeable dressing as well as protective clothing. Midwifery and medical students must receive instruction in the care of these individuals.

(d) There would appear to be no particular reason for a woman's **companion in labour** to wear protective clothing other than a gown and overshoes but it may be prudent to advise the wearing of apron and gloves before handling the baby.

(e) **Equipment and facilities:** In general, those provided for the conduct of labour in women with Hepatitis B are entirely appropriate for HIV seropositive mothers. Some special features relevant to the care of HIV positive women are as follows: There should be an arrangement for the decontamination of all equipment parts at risk of coming into direct contact with spilled body fluids, such as stethoscope heads and tocograph transducer heads (DHSS document HM(87)1). A suggested regimen is:—

   i) *Arrangements for the handling of used instruments* are a matter for local policy. Advice on transportation and decontamination of used instruments is contained in DHSS document HN(87)1.

ii) *Suction apparatus:* Suction jars for the collection of blood and body fluid; before use add a volume of 10% sodium hypochlorite solution (undiluted household bleach) equal to at least one third of the total holding volume of the jar. When work is complete or the jar is full allow it to stand for at least 30 minutes before carefully emptying the contents. Splashing must be avoided. The jar and its bung should then be bagged, labelled (e.g. BIOHAZARD) and sent for central processing in a unit equipped with autoclaving facilities. Gloves must be worn when dealing with this item.

iii) *Stethoscopes,* both adult and infant, should be cleaned using 0.1% sodium hypochlorite (1,000 ppm available chlorine; 1 in 100 dilution of household bleach) or 70% alcohol. For direct soiling of sphygmomano-meter cuffs with body fluids, treat as in (iv) below.

iv) *Airways, masks and corrugated tubing,* if not disposable, should be bagged and returned to a central processing unit for treatment in a suitable washing machine [see DHSS document HN (87)1].
Where no machine processing service is available, these items must be immersed for at least 5 minutes (dislodging entrapped air) in water at 98-100°C which is the recommended exposure to inactivate Hepatitis B virus [see DHSS document HN (87)1].

v) *Any resuscitation equipment* not suitable for heat sterilization should be packaged, labelled and transported for decontamination in accordance with local policy.

vi) *Intrauterine catheters* should not be used unless considered essential.

vii) *Fetal blood sampling* and the use of *fetal scalp electrodes* should be avoided when possible, as they inevitably provide a small open wound in a contaminated area; not all infants born to HIV positive mothers are affected. External transducers may be used.

(f)   **Cutting the cord** carries a very real risk of spurting blood and extra care must be taken.

(g)   **Episiotomy** is not contra-indicated but its repair or the repair of lacerations should only be performed by someone fully attired as in (b) above. There is a special risk of inadvertent glove puncture or needle stick injury during repair of extensive perineal injuries and it is recommended that this procedure should not be carried out by inexperienced operators in HIV-positive cases.

(h)   The **placenta and membranes** should be examined initially in the delivery room by an attendant in full protective clothing, including eye protection. Subsequent disposal should be according to local Control of Infection guidelines. Products of conception, if required for laboratory examination, must be appropriately packaged and labelled prior to transport.

(i)   **Cleaning of delivery suite:** Contamination by blood, vomit, or other body fluid should be dealt with immediately by suitably protected staff. Care should be taken to see that contamination is not spread by inadvertent treading. Spillage on floors and work surfaces is best treated by the application of chlorine releasing granules (products containing dichloroisocyanurate) *OR* covered with a paper towel which is then soaked with sodium hypochlorite solution containing 10,000 ppm available chlorine.

(j) **For direct spills of blood and body fluid:** Dichloroisocyanurate granules should be used according to the manufacturer's instruction and then mopped up with gloved hands and bagged for safe disposal.

Some hypochlorite solution (10,000 ppm available chlorine) should be freshly prepared. (Note that some brands of domestic bleach may contain less than 100,000 ppm available chlorine on manufacture and any brand will deteriorate on prolonged storage.)

Contact time for the latter should be as long as reasonably practical but not less than 15 minutes.

(k) **For routine cleaning of light contamination:** sodium hypochlorite containing 1,000 ppm available chlorine.

After disinfectant treatment, the area should be cleaned with a compatible detergent and hot water.

Mops should have detachable heads so that they can be removed for decontamination.

NOTE: Metal equipment should not be soaked in sodium hypochlorite solution becauses it causes corrosion. After swabbing, items should be thoroughly rinsed in water.

APPENDIX IV
BIBLIOGRAPHY

Allain J-P, Laurian Y, Paul DA, Senn D. Serological markers in the early stages of human immunodeficiency virus infection in haemophiliacs. *Lancet* 1986, **2**: 1233-1276.

Barré-Sinoussi F, Nugeyre MT, Cherman JC. Resistance of AIDS virus at room temperature. *Lancet* 1985, **2**: 721-722.

Borkowsky W, Krasinski K, Paul D, Moore T, Bebenroth D, Chandwani S. Human-immunodeficiency-virus infections in infants negative for anti-HIV by enzyme-linked immunoassay. *Lancet* 1987, **1**: 1168-1170.

Centers for Disease Control. Recommendations for assisting in the prevention of perinatal transmission of HTLV III and acquired immunodeficiency syndrome. *Morbidity and Mortality Weekly Report* 1985, **34**: 721-732.

Centers for Disease Control. Update: Human Immunodeficiency virus infections in health-care workers exposed to blood of infection patients. *Morbidity and Mortality Weekly Report* 1987, **36**: 285-289.

Chiodo F, Ricchi E, Costigliola P. Vertical transmission of HTLV-III. *Lancet* 1986, **1**: 739.

Department of Health and Social Security. Acquired Immune Deficiency Syndrome (AIDS): Guidance for Surgeons, Anaesthetists, Dentists and their Teams in Dealing with Patients infected with HTLV III. *DHSS Publication CMO(86)7*, 1986.

Department of Health and Social Security. Acquired Immune Deficiency Syndrome (AIDS) and Artificial Insemination: Guidance for Doctors and AI Clinics. *DHSS Publication CMO(86)12*, 1986.

Department of Health and Social Security. Decontamination of Equipment, Linen or Other Surfaces Contaminated with Hepatitis B or Human Immunodeficiency Virus. *DHSS Publication HN(87)1*, 1987.

Department of Health and Social Security. HIV Infection and Tissue and Organ Donation. *DHSS Publication CMO(87)5*, 1987.

Eglin RP. Wilkinson AR. HIV infection and pasteurisation of breast milk. *Lancet*, 1987, **1**: 1093.

Family Planning Association. AIDS (Acquired Immune Deficiency Syndrome). Family Planning and Well-Woman Services. Provisional guidelines from the Family Planning Association and the National Association of Family Planning Doctors. *Br J Fam Planning*, 1987, **13**: 11-15.

Hill WC, Bolton V, Carlson JR. Isolation of acquired immunodeficiency syndrome virus from the placenta. *Am J Obstet Gynecol* 1987, **157**: 10-11.

Infectious Diseases Society of America. Acquired immunodeficiency syndrome. *J Infect Dis* 1986, **154**: 1-9.

Mok JQ, Giaquinto C, De Rossi A, Grosch-Wörner I, Ades AE, Peckham CS. Infants born to mothers seropositive for human immunodeficiency virus. *Lancet* 1987, **1**: 1164-1168.

Pinching AJ, Jeffries DJ. AIDS and HTLV-III/LAV infection: consequences for obstetrics and perinatal medicine. *Br J Obstet Gynaecol* 1985, **92**: 1211-1217.

Rogers MF. AIDS in children: a review of the clinical, epidemiological and public health aspects. *Ped Infect Dis* 1985, **4**: 230-236.

Royal College of Nursing. Second Report of the Royal College of Nursing AIDS Working Party. *Nursing Guidelines on the Management of Patients in Hospitals and the Community Suffering from AIDS*. RCN, London 1986.

Rubinstein A. Schooling for children with acquired immune deficiency syndrome. *J Pediatr* 1986, **109**: 242-244.

Standards ad Guidelines for Cardiopulmonary Resuscitation and Emergency Cardiac Care. Part VI. Neonatal Advanced Life Support. *J Am Med Ass* 1986, **255**: 2970.

Stewart GJ, Tyler JPP, Cunningham AL, Barr JA, Driscoll GL, Gold J, Lamont BJ. Transmission of human T cell lymphotropic virus type III (HTLV III) by artificial insemination by donor. *Lancet* 1985, **2**: 581-585.

Vogt MW, Witt DJ, Craven DE. Isolation of HTLV-III/LAV from cervical secretions of women at risk for AIDS. *Lancet* 1986, **1**: 525-527.

Wofsy CB, Cohen JB, Hauer LB, Padian NS, Michaelis LB, Evans LA, Levy JA. Isolation of AIDS-associated retrovirus from genital secretions of women with antibodies to the virus. *Lancet* 1986, **1**: 527-529.

Ziegler JB, Cooper DA, Johnson RO. Postnatal transmission of AIDS-associated retrovirus from mother to infant. *Lancet 1985*, **1**: 896-898.